A Clinical Guide to Eating Disorders

A Clinical Guide to Eating Disorders

Editor: Lewis Humphries

FOSTER
ACADEMICS
www.fosteracademics.com

www.fosteracademics.com

FOSTER
ACADEMICS

Cataloging-in-Publication Data

A clinical guide to eating disorders / edited by Lewis Humphries.
p. cm.
Includes bibliographical references and index.
ISBN 978-1-63242-503-4
1. Eating disorders. 2. Appetite disorders. 3. Psychology, Pathological.
I. Humphries, Lewis.
RC552.E18 C55 2017
616.852 6--dc23

Foster Academics,
118-35 Queens Blvd., Suite 400,
Forest Hills, NY 11375, USA

ISBN 978-1-63242-503-4 (Hardback)

Printed and bound in China.

Contents

Preface

Abnormal eating habits which adversely impact human health are called eating disorders. They are often regarded as mental disorders. The major types of eating disorders include anorexia nervosa, binge eating disorder, pica, restrictive food intake disorder, rumination disorder, etc. This book unfolds the innovative aspects of this subject which will be crucial for the progress of this field in the future. Some of the diverse topics covered in the text address the varied sub-fields that fall under this subject. For all readers who are interested in this area of psychiatry, the case studies included in this book will serve as excellent guide to develop a comprehensive understanding. It will prove to be immensely beneficial to students and researchers in this field.

The researches compiled throughout the book are authentic and of high quality, combining several disciplines and from very diverse regions from around the world. Drawing on the contributions of many researchers from diverse countries, the book's objective is to provide the readers with the latest achievements in the area of research. This book will surely be a source of knowledge to all interested and researching the field.

In the end, I would like to express my deep sense of gratitude to all the authors for meeting the set deadlines in completing and submitting their research chapters. I would also like to thank the publisher for the support offered to us throughout the course of the book. Finally, I extend my sincere thanks to my family for being a constant source of inspiration and encouragement.

Editor

I'm not just fat, I'm old: has the study of body image overlooked "old talk"?

Carolyn Black Becker[1*], Phillippa C Diedrichs[2], Glen Jankowski[2] and Chelsey Werchan[1]

Abstract

Background: Research indicates that body dissatisfaction is correlated with and often predictive of both physical and mental health problems. "Fat talk," a well-studied form of body image talk in adolescents and university-aged women, has been implicated as contributing to body dissatisfaction and mediating the relationship between body dissatisfaction and other mental health problems. Limited research, however, has investigated fat talk across the female lifespan. Further, consistent with most body image research, fat talk research solely focuses on the thin dimension of idealized female attractiveness, even though other dimensions may contribute to body dissatisfaction in women.

Method: The current study investigated whether or not "old talk," a hereto un-described form of body image talk, appears to be a parallel, but distinct, form of body image talk that taps into the young dimension of the thin-young -ideal standard of female beauty. An international, internet sample of women (aged 18–87, $N = 914$) completed questionnaires aimed at assessing fat talk, old talk, body image disturbance, and eating disorder pathology.

Results: Results indicated that both fat talk and old talk were reported by women across the lifespan, although they evidenced different trajectories of frequency. Like fat talk, old talk was significantly correlated with body image disturbance and eating disorder pathology, albeit at a lower rate than fat talk in the total sample. Old talk was more highly correlated with ageing appearance anxiety than fat talk, and the correlation between old talk and body image disturbance and ED pathology increased with women's ages.

Conclusion: Results suggest that old talk is a form of body image talk that is related to but distinct from fat talk. Old talk appears to be similarly problematic to fat talk for women whose age increases their deviation from the thin-young -ideal. Further research into the phenomenon of old talk is warranted as is increased attention to fat talk across the full lifespan of women.

Keywords: Old talk, Fat talk, Body image, Body dissatisfaction, Eating disorders, Self objectification, Ageing, Ageing anxiety

Background

Substantial research indicates that body dissatisfaction broadly defined is highly correlated with, and often longitudinally predictive of, both physical and mental health problems [1,2]. For example, among adolescent girls, researchers have found that body dissatisfaction (e.g., as measured by standardized questionnaires such as the Body Shape Satisfaction Scale [3]) prospectively predicts increases in binge eating, emotional eating, stress, low self-esteem, depression, use of unhealthy weight control behaviors, decreased physical activity, and, among overweight girls, increased weight gain between 1–5 years later [4-6]. Although most research on body dissatisfaction has been conducted with females, existing research, which is largely cross-sectional, suggests that body dissatisfaction in males is associated with eating disorders (ED), steroid use, poor psychological adjustment, and exercise dependence [7].

Ageing and body image

In addition to disproportionally targeting females, past body image research also has largely focused on a narrow age range, namely adolescents and university-aged women [8]. This is despite the fact that there is little evidence to suggest that graduation from university is

* Correspondence: cbecker@trinity.edu
[1]Department of Psychology, One Trinity Place, Trinity University, San Antonio, TX 78212, USA
Full list of author information is available at the end of the article

associated with a graduation from body image concerns. The limited research on body image in older women suggests that body dissatisfaction is relatively comparable in younger and older women [8-11]. Cross-sectional research also supports a relationship between body dissatisfaction in adult women and depression, decreased quality of life, fewer pleasant feelings, increased negative feelings, increased ED pathology, and decreased self-care [12,13]. Finally, body dissatisfaction in adult women smokers prospectively predicts greater difficulty quitting smoking [14].

There are reasons to think that body dissatisfaction might actually increase as women age [8]. For example, normal ageing typically moves women's body weight/shape further away from the thin-ideal standard of female beauty in Western culture. Moreover, as women age, they encounter a variety of developmental stages that may accelerate this movement away from the thin-ideal. Some examples include pregnancy, decreased time for exercise and self-care secondary to demands of work, home, and/or childcare, menopause, and possibly the use of medications that may increase weight. Demands on young adult and midlife women to conform to the thin-ideal also have increased with the media's focus on pregnant celebrity women, who are lauded for losing weight post-pregnancy quickly and returning to their "pre-baby" bodies (e.g., http://thestir.cafemom.com/pregnancy/144512/7_celebrity_moms_whose_postbaby). Adding to this pressure is the fact that the thin-ideal is also a young-ideal. As evidence of this, there has been a proliferation of interest in, and advertising of, anti-ageing cosmetic products, pharmaceuticals and surgical procedures, all of which are marketed to women with the underlying message that a youthful, wrinkle-free appearance is ideal [15]. Similarly, models depicted in the media are predominantly thin and young, with a recent content analysis of advertisements in popular North American women's magazines concluding that 80.72% of the models were aged 18–30 years [16]. Thus, as women age, they increasingly move away not just from being thin but also from fulfilling the young element of the thin-young-ideal. Accordingly, ageing creates new opportunities for discrepancies between women's bodies and cultural beauty ideals.

Indeed, cross-sectional research supports a relationship between ageing anxiety and both body dissatisfaction and EDs [17]. As such, the relative stability of body dissatisfaction across age groups is, in some ways, surprising. Some evidence, however, suggests that older women may more frequently employ cognitive strategies to partially offset their increasing distance from our societies' conceptualization of the ideal woman [8,11,12]. It also may be that the nature of women's body image concerns change and that they have not been adequately assessed by approaches that were developed with, and for, younger women. Lastly, there may be cohort effects. More specifically, researchers may increasingly find higher levels of body dissatisfaction in older women over time as these women have grown up in a more toxic body image climate than those of previous generations.

We should note that although most research suggests that cross-sectional samples across the female lifespan report similar levels of body dissatisfaction on standardized measures, a few studies indicate that body dissatisfaction is slightly lower in some (but not all) domains for women in older adulthood (i.e., over age 60) [8,13,18-20]. For instance, in a large cross-sectional sample of women over 50, being older was associated with decreased concern in certain facets of body image (e.g., that weight or shape negatively affected life, lesser importance of weight or body shape on self-perception), but not others (e.g. being moderately to extremely upset with gaining five pounds [18]). In summary, women across the lifespan appear to report similarly elevated levels of dissatisfaction with their bodies, although women in older adulthood (60 years and older) may report less dissatisfaction in some domains such as a perception that weight and shape negatively affected life, in comparison to younger women [18].

Fat talk and old talk

Numerous sociocultural, intrapersonal and interpersonal factors contribute to girls and women's body dissatisfaction. One factor that has received increasing attention is "fat talk" (e.g., "I'm so fat," "Wow, you look great, have you lost weight?"). The term fat talk was coined by Nichter and Vuckovic [21,22] to describe the body image talk in which pre- and adolescent girls engage when talking about the size and shape of their bodies. Nichter and Vukovic reported that this population used fat talk for impression management (i.e., to increase social likeability and decrease perceptions of arrogance). Fat talk is hypothesized to increase a sense of inter-connectedness between girls and women; yet at the same time, fat talk reinforces the thin-ideal and decreases the opportunity for girls to interact in more meaningful ways.

Empirical research has since documented that fat talk also is common in college-aged women [23,24] and pernicious. In cross-sectional samples, fat talk is associated with body dissatisfaction, drive for thinness, internalization of the thin-ideal, and ED pathology [23-25]. Clarke, Murnen, and Smolak [26] found that fat talk predicted unique variance in ED symptoms and body shame. Further, Stice, Maxfield and Wells [27] found that a mere 3–5 minutes of exposure to fat talk significantly increased body dissatisfaction among undergraduate women, as compared to exposure to non-appearance -related conversations. Finally, Arroyo and Harwood [28] found evidence that fat talk explains a significant amount of variance in body dissatisfaction, perceived pressure to be thin and depression. This research also found that FT longitudinally mediated the relationship between negative body image and broader mental health concerns.

To our knowledge, only one study examined fat talk in an older sample (i.e., *M* age = 45). Martz, Petroff, Curtin, and Bazzini [29] found that women reported that, in their own lives, situations involving fat talk were significantly more likely to occur as compared to situations involving self-accepting or positive body talk. Thirty-one percent of women reported high exposure to fat talk and the mean rating of fat talk exposure was 2.74 with a score of 3 being equated to "usually". Although Martz et al. [29] comment that these frequencies seem relatively low, the findings by Stice et al. [27] suggest that fairly low levels of exposure to fat talk can have a significant, negative effect. Indeed, Stice et al. [27] stated that it was "noteworthy that such a brief and subtle manipulation" yielded an effect of medium size (p. 113).

In 2008, the Tri Delta sorority launched Fat Talk Free® Week, aimed at raising awareness of fat talk and encouraging people to stop fat talk. Since 2008, this advocacy campaign has become both annual and international, and various locations have been declared Fat Talk Free® Zones. In 2011, the owner of a pilates studio that was a dedicated Fat Talk Free® Zone contacted the first author and asked what she was supposed to do about problematic "old talk" (e.g., "I look so old", "Look at these wrinkles", "Do you want to come to a Botox party?"), in which women of a variety of ages engaged (e.g., women in their 30's, 40's and older). In response to this, we began listening to conversations around us and in the media. We also searched the literature for any references to old or ageing talk and its relationship to body image. Although we observed the phenomenon described by the studio owner, we were unable to find any social science literature specifically pertaining to this form of body talk behavior. We hypothesized that old talk is a distinct but, until now, unstudied form of body image talk, and therefore concluded that it was worthy of at least a preliminary investigation.

Current study

The primary aim of this mixed-methods study was to a) assess the self-reported frequency of old talk, b) gain a preliminary understanding of the content of old talk, and c) investigate whether it, like fat talk, is associated with negative body image, self-objectification, and ED pathology. Given that body image is multi-dimensional, we chose to assess several different facets of body image that have been studied in connection to fat talk including body satisfaction, thin-ideal internalization, drive for thinness as well as the related construct of self-objectification. We also assessed anxiety related to aging appearance. Because only one paper has examined fat talk in a broad age range and we needed to study old talk across the female adult lifespan, we also sought to investigate fat talk in the same sample and to compare the two forms of body image talk. Finally, since the overwhelming majority of fat talk research has been conducted within the United States (USA), we expanded the geographical boundaries of our study to the United Kingdom (UK) and Australia. We outline our specific hypotheses for this study below.

With regards to fat talk we hypothesized that: 1) fat talk would be a common occurrence (i.e., that we would find fat talk across all ages, and rates of fat talk would remain largely unchanged across age groups), 2) consistent with Salk and Englen-Maddox's [24] failure to find a correlation between fat talk and weight, we would find fat talk across women of all body weights, 3) we would find a third person effect for frequency of fat talk in friends, family and the media based on Salk and Englen-Maddox's [24] finding the participants reported more fat talk in others versus themselves.

With regards to old talk, we hypothesized that: 1) participants would report engaging in old talk, though at a lower rate than fat talk since younger women naturally conform to the young part of the thin-young-ideal, 2) that old talk would predominantly occur among women aged 30 and older and would increase significantly with age, 3) that we would find third person effects for friends, family and the media.

Regarding correlations with body image, self-objectification, and ED related variables, we hypothesized that: 1) since both fat talk and old talk represent some degree of buy-in to the thin-young-ideal, both would be significantly correlated with body image, self-objectification, and ED pathology measures, 2) fat talk and old talk would correlate with each other, but not perfectly, suggesting that fat talk and old talk are related but not identical constructs, 3) we would consistently find higher correlations with fat talk, as compared to old talk, for all body image, self-objectification, and ED measures except appearance ageing anxiety, which would correlate more closely with old talk. The rationale for hypothesis one is that both are likely associated with internalization of the thin-young ideal. We had no hypotheses about the qualitative data. Our primary goal was to determine if we found similar fat talk content to that reported by Salk and Englen-Maddox [24] in their mixed-methods fat talk study with college women and to see if old talk content was similar to what we found for fat talk or not.

Methods

Participants

A snowballing sample of adult women from the USA, UK and Australia was recruited to complete an anonymous, online questionnaire. A total of 914 women, aged 18–87 years ($M = 36.80$, $SD = 13.48$) consented to take part in the study and completed at least one portion of the questionnaire. Table 1 presents a demographic summary of participants' age, body mass index, education and ethnicity by country of residence. Demographic information was not available for women who did not report their country of residence as these questions were grouped together at the very end of the questionnaire.

Procedure

On authors' request, community organizations and workplaces with large female populations (e.g., universities, YWCA) distributed a standardized email inviting women to complete a brief online questionnaire titled "Women's Conversations and Opinions about Themselves". Similarly worded invitations also were posted on internet forums (e.g., Mumsnet, BubHub) and social networking websites (e.g., Facebook) and emailed to authors' contacts. All emails and posts requested that women forward the study invitation to their own social networks.

The recruitment email described the study purpose as exploring topics that women frequently discuss with other women and how this relates to their health and well-being. After providing consent, participants completed measures online in the order that they are described below. Upon completion, participants could enter a prize draw to win a £50/$80 Amazon gift voucher. Ethical approval to conduct the study was granted by the internal review boards at the authors' respective institutions.

Measures

Demographic information

Participants reported their age, height, weight, country of residence, highest level of education achieved and ethnicity. Body Mass Index (BMI) was calculated by dividing self-reported weight (kilograms) by height^2 (meters). Although gathering participant's height and weight data via self-report is not optimal, as this was a survey study we were unable to assess these constructs more objectively. Nonetheless, research has shown that self-report weights are reasonably accurate [30].

Fat talk

To assess the fat talk content, participants completed an imagined conversation script between themselves and a specific friend, in accordance with Salk and Engeln-Maddox [24]. The conversation began with a friend saying *"Ugh, I feel so fat"*. The participant then recorded her initial response to her friend in an open-ended response box, followed by a response from her friend and a final response from the participant.

To measure frequency of fat talk, participants received the following definition which included 9 fat talk examples (e.g., "she would be prettier if she lost weight," "do I look fat in this?"): *"The term "fat talk" is used to describe any speech that implicitly or explicitly reinforces or endorses the thin-ideal standard of female beauty that*

Table 1 Participant demographics

	USA		UK		Australia		Elsewhere	
	($n = 367$)		($n = 224$)		($n = 168$)		($n = 22$)	
	M	*SD*	*M*	*SD*	*M*	*SD*	*M*	*SD*
Age	39.41	14.37	32.28	11.75	37.42	12.21	34.82	12.67
Body Mass Index	24.09	4.68	24.69	6.31	25.48	5.63	23.80	4.01
	n	%	n	%	n	%	n	%
Education[a]								
Some high school	2	0.5	0	0	5	2.60	0	0
High school	27	7.4	48	21.52	20	11.90	6	30.0
Diploma/ Associate's Degree	20	5.4	23	10.31	35	21.21	0	0
Undergraduate	142	38.8	95	42.60	70	41.67	7	35.0
Postgraduate	175	47.9	57	25.57	38	22.62	7	35.0
Ethnicity[b]								
White	312	85.7	210	93.8	153	91.1	18	81.1
Other	52	14.3	14	6.2	15	8.9	4	18.1

a. Education indicates highest level of education completed. Frequencies (%) calculated with available data on a within country basis.
b. Because we had an international sample and the vast majority of participants identified as White, for brevity we collapsed all other ethnic groups into 'Other'.

is promoted in western culture. Fat talk can appear to be either critical (e.g., "She's too fat to wear that skirt") or seemingly complimentary (e.g., "I wish I was as thin as you")." Consistent with Salk and Engeln-Maddox's methodology [24], participants next responded to three items on a 5-point Likert scale (1 = never or it's extremely rare; 5 = it's extremely common) to indicate how often they personally engage in fat talk, how often their female friends and family engage in fat talk, and how often they see or hear fat talk in the media.

We also administered a slightly modified version of the Fat Talk Scale [26]. This scale includes 9 scenarios in which a woman is talking to a female friend and fat talk arises (e.g., *"Anna and her friends are taking a workout class together. While changing into their workout clothes, one of Anna's friends clutches her stomach and says she looks so fat. Her other friend says she hates her thighs. Anna responds with something she hates about her own body."*). Participants indicated on a 5-point Likert scale (1 = never; 5 = always) the extent to which they would respond in the way Anna responded. We modified scenarios that appeared exclusively aimed at younger women (e.g., one that included walking to class) to be more age neutral. Reliability for the Fat Talk Scale in this study was good (*Cronbach's* $\alpha = .92$); previous research supports its test re-test reliability and validity [26].

Old Talk

To assess the old talk content, participants completed another imagined conversation script between themselves and a specific friend who begins by saying *"Ugh, look at these wrinkles. I can't believe how old I look"*. The response format was consistent with the fat talk conversation task described above.

To measure frequency of old talk, participants received the following definition of old talk along with 9 old talk examples: *"The term "old talk" is used to describe any speech that implicitly or explicitly reinforces or endorses the young (and still thin) -ideal standard of female beauty that is promoted in western culture. Old talk can appear to be either critical (e.g., "She's looking really old.") or seemingly complimentary (e.g., "You so don't look your age! Tell me your secret.")."* Participants separately rated on a 5-point Likert scale (1 = never or it's extremely rare; 5 = it's extremely common) how often they personally engage in old talk, how often their female friends and family engage in old talk, and how often they see or hear old talk in the media.

Based upon the Fat Talk Scale [26], we created an Old Talk Scale for this study. This scale included 9 scenarios in which a woman named Anna is talking to female friends and old talk arises (see Appendix A for Old Talk Scale). Scenarios were based on conversations observed by the authors or pilates instructor mentioned above. Participants indicated on a 5-point Likert scale (1 = never; 5 = always) the extent to which they would respond as Anna did in each scenario. Higher scores indicate a greater tendency to engage in old talk. Reliability for the Old Talk Scale was good (*Cronbach's* $\alpha = .88$).

Thin-ideal Internalization

To assess thin-ideal internalization, the internalization-general (9 items; e.g., "I compare my body to the bodies of people who are on TV"; 1 = definitely disagree, 5 = definitely agree) and internalization-athlete (5 items; e.g., "I compare my body to that of people in "good shape"; 1 = definitely disagree, 5 = definitely agree) subscales of the Sociocultural Attitudes Towards Appearance Questionnaire-3 (SATAQ-3) [31] were administered. Higher scores indicate greater internalization of cultural beauty ideals. The SATAQ-3 is widely used and has good convergent validity [31]. Reliability for the subscales was good (*Cronbach's* $\alpha = .93$; .84).

Body areas satisfaction

The Body Areas Satisfaction subscale of the Multidimensional Body Self Relations Questionnaire (MBSRQ) [32] assessed women's satisfaction with discrete body parts. Participants rated their satisfaction with 9 aspects of appearance (e.g., face, mid torso, weight) on a 5-point Likert scale (1 = very dissatisfied, 5 = very satisfied). Significant data supports the reliability and validity of the MBSRQ [32]. Higher scores indicate greater body satisfaction. Reliability was good in this sample (*Cronbach's* $\alpha = .85$)

Self-objectification

The Self-Objectification Questionnaire [33] assessed the extent to which women focus on appearance-based aspects of their bodies in comparison to competence-based aspects. Participants ranked body attributes in order of perceived importance to physical self-concept (1 = most important, 9 = least important). Scores were calculated by computing a difference score between the sum of the ranks for appearance-based items (e.g., physical attractiveness, weight) and those for competence-based items (e.g., fitness, health), with higher scores indicate greater levels of self-objectification. Previous research has demonstrated that this scale has acceptable construct validity [33].

Ageing appearance anxiety

The Physical Appearance subscale of the Anxiety about Aging Scale [34] assessed concern about the effects of ageing on appearance (5 items; e.g., "When I look in the mirror, it bothers me to see how my looks have changed with age; 1 = strongly disagree, 5 = strongly agree). In our review of the aging literature, we found this to be the most widely used scale. Lasher and Faulkender [34] found good internal consistency for this measure, which has high face validity. Higher scores indicate greater ageing anxiety and the scale had good reliability in this study (*Cronbach's* $\alpha = .77$).

Drive for thinness

The Drive for Thinness subscale from the well validated Eating Disorder Inventory-2 [35,36] assessed participants' preoccupation with weight and dieting (7 items; e.g., "I think about dieting"; 1 = never, 6 = always). Higher scores indicate greater drive for thinness. The scale had good reliability in this sample (*Cronbach's* $\alpha = .83$).

Eating disorder pathology

Diagnostic items from the Eating Disorders Examination-Questionnaire [37] assessed ED pathology (12 items; e.g., "Over the past 28 days, how many times have you made yourself sick (vomit) as a means of controlling your shape or weight?"). Higher scores indicate greater eating pathology. Research supports the two week test-retest reliability, internal consistency, and temporal stability of the EDE-Q [38,39]. The scale had good reliability (*Cronbach's* $\alpha = .79$).

Results

Because our sample was substantially more geographically diverse than other studies in this area, we examined if there were any differences between the main countries in our study prior to treating the sample as a unified group. For this analysis, we removed participants who resided in a country other than the USA, UK or Australia ($n = 22$), as well as participants who did not report country of residence ($n = 133$). Preliminary analyses indicated that countries differed with respect to age and BMI, thus we co-varied these variables in the between-country analyses. Results indicated that participants from all countries were equally likely to engage in fat talk, F (2, 756) = 2.30, $p = .831$, $\eta_p^2 = .006$. We similarly found no significant differences in reported old talk engagement and participant's country of residence, $F(2, 730) = 2.50$, $p = .084$, $\eta_p^2 = .007$.

Fat talk content

Responses to the fat talk conversation were coded and analyzed thematically by the third and fourth author in accordance with the procedure outlined by Salk and Engeln-Maddox [24]. To determine if the seven themes observed by Salk and Engeln-Maddox [24]. (*denial, empathy, probing, evidence, causes, action together, I'm fat you're not*) captured the content of our data, we attempted to code conversations from the first 70 participants into these themes. Overall, the themes fit the data well (i.e., most responses were easily coded into the original seven themes), although three new themes were identified; *healthy ideal, disengagement* and *discount*. Table 2 provides a summary of the analysis of fat talk conversations.

The coders next analyzed all data by first coding participants' initial responses into one of three dominant themes (*denial, probing, empathy).* The most common initial response to a friend engaging in fat talk was *denial* (63.9%), followed by *probing* (13.1%) and *empathy* (12.65%). A minority of initial responses (10.35%) did not fit into these themes. Inter-rater reliability (IRR) for the coding of initial responses was good (*Cohen's kappa* = .81).

Secondly, the entire conversation for each participant was coded into the full set of 10 themes, with each conversation being coded into as many relevant themes as needed to adequately describe the data. The most common response types across the entire conversation were *denial* (64.75%), *evidence* (50.5%), *discount* (28.7%), *action (*26.7%) and *empathy* (23.15%). IRR was acceptable for all themes (*Cohen's kappa* ≥ .70).

Frequency of fat talk

As hypothesized, an overwhelming majority (81%) of the total sample reported engaging in at least occasional fat talk. Among the 881 who responded to this item, 33% reported frequently engaging in fat talk (score 4 or 5; see Table 3). The mean rating of fat talk was 2.86 ($SD = 1.23$).

Because our sample included a much more diverse range of ages and weights than most previous studies of fat talk, we examined if these factors were associated with differences in fat talk. We divided participants into four main age groups (18–29 years, $n = 292$; 30–45 years, $n = 293$; 46–60 years, $n = 141$; and 61 and older, $n = 55$) and excluded those who did not report age ($n = 133$). Groups were created with the following concerns in mind: not wanting to create too many groups, having ages that roughly held together in terms of life stages, and not creating groups with very small samples. We also consulted a life span developmental psychologist for advice in creating the groups as well as the lifespan literature [40]. Preliminary analyses indicated that BMI differed for the different age groups. Thus we co-varied BMI.

In contrast to our hypothesis, we found a significant difference in frequency of engaging in fat talk based on age, F (3, 753) = 3.98, $p = .008$, $\eta_p^2 = .016$. Mean ratings indicated that engagement in fat talk slowly decreased as participant age increased (see Table 3), although rates of at least occasional fat talk remained stable across age group (82-86%). As can be seen in Table 3 fat talk did not noticeably change until women reached the oldest age bracket (> 61 years), and post-hoc analyses indicated

Table 2 Fat talk content thematic analysis summary

Theme	Definition	Example responses	Initial responses %	Entire conversation %	*Kappa*
Denial	Participant denies that friend is fat	*"You're not fat at all."*	63.9	64.75	.85
Empathy	Participant indicates that she or others can relate to feeling fat and being upset	*"Ah I know how you feel." "I can totally understand the feeling."*	12.65	23.15	.78
Probing	Participant questions friend as to why she feels fat	*"What makes you feel like this?" "Why what's wrong?"*	13.10	15.75	.84
Evidence	Friend provides evidence to support the statement that she is actually fat	*"Yes I am. Look at this (then grabs her love handles)."*	-	50.5	.70
Causes	Participant discusses or inquires about the causes contributing to friend's belief	*"You need to stop watching these dumb rom coms." "Have you not been exercising lately? Or is it PMS?"*	-	11.0	.82
Action	Participant suggests or prompts plan of action	*"Well have you tried eating better?"*	-	26.7	.84
I'm fat, you're not	Participant disagrees by commenting on her own fatness	*"I don't think you are fat, but I am."*	-	6.75	.75
Healthy Ideal	Participant actively promotes health instead of appearance	*"The important thing is that you feel healthy and happy."*	-	4.5	.77
Discount	Participant or friend rejects the other's denial that they are not fat	*"Whatever, you're only saying that because you have to."*	-	28.7	.89
Disengage	Participant actively dismisses and attempts to stop the fat talk	*"Don't say that!"*	-	13.0	.90

Note: Cohen's kappa coefficients reported here were calculated for the analysis in which the coders analyzed the entire conversation. Kappa for initial response coding was .81.

Table 3 Frequencies and means for fat talk and old talk

	None/Rare %	Occasionally %	Sometimes %	Quite often %	Extremely common %	*M (SD)*
Self Fat Talk						
Total Sample	16	26	25	22	11	2.86 (1.24)
18–29 Years	15	23	24	23	15	2.99 (1.30)[a]
30–45 Years	15	28	24	24	10	2.86 (1.21)[ab]
46–60 Years	18	28	21	21	11	2.79 (1.29)[ab]
61+ Years	16	35	35	12	2	2.49 (0.98)[b]
Underweight	19	24	21	14	21	2.98 (1.44)[ab]
Normal Weight	16	30	24	21	9	2.77 (1.21)[a]
Overweight	9	25	27	24	15	3.12 (1.21)[b]
Obese	21	18	24	25	11	2.88 (1.25)[ab]
F&F Fat Talk	5	20	27	37	12	3.33 (1.06)
Media Fat Talk	1	5	12	38	45	4.21 (0.89)
Old Talk						
Total Sample	34	30	22	12	3	2.21 (1.12)
18–29 Years	52	29	15	3	1	1.17 (0.89)[a]
30–45 Years	27	29	24	24	4	2.40 (1.16)[b]
46–60 Years	14	31	30	17	7	2.71 (1.11)[c]
61+ Years	9	33	33	26	0	2.72 (0.94)[c]
F&F Old Talk	16	35	28	17	4	2.57 (1.07)
Media Old Talk	3	14	24	39	20	3.59 (1.06)

Note: Subgroupings with different superscripts differ significantly from one another at $p < .05$. Subgroupings with the same superscripts did not differ significantly from one another. *F&F Fat Talk*, Friends and Family Fat Talk. *F&F Old Talk*, Friends and Family Old Talk.

that only the youngest and oldest age groups significantly differed. Thus our hypothesis that fat talk would remain largely unchanged across age groups was mostly, but not fully, supported.

To analyze differences by weight, we used traditional BMI cut-off points to split our sample into underweight (BMI <18.5, $n = 42$), normal weight (BMI = 18.5-24.9, $n = 452$), overweight (BMI = 25–29.9, $n = 158$) and obese categories (30+, $n = 115$). See Table 3 for frequencies and means. Preliminary analyses indicated that BMI groups differed with respect to age, which we co-varied. Results indicated that BMI groups differed significantly in self-fat talk frequency, F (3, 753) = 4.02, $p = .007$, $\eta_p^2 = .016$. Mean ratings indicated that the overweight group engaged in the most fat talk whereas the normal weight group engaged in the least. Post-hoc analyses indicated that only these two groups differed significantly, and an overwhelming majority of all groups reported at least occasional fat talk (79% - 91%). Thus our hypothesis that fat talk would occur equally across women of all weights was largely, but not fully, supported.

Given the missing age data for 133 participants, the fact that most sub-groups did not differ from one another in age and BMI analyses, and our desire to avoid over-analyzing our data, we examined reported frequency that female friends and family engage in fat talk (F&F FT) and media fat talk for the total sample only. For F&F FT, 96% of participants responding to this question ($n = 878$) reported at least occasional fat talk. As hypothesized, we found a third person effect, with mean F&F FT frequency being greater compared to self, t (877) = 11.81, $p < .001$. For media fat talk, 99% of participants reported exposure to at least occasional media fat talk. Consistent with our third person effect hypothesis, mean fat talk significantly rose from self to media, t (878) = 28.36, $p < .001$.

Old talk content

Responses to old talk conversation were coded and analyzed thematically in accordance with the procedure described above for fat talk. To determine if the ten themes observed in the fat talk conversations (*denial, empathy, probing, evidence, causes, action, I'm old you're not, healthy ideal, discount* and *disengage*) captured the content of the old talk conversations, we attempted to code the old talk conversations from the first 70 participants into these themes. Overall, the themes fit the data well (i.e., most responses were easily coded into the 10 fat talk themes); *probing* and *healthy ideal,* however, occurred in a minority of cases (< 2.15%) and were therefore removed. Additionally, one new theme was identified; *ageing is natural and positive.* Table 4 provides a summary of the analysis of old talk conversations.

The coders then analyzed the full dataset by first coding participants' initial responses into one of three dominant themes (*denial, empathy, ageing is natural and positive).* The most common initial response to a friend engaging in old talk was *denial* (60.65%), followed by *ageing is natural and positive* (18.15%) and *empathy* (13.45%). A minority of initial responses (7.75%) did not fit into these themes. IRR for initial response coding was good (*kappa* = .83).

The entire conversation for each participant was then coded into the full set of nine themes. The most common response types across the entire conversation were *denial* (51.5%), *evidence* (35.35%), *ageing is natural and positive* (28.7%), *discount* (23.75%) and *action (*15.2%). IRR was acceptable for all themes coded across entire conversations (*Cohen's kappa* ≥ .71).

Frequency of old talk

We repeated the major fat talk analyses for old talk frequency, with the exception of the BMI analyses because that was not part of our original set of hypotheses or research design. Of the 830 participants who responded to the self-old talk question, as hypothesized, the majority of women (66%) reported engaging in old talk (see Table 3). Although this is lower than that for fat talk (also consistent with our hypotheses), it still represents the majority of participants. In the total sample, the rate of frequent old talk (score 4 or 5) was lower (15%) than the rate of frequent FT (33%). The mean rating for self-old talk was 2.21 ($SD = 1.12$).

As hypothesized, the ANCOVA for age, F (3, 753) = 46.33, $p < .001$, $\eta_p^2 = .015$, was highly significant. Frequency of old talk steadily increased as participant age increased. Additionally, the oldest two age groups reported engaging in old talk at a similar or greater frequency than fat talk (see Table 3). Post-hoc tests indicated that the youngest group differed significantly from each of the three older age groups (in ascending order: t (583) = −8.04, $p < .001$; t (431) = −10.05, $p < .001$; t (345) = −7.81, $p < .001$), and that the second youngest age group differed from the two oldest age groups (in ascending order, t (432) = −2.62, $p = .009$; t (346) = −2.03, $p = .04$). In summary, our hypothesis that frequency of old talk increases with age was supported. Surprisingly, however, almost 50% of the youngest age group also reported engaging in at least occasional old talk.

With regards to friends and family old talk (F&F OT), an overwhelming majority (84%) of participants reported at least occasional F&F OT, and we found a significant third person effect, t (826) = −10.88, $p < .001$. As with fat talk, we see a pronounced rise in frequency in response to the media old talk question. Ninety-seven percent of participants reported exposure to at least occasional media old talk, and 59% frequent. Media old talk differed

Table 4 Old talk content thematic analysis summary

Theme	Definition	Example responses	Initial responses %	Entire conversation %	*Kappa*
Denial	Participant denies that friend is old	*"You don't look old at all!"*	60.65	51.5	.84
Empathy	Participant indicates that she and others can relate to feeling old and concerned about ageing appearance	*"I know, I feel the same, it just catches up with you when you aren't looking and it's only going to get worse."*	13.45	14.75	.75
Ageing is natural and positive	Participant implies that ageing is natural, positive and/ or inevitable	*"Aging is natural and beautiful.... I wish I had wrinkles, they make you look wise.*	18.15	28.7	.75
Evidence	Friend provides evidence to support the statement that she is actually old	*"I disagree, LOOK at them."*	-	35.35	.74
Causes	Participant discusses or inquires about the causes contributing to friend's belief that she is old and showing visible signs of ageing	*"It's from smiling and laughing too much"*	-	4.35	.92
Action	Participant suggests or prompts plan of action to address feelings	*"If you're so worried, get some decent anti-wrinkle cream, nothing to lose!"*	-	15.2	.80
I'm old, you're not	Participant disagrees by commenting on her own signs of ageing	*"That is so not bad. Look at my wrinkles"*	-	8.9	.84
Discount	Participant or friend rejects the other's denial that they are not old	*"Yes I do, look at these!"*	-	23.75	.71
Disengage	Participant actively dismisses and tries to stop the old talk	*"Girl, don't even go there. You are gorgeous."*	-	5.85	.90

Note: Cohen's kappa coefficients reported here were calculated for the analysis in which the coders analyzed the entire conversation. Kappa for initial response coding was .83.

significantly as compared to self-old talk, t (829) = −29.56, $p < .001$.

Relationships between fat talk, old talk, body image and ED pathology

The mean fat talk and old talk scale scores were 21.61 (SD = 8.13) and 15.8 (SD = 6.28) respectively. As hypothesized, scores on the fat talk and old talk scales were significantly, but *not* perfectly, correlated, $r = .54$, $n = 776$, $p < .001$ (two tailed: see Table 5). This suggests that fat talk and old talk are related, but distinct phenomena. Also as hypothesized, the fat talk scale was significantly correlated with thin-ideal internalization (both general and athlete), body areas satisfaction (negative correlation), self objectification, physical appearance aging anxiety, drive for thinness and ED pathology (r's range from .23-.67; all $p < .001$; see Table 5). The same was found for the old talk scale (r's range from .23-.47; all $p < .001$; see Table 5). Consistent with our hypothesis, correlations for the fat talk scale were larger than those found for the old talk scale, with the exception of the appearance ageing anxiety.

Based on the finding that old talk frequency was most common in the two oldest age groups, we also examined correlations in this subsample (see Table 5). As with the

Table 5 Correlations between fat talk & old talk scales and measures of body image and eating disorder pathology

	Total sample		Ages 46+	
	Fat talk scale	Old talk scale	Fat talk scale	Old talk scale
Old Talk Scale	.535*		.719*	
SATAQ-3 General Intern	.497*	.331*	.452*	.459*
SATAQ-3 Athlete Intern	.316*	.271*	.312*	.346*
Body Areas Satisfaction[a]	-.528*	-.385*	-.522*	-.402*
Self Objectification	.441*	.232*	.430*	.340*
Appearance Ageing Anxiety	.230*	.474*	.312*	.461*
EDI Drive for Thinness	.668*	.387*	.629*	.513*
EDE-Q ED Pathology	.540*	.385*	.612*	.603*

a Body Areas Satisfaction: Higher scores are better. * $p < .001$.

total sample, all correlations were highly significant ($p < .001$). Interestingly, the fat talk and old talk scales became more correlated in this subgroup. Further, in contrast to the total sample, old talk correlations were mostly equivalent to, or greater than, those found for fat talk for thin-ideal internalization (general and athlete) and ED pathology. Finally, with the exception of appearance ageing anxiety, all correlations increased for the old talk scale in this subsample relative to the general sample.

Discussion

Research indicates that body dissatisfaction is associated with a range of physical and mental health problems. As such, identifying factors that are associated with and may play a role in causing, sustaining, or deepening body dissatisfaction is an important public health issue. Even more critical is the identification of factors that are modifiable and therefore potentially important targets for body image interventions. Previous research implicates fat talk as a factor that not only is associated with body dissatisfaction and ED pathology, but also increases body dissatisfaction when experimentally manipulated. This study contributes to the existing literature by exploring fat talk among women from three countries across the lifespan. Our findings also suggest that researchers need to broaden their study of body image talk to include old talk, particularly when studying midlife and older adult women.

In contrast to existing literature that has typically focused on fat talk as a behavior of adolescents and young women, we found that women of all ages reported engaging in at least some fat talk, with rates of occasional fat talk remaining at a constant 82-85% across our four age groups. Although frequency of fat talk did gradually decrease in the older age groups, the reduction was non-significant except when the youngest and oldest groups were compared. These results suggest that fat talk research needs to include, at minimum, women through the full midlife stage. Moreover, because no body image study has yet followed midlife and older women over a significant period of time, it remains unclear to what degree current findings represent cohort effects. More specifically, it may be that lower rates of fat talk in the very oldest age group represent a generation difference and that women who are currently in their 20s will sustain their current levels of fat talk as they age.

Results for old talk across the ages showed a different pattern than those for fat talk. First, as hypothesized, overall rates of old talk were lower than that for fat talk, with 66% of women reporting at least occasional old talk. Second, whereas rates of fat talk slowly decreased as women aged, rates of old talk increased over the lifespan. The different trajectories of fat talk and old talk across the lifespan provide support for the notion that fat talk and old talk are distinct constructs. They also suggest that when women are young, the most salient feature of the thin-young-ideal is thinness. In contrast, when women are in mid-life both thinness and youth appear to be of concern. Finally, when women enter older adulthood youth appears to become more salient than thinness. Having said this, fat talk was still common among the eldest sub-group, and almost 50% of the youngest age group reported periodic old talk. This suggests that in all ages we should examine effects of the thin-young-ideal, and not just focus on the thin aspect of ideal female beauty.

In contrast to our hypothesis that there would be no differences in fat talk based on body weight, we found a significant difference based on BMI. Although women across all weight categories reported high levels of at least occasional FT (79-91%), frequency of fat talk was highest in our overweight group, which differed significantly from the normal weight group. This contrasts to research with younger women and adolescent girls. Nichter [22] described fat talk as something that almost exclusively occurs among underweight and normal weight adolescent girls. Our findings are, however, consistent with the only other study to examine adult women. Martz et al. [29] found that obese participants reported the greatest pressure to engage in fat talk.

As hypothesized, we found a third person effect [41] for the perceived extent to which both friends and family and the media engage in both fat talk and old talk. This means that women are likely to report that other people engage in significantly more fat talk and old talk then they themselves do. Rates for media fat talk and media old talk were both extremely high. In contrast to extensive research examining effects of idealized media images on body image and health, there is little research that has examined media fat talk and none for media old talk. Given findings of Stice and colleagues [27], in which exposure to a low dose of fat talk by a confederate produced significant worsening of body satisfaction, we suggest that research is needed to determine effects, if any, of media fat talk and media old talk.

As expected, fat talk and old talk scales were significantly correlated with each other, albeit not perfectly. Again, this suggests that the scales tapped into related but different constructs. Both scales also were significantly correlated with all body image and ED pathology measures included in this study. Women who reported greater levels of fat talk and old talk were also more likely to report higher levels of thin-ideal internalization, self-objectification, appearance ageing anxiety, drive for thinness and ED pathology as well as decreased body satisfaction. As hypothesized, fat talk was more strongly related to all body image and ED measures, with the exception of the ageing appearance anxiety, which was more highly correlated with the old talk scale. When we examined the same correlations among women 46 years and older, who reported engaging in the most old talk, we found that almost every correlation for old talk increased. This suggests that old talk is more strongly linked to body image and ED disturbance when it is examined in the population for which it is most salient.

This study has several limitations. First, we used convenience, snowball sampling versus probability samplings. Second, a majority of the women were under 45 years of age. Third, our reliance on internet sampling means the study could have selection bias particularly with respect to socio-economic status (SES) as internet access may be a proxy for SES. Fourth, we relied on self-report. Although this methodology is common in fat talk studies, future research should include other methodologies.

Conclusion

This study provides a significant contribution regarding body image talk among women, and suggests that, due to its prevalence and association with body image and ED pathology, old talk should be addressed in future body image research, particularly among women in mid-older life. Additionally, results suggest that body image programs targeting mid-life and older women may benefit from addressing a) the thin *and* young aspects of idealized female beauty and b) the role of old talk and fat talk in perpetuating unhelpful beauty ideals and appearance-related distress. Finally, results suggest that calls for greater body size diversity in media imagery to promote positive body image (e.g., Australian Government [42]) should also be accompanied by calls to reduce discourse that stigmatizes and reinforces unhelpful beauty ideals in relation to age.

Appendix A

Old talk scale

Below are some scenarios in which women express and respond to aging concerns. Please read each scenario and then answer the corresponding question* by circling Never (=1), seldom , sometimes, often, or always (=5). (*The corresponding question for each item is "Please indicate the extent to which you would respond the way Anna did in this situation.").

1. Anna is having a bad day. She does not feel herself and is somewhat down. While walking to a meeting, a female co-worker says that she looks nice today. Anna groans and says "You obviously aren't looking at my face – I think I developed new wrinkles overnight. I look so old and tired."
2. Anna and her friends are taking a workout class together. While changing into their workout clothes, one of Anna's friends looks in the mirror and says "I really need to start Botox." Her other friend says she is thinking about getting her teeth whitened and dermabrasion to even out her skin tone. Anna responds with something she hates about her own body.
3. Anna is eating lunch with her friends and decides to have dessert. As she finishes her dessert, she makes a comment like "I can't believe I did that. My belly is so huge compared to when I was younger. I hate it but I can't seem to fix it."
4. Anna and her friend are walking to their car after watching a movie. Anna comments that the lead actress looks amazing for her age and says "I wish I could look even half that good these days. I wonder what she does to look that good. I hate getting older."
5. Anna is shopping with her friend Emily. Anna is at the cosmetics counter and asks Emily "what do you use on your skin. I need something that will make me look younger. I keep trying different things but nothing works." Emily suggests checking out a recent fashion magazine review of anti-aging products.
6. Anna is hanging out with a friend when she looks in the mirror and says "I don't think I can wear a swimsuit this year. I have developed a middle aged body and I just can't seem to accept it."
7. Anna is talking with a friend about dating. Anna says "I might as well give up. No one wants to go out with someone as old as me." Anna's friend responds she is thinking of getting plastic surgery because "a facelift will hurt less than seeing John start looking at younger girls."
8. Anna is taking a workout class with a friend when a substitute teacher enters the room. Anna's friend states – "That can't be our teacher – she's too old to be teaching a class like this."
9. Anna's friend Emily really feels as though she looks older than she likes. Emily turns to Anna and says "This is a secret, but I am really thinking about getting a face and neck lift. I think it's the only way I am going to feel better about myself." Anna says "I know what you mean. I don't feel old. I just wish I looked as young as I feel."

How old did you think Anna was as you completed this scale?

Competing interests

The authors have no competing interests to report.

Author contributions

CBB created idea for study, collaborated in the study design, analyzed quantitative data, wrote a majority of the first draft, and edited the manuscript. PD collaborated in the study design, created and managed the online survey, cleaned the data, supervised GJ and CW in the coding and analysis of the qualitative data, contributed to the writing of the first draft, and edited the manuscript. GJ collaborated in the study design, coded and analyzed the qualitative data, contributed to the writing of the first draft and edited the manuscript. CW coded and analyzed the qualitative data, contributed to the writing of the first draft and edited the manuscript. All authors read and approved the final manuscript.

Acknowledgements
The authors acknowledge Karine Berthou and the Succeed Foundation for financial support of this study as well as assistance in promoting the study. The authors also thank Aida Zorilla for her observations and support.

Author details
[1]Department of Psychology, One Trinity Place, Trinity University, San Antonio, TX 78212, USA. [2]Center for Appearance Research, University of the West of England, Coldharbour Lane, Bristol BS16 1QY, UK.

References

1. Haines J, Neumark-Sztainer D: **Prevention of obesity and eating disorders: a consideration of shared risk factors.** *Health Educ Res* 2006, **21**:770–782.
2. Paxton S: *Research review of body image programs: an overview of body image dissatisfaction prevention programs.* Melbourne, Victoria: Prepared for the Victorian Government Department of Human Services; 2002.
3. Pingitore R, Spring B, Garfield D: **Gender differences in body satisfaction.** *Obes Res* 1997, **5**:402–409.
4. Johnson F, Wardle J: **Dietary restraint, body dissatisfaction, and psychological distress: a prospective analysis.** *J Abnorm Psychol* 2005, **114**:119–125.
5. Neumark-Sztainer D, Paxton SJ, Hannan PJ, Haines J, Story M: **Does body satisfaction matter? Five-year longitudinal associations between body satisfaction and health behaviors in adolescent females and males.** *J Adolesc Health* 2006, **39**:244–251.
6. Van den Berg P, Neumark-Stzainer D: **Fat 'n' happy 5 years later: is it bad for overweight girls to like their bodies.** *J Adolesc Health* 2007, **41**:415–417.
7. McCabe M, Ricciardelli L: **Body image dissatisfaction among males across the lifespan: a review of past literature.** *J Psychosom Res* 2004, **56**:675–685.
8. Tiggemann M: **Body image across the life span: stability and change.** *Body Image* 2004, **1**:29–41.
9. Grippo KP, Hill MS: **Self-objectification, habitual body monitoring, and body dissatisfaction in older European American women: exploring age and feminism as moderators.** *Body Image* 2008, **5**:173–182.
10. Pruis TA, Janowsky JS: **Assessment of body image in younger and older women.** *J General Psychol* 2010, **137**:225–238.
11. Webster J, Tiggemann MJ: **The relationship between women's body satisfaction and self-image across the life span: the role of cognitive control.** *Genetic Psychol* 2003, **164**:241–252.
12. McLean SA, Paxton SJ, Wertheim EH: **Factors associated with body dissatisfaction and disordered eating in women in midlife.** *Int J Eat Disord* 2010, **43**:527–536.
13. Reboussin BA, Rejeski WJ, Martin KA, Callahan K, Dunn AL, King AC, Sallis JF: **Correlates of satisfaction with body function and body appearance in middle- and older aged adults: the activity counseling trial (ACT).** *Psychol Health* 2000, **15**:239–254.
14. King TK, Matacin M, White KS, Marcus BH: **A prospective examination of body image and smoking cessation in women.** *Body Image* 2005, **2**:19–28.
15. Smirnova MH: **A will to youth: the woman's anti-aging elixir.** *Soc Sci Med*, . in press.
16. Wasylkiw L, Emms AA, Poirier KF: **Are all models created equal? A content analysis of women in advertisements of fitness versus fashion magazines.** *Body Image* 2009, **6**:137–140.
17. Slevec JH, Tiggemann M: **Predictors of body dissatisfaction and disordered eating in middle-aged women.** *Clin Psychol Rev* 2011, **31**:515–524.
18. Gagne DA, Von Holle A, Brownley KA, Runfola CD, Hofmeier S, Branch KE, Bulik CM: **Eating disorder symptoms and weight and shape concerns in a large web-based convenience sample of women ages 50 and above: results of the gender and body image (GABI) study.** *Int J Eat Disord* 2012, **45**:832–844.
19. Lewis DM, Cachelin FM: **Body image, body dissatisfaction, and eating attitudes in midlife and elderly women.** *Eat Disord* 2001, **9**:29–39.
20. Oberg P, Tornstam L: **Body images among men and women of different ages.** *Ageing Soc* 1999, **19**:629–644.
21. Nichter M, Vuckovic N: **Fat talk.** In *Many mirrors: body image and social relation.* Edited by Sault N. New Jersey: Rutgers University Press; 1994:109–131.
22. Nichter M: *Fat talk.* Cambridge, MA: Harvard University Press; 2000.
23. Ousley L, Cordero ED, White S: **Fat talk among college students: how undergraduates communicate regarding food and body weight, shape and appearance.** *Eat Disord* 2008, **16**:73–84.
24. Salk RH, Engeln-Maddox R: **"If you're fat, then I'm humongous!": frequency, content, and impact of fat talk among college women.** *Psych Women Q* 2011, **35**:18–28.
25. Warren CS, Holland S, Billings H, Parker A: **The relationships between fat talk, body dissatisfaction, and drive for thinness: perceived stress as a moderator.** *Body Image* 2012, **9**:358–364.
26. Clarke PM, Murnen SK, Smolak L: **Development and psychometric evaluation of a quantitative measure of "fat talk.** *Body Image* 2010, **7**:1–7.
27. Stice E, Maxfield J, Wells T: **Adverse effects of social pressure to be thin on young women: an experimental investigation of the effects of "fat talk".** *Int J Eat Disord* 2003, **34**:108–117.
28. Arroyo A, Harwood J: **Exploring the causes and consequences of engaging in fat talk.** *J Appl Commun Res* 2012, **40**:167–187.
29. Martz DM, Petroff AB, Curtin L, Bazzini DG: **Gender differences in fat talk among American adults: results from the psychology of size survey.** *Sex Roles* 2009, **61**:34–41.
30. Stunkard AJ, Albaum JM: **The accuracy of self-reported weights.** *Am J Clin Nutr* 1981, **34**:1593–1599.
31. Thompson JK, Van denBerg P, Roehrig M, Guarda AS, Heinberg LJ: **The sociocultural attitudes towards appearance scale-3 (SATAQ-3): development and validation.** *Int J Eat Disord* 2004, **35**:293–304.
32. Brown TA, Cash TF, Mikulka PJ: **Attitudinal body image assessment: factor analysis of the Body Self-Relations Questionnaire.** *J Pers Assess* 1990, **55**:135–144.
33. Noll SM, Fredrickson BL: **A meditational model linking self-objectification, body shame and disordered eating.** *Psych Women Q* 1998, **22**:623–636.
34. Lasher KP, Faulkender PJ: **Measurement of aging anxiety: development of the Anxiety about Aging Scale.** *Int J Aging Hum Dev* 1993, **37**:247–259.
35. Garner DM: *Eating Disorder Inventory-2: professional manual.* Florida: Psychological Assessment Resources Inc; 1991.
36. Anderson DA, Lundgren JD, Shapiro JR, Paulosky CA: **Assessment of eating disorders: Review and recommendations for clinical use.** *Behav Modif* 2004, **28**:763–782.
37. Fairburn CG, Beglin SJ: **Assessment of eating disorder psychopathology: interview or self-report questionnaire?** *Int J Eat Disord* 1993, **16**:363–370.
38. Luce KH, Crowther JH: **The reliability of the eating disorder examination-self-report questionnaire version (EDE-Q).** *Int J Eat Disord* 1999, **25**:349–351.
39. Mond JM, Hay PJ, Rodgers B, Owen C, Beumont PJV: **Temporal stability of the eating disorder examination questionnaire.** *Int J Eat Disord* 2004, **36**:195–203.
40. Levinson DJ: *Seasons of a Man's Life.* New York: Knopf; 1985.
41. Price V, Tewksbury D: **Measuring the third-person effect of news: the impact of question order, contrast, and knowledge.** *Int J Pub Opinion Res* 1996, **8**:120–141.
42. Australian Government: *Voluntary industry code of conduct on body image;* 2010. http://www.youth.gov.au/.

2

Optimizing prediction of binge eating episodes: a comparison approach to test alternative conceptualizations of the affect regulation model

Matthew Fuller-Tyszkiewicz[1*], Ben Richardson[1], Helen Skouteris[1], David Austin[1], David Castle[2,3], Lucy Busija[4], Britt Klein[5,6], Millicent Holmes[1] and Jaclyn Broadbent[1]

Abstract

Background: Although a wealth of studies have tested the link between negative mood states and likelihood of a subsequent binge eating episode, the assumption that this relationship follows a typical linear dose–response pattern (i.e., that risk of a binge episode increases in proportion to level of negative mood) has not been challenged. The present study demonstrates the applicability of an alternative, non-linear conceptualization of this relationship, in which the strength of association between negative mood and probability of a binge episode increases above a threshold value for the mood variable relative to the slope below this threshold value (threshold dose response model).

Methods: A sample of 93 women aged 18 to 40 completed an online survey at random intervals seven times per day for a period of one week. Participants self-reported their current mood state and whether they had recently engaged in an eating episode symptomatic of a binge.

Results: As hypothesized, the threshold approach was a better predictor than the linear dose–response modeling of likelihood of a binge episode. The superiority of the threshold approach was found even at low levels of negative mood (3 out of 10, with higher scores reflecting more negative mood). Additionally, severity of negative mood beyond this threshold value appears to be useful for predicting time to onset of a binge episode.

Conclusions: Present findings suggest that simple dose–response formulations for the association between negative mood and onset of binge episodes miss vital aspects of this relationship. Most notably, the impact of mood on binge eating appears to depend on whether a threshold value of negative mood has been breached, and elevation in mood beyond this point may be useful for clinicians and researchers to identify time to onset.

Keywords: Threshold modeling, Binge eating, Negative mood, Intensive longitudinal design, Experience sampling

Background

Binge eating, which is characterized by rapid overconsumption of food and a sense of loss of control over eating [1], is a common feature of eating disorders, such as bulimia nervosa, anorexia nervosa-binge/purge subtype, and eating disorder not otherwise specified. Furthermore, it is the key symptom of Binge Eating Disorder, recently defined in the DSM-V [2]. Given its known links to a range of health consequences, including obesity, gastrointestinal problems, and Type II diabetes [3,4], understanding of the antecedents (both distal and proximate) for binge eating is crucial for developing effective treatment solutions. This study proposes a novel modeling technique (threshold modeling) that may be used to better understand the role that negative mood states play in the onset of binge eating episodes.

The affect regulation model [5,6] proposes that individuals binge eat in order to reduce severe and potentially chronic states of negative mood (e.g., through distraction or release of neurotransmitters, such as serotonin, that alleviate negative mood). One way of interpreting this model is

* Correspondence: matthewf@deakin.edu.au
[1]School of Psychology, Deakin University, 221 Burwood Highway, Burwood, VIC 3125, Australia
Full list of author information is available at the end of the article

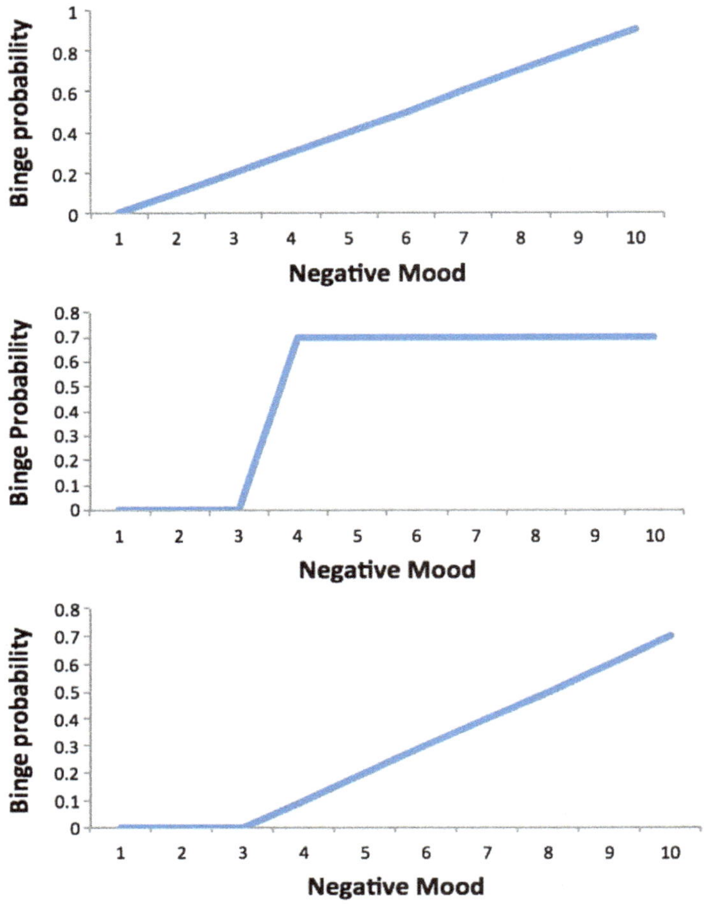

Figure 1 Alternative conceptualisations of the relationship between negative mood and likelihood of a binge eating episode.

as a linearized relationship, such that as the severity of negative mood increases, so too will the likelihood of a binge episode (see the top panel of Figure 1). Indeed, this is the most common modeling approach in the literature, and these studies have generally found negative mood severity to be predictive of a binge event [5].

However, the relationship between negative mood and risk of binge eating predicted in the affect regulation model does not necessarily have to be linear. In particular, it could be that there is some level or 'threshold' of negative affect that must be surpassed before a coping response (i.e., binge eating) is triggered. That is, once a 'comfortable' level of negative mood is breached, the individual is highly likely to binge, whereas any negative mood state below this threshold is highly unlikely to produce a binge. Increases beyond this threshold may have one of several consequences. First, subsequent increases beyond the threshold may have negligible impact on likelihood of a binge as the act of crossing the threshold is decisive in predicting onset (we will call this the *threshold + stability model*; see middle panel in Figure 1). For instance, supposing that an individual's threshold value is 3 out of 10 on a negative mood scale, a mood rating of 9 is just as likely (barring measurement error) to result in a binge as a mood rating of 4, since both exceed the level of negative mood with which the individual is comfortable. An alternative, and more probable, scenario is that the extent to which negative mood exceeds the threshold further increases the likelihood of a binge episode as there is greater impetus to reduce negative feelings (the *threshold + dose response model*; see bottom panel in Figure 1). To the authors' knowledge, neither of these threshold approaches has been tested previously in relation to binge eating.

The nature of the mood-binge eating relationship is an important issue that has both theoretical and practical implications. For example, if either of the threshold models is correct, severity of negative mood may be more predictive of time to onset than simply likelihood of a binge episode. That is, although the relationship between negative mood and time to onset of a binge would be linear – negative mood steadily increases as time to onset reduces – the actual point at which the binge becomes likely occurs earlier, at a lower level of negative mood. This is important for timely intervention which could be cued to occur once the threshold of negative mood is surpassed rather than waiting until negative mood has increased to a high level, at which point the binge eating episode is imminent.

The present study used the experience sampling method (ESM [7]) to explore the nature of the negative mood-binge relationship by: (1) comparing the severity and threshold approaches for modeling the relationship between negative mood and binge eating, and (2) evaluating the extent to which severity of negative mood predicts time to onset of a binge episode. ESM was used in preference for experimental designs in order to monitor mood and binge eating symptoms in a more ecologically valid manner [8], and to also allow for multiple assessment points in order to better ascertain the time course from trigger (elevated negative mood) to event (binge episode) [8,9].

Superiority was operationalized as the model that exhibited the strongest effect of mood on binge eating. In addition, we predicted that shape of the severity-time to onset relationship would be negative and log-linear, such that more extreme negative mood would be associated with shorter times to onset for a binge.

Methods

Participants

Following ethics approval from the university's Human Research Ethics Committee, participants were recruited via brief presentations at the beginning of tutorials and lectures in numerous classes at a large metropolitan university in Melbourne, Australia. The presentations emphasized that the study aim was to evaluate mood and eating experiences of women over a typical week. Participation was not limited to those with a current diagnosis or prior history of an eating disorder. Recruitment was limited to women in order to be consistent with the majority of prior studies investigating the affect regulation model from an experience sampling framework [5].

A total of 93 women agreed to participate, which is considerably greater than the average number of participants in previous ESM studies (Mean number = 28.7 participants, [5]). They had an age range of 18 to 40 years ($M = 24.72$, $SD = 4.15$). The average self-reported body mass indices (BMI = kg/m^2) was 24.12 ($SD = 4.39$). Applying National Institute of Health [10] guidelines for classifying BMI categories, 3 (3.2%) participants were underweight (BMI < 18.5), 58 (62.4%) were in the normal weight category (BMI = 18.5 to 24.9), 27 (29%) were overweight (BMI = 25 – 29.9), and 5 (5.4%) were obese (BMI ≥30).

Instruments

Trait measures (Phase 1: Pre-daily diary)

Demographics This questionnaire obtained information concerning the participants' age, height and weight.

Dietary restraint The restrained eating behavior subscale of the Dutch Eating Behaviour Questionnaire (DEBQ [11]) was used to evaluate how often participants employed different dietary restraint behaviours (e.g., "Do you try to eat less at meal times than you would like to eat?"). Items from the DEBQ were rated on a 5-point Likert scale, ranging from 1 (*never*) to 5 *(very often)*, and averaged to form a single index of dietary restraint. The DEBQ has been shown to have good internal consistency, concurrent validity, and factorial validity [11-13]. Cronbach's alpha for the current sample was .92. The questionnaire was included in order to evaluate the level of eating pathology in order to provide context for the results.

State-based measures (Phase 2: Daily diary)

Negative mood The two negative mood items from the Trait Affect Scale (TAS (Blore, J., Subjective wellbeing: an assessment of competing theories, unpublished thesis)) [14] were used to measure negative state affect. The items were modified so that participants were required to indicate how they felt "right now" instead of "in general". Items were rated on an 11-point Likert scale ranging from 0 (*not at all)* to 10 (*extremely*). Item scores were averaged so that the possible score range was 0 to 10, with higher scores reflecting greater negative mood. Previous research has shown this measure to be sensitive to moment-by-moment fluctuations in mood [Blore, J., Subjective wellbeing: an assessment of competing theories, unpublished thesis], and to correlate with other state-based constructs such as body dissatisfaction (e.g., (Blore, J., Subjective wellbeing: an assessment of competing theories, unpublished thesis)) [14]. Using Geldhof, Preacher, and Zyphur's [15] method for calculating internal consistency of state-based scales in a multi-level framework, the maximal reliability for the negative mood states scale in the present study was estimated as .92.

Binge eating Participants were asked whether they had consumed food since their previous assessment. An answer of 'Yes' was followed up with six items derived from the Questionnaire for Eating and Weight Patterns – Revised (QEWP-R [16,17]) to determine whether they had engaged in a binge eating episode. Participants received the following items reflecting DSM symptoms of a binge episode (preceded by the stem *'Did you experience...'*): (a) rapid consumption of food, (b) eating until uncomfortably full, (c) eating despite not being hungry, (d) eating large quantities of food (relative to your usual meal size), (e) eating alone, or (f) feeling guilt and shame after eating.

Responses for these items were assigned a value of 1 for 'Yes' and 0 for 'No', so that possible scores for binge eating ranged from 0 to 6. An eating episode was classified as a probable case of binge eating if the participant reported three or more of the six symptoms listed above [1].

Procedure

Interested participants registered for the study by following a web link (presented in recruitment presentations) that directed them to a Plain Language Statement (PLS). Those who agreed to participate were directed to a subsequent webpage to complete the baseline questionnaire. At the completion of this web-based survey, participants provided mobile phone contact details to enable the researchers to text them notifications seven times per day for a period of one week. This was automated using Red Oxygen, a bulk SMS website.

To reduce the threat of response sets due to a predictable notification schedule [18], notifications were scheduled at random intervals each day between the hours of 10 am and 8 pm, with a minimum of 1 hour between notifications. Each notification contained a web link prompting participants to complete the state-based measures. The web-survey was designed to rescale to an appropriate size for smartphones so that participants could complete the survey via either their phone or computer. Hour and date of survey completion were recorded for all samplings. At the end of the 7-day testing period, participants were mailed a $20 gift voucher as an honorarium.

Data analytic strategy

Compliance to experience sampling protocol

Given the large number of assessment points used in a typical experience sampling study, it is common for participants to fail to complete some of their allotted assessments. Although missing data may lower study power, generalizability of results remain valid provided missingness is not meaningfully linked to individual difference factors [7]. Consequently, number of assessments completed (out of a total of 49) was correlated against BMI and dietary restraint, two variables that are highly relevant to the study of binge eating [19,20].

Threshold modeling

Hypothesis 1 was tested using logistic regression with standard errors adjusted for clustering by individual. Occurrence of a probable binge episode (coded as 'Yes' for binge symptoms scores greater than or equal to 3, and 'No' for scores less than 3) was regressed onto negative mood states, first as a continuous variable (the traditional approach), and then as a categorical variable reflecting whether a negative mood score met/exceeded a prescribed threshold value (i.e., the threshold + dose response approach). As the goal was to demonstrate the value of the threshold approach rather than derive a singular threshold value, we trialed all values of negative mood as thresholds, excluding the minimum (0) and maximum (10) values. In all models, binge eating was regressed onto the negative mood variable from the preceding assessment point in order to establish temporal precedence of the predictor variable. Moreover, time interval between assessment points was included as a covariate to control for differences in time intervals produced by the random assessment schedule. The superiority of the threshold + dose response model or the traditional model was based on which version of the predictor variable had a stronger effect size for predicting binge eating. Effect size was reported in odds ratios given that the outcome measure was dichotomous.

Time to onset modeling

Survival analysis was used to evaluate the extent to which level of negative mood predicted time to onset of a binge episode. Initially, a Cox proportional hazard model [21] was fitted, with negative mood as a continuous predictor; a variable to represent censoring due to completion of testing period before the onset of a binge, and participant ID as a grouping variable to allow for multiple outcomes of the same type (i.e., a binge) within the same person while correcting for non-independence that this introduces [22]. After establishing the strength and direction of linear association between severity of negative mood and time to onset, a subsequent model was run, with the same configurations as the first, with the exception that the negative mood variable was dummy coded so that more severe negative mood was compared against a less severe reference group. These dummy coded variables were introduced into the model as predictors of time to onset instead of the continuous mood variable in order to illustrate the extent to which increasing negative mood beyond a threshold level hastened the onset of a binge.

Results

Data cleaning and descriptives

Data were screened for patterns of missingness, presence of outliers and non-normality, and evidence of systematic bias in compliance with the experience sampling component of the study. Less than 2% missing data was found for Phase 1 (trait based measures), and dealt with using expectation maximization. On average participants completed over 80% of the experience sampling assessment points ($M = 39.94$ assessments, $SD = 7.39$, range 19–49). Individual differences in the number of Phase 2 random assessments completed were not associated reliably with BMI ($r = -.05$, $p = .635$) or dietary restraint ($r = -.07$, $p = .497$). There were no outliers or evidence of non-normality in any variable. Moreover, levels of dietary restraint ($M = 28.78$, $SD = 8.99$, possible range = 10–50) were moderate for the sample as a whole and showed considerable variability around this mean, ensuring coverage of the spectrum of severity for eating disturbances.

As may be expected given that ESM samples randomly many times per day, the prevalence of episodes of binge eating was relatively infrequent compared to the total number of assessments, occurring in 149 of 3714 assessments (4% overall across all participants). Thirty-one out of 93 participants (33%) reported at least one binge episode and, of those who reported a binge episode, the average number of binge episodes was 3.06 ($SD = 2.46$, range = 1 to 9 binge episodes). The proportion of cases that met the cut-off for the various thresholds for negative mood declined linearly, such that 94% of assessment points included a negative mood score of 1 or more, whereas only 3% of assessments included negative mood scores of 10 (see the left-hand column in Table 1).

Threshold modelling

As shown in Table 1, the association between negative mood and binge outcome was statistically significant, although the effect size was negligible when using the traditional approach of modeling negative mood as a continuous variable (odds ratio, OR = 1.25, $p = .001$). In contrast, the threshold approach more accurately predicted onset of a binge, with a linear trend in effect sizes from threshold 3 (comparing negative mood scores of 0–2 against 3–10) onwards. From threshold 6 (comparing negative mood scores of 0–5 against 6–10) onwards, the threshold approach had an effect that was at least three times as strong in predicting onset of a binge episode than the traditional approach.

Time to onset modeling

Survival analysis established a negative log-linear association between level of negative mood and time to onset of a binge episode ($B = -.93$, $p = .035$), indicating that extreme negative mood states were temporally closer than low negative mood states to binge onset. In subsequent modeling, negative mood was dummy coded with scores of 5 (representing the midpoint on the negative mood scale) used as a reference category and values of 6 to 10 used as target group. Results of this additional analysis showed that the extent of negative mood generally heightened the onset time for a binge, with the exception of negative mood values of 9; negative mood 6 vs. 5: $B = -.31$, $p = .020$, negative mood 7 vs. 5: $B = -.25$, $p = .039$, negative mood 8 vs. 5: $B = -.31$, $p = .086$, negative mood 9 vs. 5: $B = .13$, $p = .273$, negative mood 10 vs. 5: $B = -.16$, $p = .346$.

Table 1 Effect sizes (Odds Ratios) for the relationship between negative mood and binge eating

Predictor	% above	Odds ratio	*p* value
Traditional	n/a	1.25	.001
Threshold 1	93.8%	2.91	.038
Threshold 2	82.9%	2.37	.023
Threshold 3	56.1%	1.68	.055
Threshold 4	40.1%	1.93	.022
Threshold 5	27.8%	2.38	.003
Threshold 6	15.5%	3.68	.000
Threshold 7	8.5%	3.97	.000
Threshold 8	4.7%	4.46	.002
Threshold 9	2.8%	5.58	.002

Notes: % above = proportion of assessment points (across all participants) that met or exceeded the threshold cut-value. n/a = not applicable.

Discussion

Overview of findings

Although a growing body of literature has documented the influence of negative mood states on binge eating [5], there has been limited discussion of how different modeling approaches serve to optimize prediction of binge eating. Therefore, the present study utilized the experience sampling method [7] to test alternate models of the nature of the negative mood-binge eating relationship. In particular, we tested whether the negative mood-binge eating relationship is best characterized as (i) linear or (ii) a threshold. If the latter is correct, surpassing this threshold will serve to increase both (i) risk of binge eating and (ii) subsequent negative mood. Given this, we also tested whether increased negative mood beyond the threshold predicts time to onset of the binge episode; that is, that severity of negative mood can be used to estimate time to onset of a binge.

Our findings offer support for both of our predictions. Whether or not an individual exceeded a threshold value proved to be a better predictor than the severity of negative mood for likelihood of a subsequent binge episode for all thresholds. Once the cut-point reached 6 out of 10 on the negative mood scale, the threshold version of negative mood was approximately three times stronger in predicting binge occurrence than the traditional approach of modeling negative mood severity (i.e., using mood as a continuous predictor). Model effect sizes were further optimized as the cut-point was increased.

The fact that the odds ratios continued to increase monotonically with the rising threshold cut-off rather than stabilizing or reducing may be explained in several ways. First, it may be that exceeding a threshold makes the binge outcome likely, but that continued and intensifying negative mood enhances the likelihood of a binge in much the same way that threshold dose–response models in toxicology predict that whereas sub-threshold doses of a carcinogen may have negligible and possibly contrary effects on health, once exposure exceeds the threshold, health risk is proportional to level of exposure [23,24]. Consistent with the affect regulation model [5,6], an individual when faced with negative emotional states may seek healthy solutions initially but, discouraged by continued or exacerbated symptoms, may then escalate to more unhealthy, distracting solutions, such as binge eating.

A second possible explanation for the increasing odds of a binge as the cut-point increases has to do with the timing between exposure to negative mood and onset of binge. In the survival analysis, time to onset hastened as severity of negative mood increased. Thus, whereas a negative mood state of 8 out of 10 may indicate an imminent binge episode, a moderate negative mood state (such as 6 out of 10) may allow sufficient lead time for intervening events to distract the individual, thus preventing a binge episode. Indeed, the odds of a binge episode at lower levels of negative mood may be attenuated due to naturally occurring interventions, such as presence of others, work or family responsibilities, that may take precedence and/or make it difficult or undesirable to binge. This latter (timing-based) explanation is consistent with prior studies that have shown that binge eating is preceded by a period of escalating negative mood. Crosby et al. [25] found that binge episodes were most common on days in which individuals experienced either stable elevated negative mood or consistently rising negative mood throughout the day. Similarly, Smyth et al. [26] demonstrated a steady rise in negative mood in a 6 hour period that peaked immediately prior to a binge episode.

The present findings show statistical superiority of the threshold approach for modeling likelihood of a binge. This approach may also have an advantage in interpretability over the severity approach. In the severity approach used in the present study, negative mood states were modeled as group-mean centred predictors, meaning that the substantive research question is whether deviations in self-reported mood state above one's own usual mood state increase the likelihood of a binge eating episode. The interpretive adequacy of this approach then depends on: (1) the average mood state of the individual over the testing period; (2) the extent to which they fluctuate around this mean; and (3) how far they deviate from their mean. In the present study, 52% of participants had an average negative mood score of 3 or below. Such a low average score would mean that many instances in which the individual exceeds their average negative mood would still be comfortable levels of negative mood that are unlikely to distress them or prompt strategies such as overeating. In contrast, the threshold value can be seen to be more meaningfully interpreted as it is the level of negative mood beyond which a binge episode becomes increasingly likely.

Implications of findings for future research and clinical practice

These findings have potential implications for treatment of binge eating. While, on the one hand, extreme negative mood states (when modeled as a threshold) are the best predictor of likelihood of a binge, it may be prudent to intervene once a patient exceeds a moderate level of negative mood for several related reasons. First, even at a threshold of 6, the mood-binge eating relationship is strong [27]. Second, as there appears to be a greater temporal gap between experience of moderate negative mood and a binge than there is between severe negative mood and bingeing, there is more time to intervene. Also, it is possible that reducing moderate negative mood to a sub-threshold level is easier than attempting to reduce severe negative mood. Third, with the advent of self-guided e-health technologies, such as interactive websites and smartphone apps that monitor risk and provide early warning signals for target event [28], the increase in false positives produced by using a less accurate threshold value may be justified if treatment is not dependent upon consultation with a clinician. As an app is more cost-effective than a therapy session and does not burden the health system with unnecessary appointments [28], a conservative approach (erring on the side of action instead of inaction) may have benefits that outweigh costs. Furthermore, the alternative – setting an extreme threshold – may increase specificity at the expense of sensitivity, as it may be that some episodes of binge eating arise when the individual's negative mood state is only moderate.

Given that negative mood states are a common feature of many psychological disorders, including depression and bipolar disorder, this threshold model may have broader applicability for predicting symptoms of psychological disorder other than binge eating. Future research should evaluate the generalizability of our threshold approach for predicting onset of other events of clinical importance.

Limitations

Our findings should be considered within the context of several limitations of the study. First, as effect sizes were used to compare models, it is possible that the difference in model performance (linear vs threshold) is somewhat overstated in the present study. After all, odds ratios in logistic regression analyses will be larger for categorical (threshold model) than continuous predictors (linear model). It is encouraging then, that even with this potential bias, the strength of association increased substantially as the threshold negative mood level was elevated.

Second, the method used in the present study to assess binge episodes does not definitively diagnose a binge episode. In particular, two key aspects of binge eating (quantity consumed and perceived loss of control) may not have been captured optimally. Quantity of food was assessed by self-report rather than objectively, and the five symptoms of binge eating used in the present study correspond well with perceived loss of control during eating [29], but do not explicitly ask about loss of control. Thus, it is possible that the present measure detects related, yet distinct eating behaviors, such as dysregulated or emotional eating, instead of binge eating.

A related concern is that although the sample appeared to cover the spectrum of severity of dietary restraint, formal diagnoses of eating disorders were not conducted, and given that a convenience sample of university students was recruited, it is likely that many of the participants would not meet criteria for an eating disorder diagnosis. Similarly, although we exclusively recruited women in order to be consistent with previous literature [5], binge eating is also common among men [30]. As such, it is possible that the frequency of binge eating episodes and the strength of association between negative mood and binge eating onset is weaker in the present study than would be anticipated for a clinical population that sampled both men and women. It is encouraging then, that this association yielded strong effects even in this non-clinical sample. Nevertheless, future research is needed to validate present models in a clinical sample, and this should include objective measures of binge eating occurrence.

Conclusion

The present findings clearly support a threshold approach for modeling the influence of negative mood on likelihood of a binge episode. Even at low threshold values, this approach clearly outperformed the traditional, severity approach for predicting negative mood studies. However, the findings suggest that severity of negative mood may be more usefully employed to predict time to onset of a binge episode. Although likelihood of a binge and time to onset were strongest and shortest, respectively, at highest levels of negative mood, we argue that there is need to intervene at even moderate levels of negative mood because moderate levels were also strongly predictive of a binge outcome and, importantly, this allows more time to prevent the binge episode. This information could be used in the development of a smartphone app that seeks to disrupt the connection between negative mood and binge eating. A useful next step for future research would be to evaluate the efficacy of intervening at different threshold values for reducing the frequency of binge episodes.

Competing interests
The authors declare that they have no competing interests.

Authors' contributions
MFT, BR, and LB conducted all analyses and wrote the Results section. MH, HS, and JB contributed to conception of the project. DA, DC, and BK made significant contributions to interpretation of findings in light of study implications, as based on their clinical experience. All authors contributed to drafting and revision of the manuscript. All authors read and approved the final manuscript.

Acknowledgements
The authors would like to thank the reviewers for their valuable input in shaping this manuscript. There were no funding sources for this project.

Author details
[1]School of Psychology, Deakin University, 221 Burwood Highway, Burwood, VIC 3125, Australia. [2]Psychiatry Department, University of Melbourne, Melbourne, VIC, Australia. [3]St Vincent's Hospital, Melbourne, VIC, Australia. [4]Faculty of Health, Deakin University, Burwood, Australia. [5]DVC-Research & Innovation Portfolio; the School of Health Sciences; and the Collaborative Research Network, Federation University, Ballarat, Australia. [6]National Institute for Mental Health Research, The Australian National University, Canberra, Australia.

References

1. Latner JD, Clyne C: **The diagnostic validity of the criteria for binge eating disorder.** *Int J Eat Disord* 2008, **41**:1–14.
2. American Psychiatric Association: *Diagnostic and Statistical Manual of Mental Disorders.* 5th edition. Arlington, VA: American Psychiatric Publishing; 2013.
3. Johnson JG, Spitzer RL, Williams JB: **Health problems, impairment and illnesses associated with bulimia nervosa and binge eating disorder among primary care and obstetric gynaecology patients.** *Psychol Med* 2001, **31**:1455–1466.
4. Yanovski SZ: **Binge eating disorder and obesity in 2003: could treating an eating disorder have a positive effect on the obesity epidemic?** *Int J Eat Disord* 2003, **34**:S117–S120.
5. Haedt-Matt AA, Keel PK: **Revisiting the affect regulation model of binge eating: a meta-analysis of studies using ecological momentary assessment.** *Psychol Bull* 2011, **137**:660–681.
6. Hawkins RC, Clement PF: **Binge eating: measurement problems and a conceptual model.** In *The Binge Purge Syndrome: Diagnosis, Treatment, and Research.* Edited by Hawkins RC, Fremouw WJ, Clement PF. New York: Springer; 1984:229–251.
7. Bolger N, Laurenceau JP: *Intensive Longitudinal Methods: An Introduction to Diary and Experience Sampling Research.* New York: Guilford Press; 2013.
8. Beal DJ, Weiss HM: **Methods of ecological momentary assessment in organizational research.** *Organ Res Methods* 2003, **6**:440–464.
9. Bolger N, Davis A, Rafaeli E: **Diary methods: capturing life as it is lived.** *Annu Rev Psychol* 2003, **54**:579–616.
10. National Institute of Health: *Clinical Guidelines on the Identification, Evaluation, and Treatment of Overweight and Obesity in Adults: Executive Summary.* [www.nhlbi.nih.gov/guidelines/obesity/ob_exsum.pdf]
11. Van Strien T, Fritjers JER, Berger GPA, Defares PB: **The Dutch Eating Behavior Questionnaire (DEBQ) for assessment of restrained, emotional, and external eating behavior.** *Int J Eat Disord* 1986, **5**:295–315.
12. Van Strien T: **The concurrent validity of a classification of dieters with low versus high susceptibility toward failure of restraint.** *Addict Behav* 1997, **22**:587–597.
13. Wardle J: **Eating style: a validation of the Dutch eating behavior questionnaire in normal subjects and women with eating disorders.** *J Psychosom Res* 1987, **31**:161–169.
14. Colautti L, Fuller-Tyszkiewicz M, Skouteris H, McCabe M, Blackburn S, Wyett E: **Accounting for fluctuations in body dissatisfaction.** *Body Image* 2011, **8**:315–321.
15. Geldhof GJ, Preacher KJ, Zyphur MJ: **Reliability estimation in a multilevel confirmatory factor analysis framework.** *Psychol Methods* 2014, **19**:72–91.
16. Nangle DW, Johnson WG, Carr-Nangle RE, Engler LB: **Binge eating disorder and the proposed DSM-IV criteria: psychometric analysis of the Questionnaire of Eating and Weight Patterns.** *Int J Eat Disord* 1994, **16**:147–157.

17. Yanovski SZ: **Binge eating disorder: current knowledge and future directions.** *Obes Res* 1993, **1**:306–324.
18. Napa Scollon C, Kim-Prieto C, Diener E: **Experience sampling: promises and pitfalls, strengths and weaknesses.** *J Happiness Stud* 2003, **4**:5–34.
19. Guss JL, Kissileff HR, Devlin MJ, Zimmerli E, Walsh T: **Binge size increases with body mass index in women with binge-eating disorder.** *Obes Res* 2002, **10**:1021–1029.
20. Johnson F, Pratt M, Wardle J: **Dietary restraint and self-regulation in eating behavior.** *Int J Obes (Lond)* 2012, **36**:665–674.
21. Breslow NE: **Analysis of survival data under the proportional hazards model.** *Int Stat Rev* 1975, **43**:45–57.
22. Galbraith S, Daniel A, Vissel B: **A study of clustered data and approaches to its analysis.** *J Neurosci* 2010, **30**:10601–10608.
23. Calabrese EJ, Baldwin LA: **The hermetic dose–response model is more common than the threshold model in toxicology.** *Toxicol Sci* 2003, **71**:246–250.
24. Cox C: **Threshold dose–response models in toxicology.** *Biometrics* 1987, **43**:511–523.
25. Crosby RD, Wonderlich SA, Engel SG, Simonich H, Smyth J, Mitchell JE: **Daily mood patterns and bulimic behaviors in the natural environment.** *Behav Res Ther* 2009, **47**:181–188.
26. Smyth J, Wonderlich S, Heron K, Sliwinski M, Crosby R, Mitchell J, Engel S: **Daily and momentary mood and stress predict binge eating and vomiting in bulimia nervosa patients in the natural environment.** *J Consult Clin Psychol* 2007, **75**:629–638.
27. Ferguson CJ: **An effect size primer: a guide for clinicians and researchers.** *Prof Psychol-Res Pr* 2009, **40**:532–538.
28. Kelly J, Gooding P, Pratt D, Ainsworth J, Welford M, Tarrier N: **Intelligent real-time therapy: harnessing the power of machine learning to optimize the delivery of momentary cognitive-behavioural interventions.** *J Ment Health* 2012, **21**:404–414.
29. White MA, Grilo CM: **Diagnostic efficiency of DSM-IV indicators for binge eating episodes.** *J Consult Clin Psychol* 2011, **79**:75–83.
30. Striegel-Moore R, Franko D: **Should binge eating disorder be included in the DSM-V? A critical review of the state of the evidence.** *Annu Rev Clin Psychol* 2008, **4**:305–324.

3

Eating disorder subtypes differ in their rates of psychosocial improvement over treatment

Allison C Kelly[1*] and Jacqueline C Carter[2]

Abstract

Background: Individuals with Anorexia Nervosa (AN) are renowned for their poor short- and long-term treatment outcomes. To gain more insight into the reasons for these poor outcomes, the present study compared patients with AN-R (restrictive subtype), AN-BP (binge-purge subtype), bulimia nervosa (BN), and eating disorder not otherwise specified (EDNOS) over 12 weeks of specialized eating disorders treatment.
Eighty-nine patients completed the Eating Disorder Examination- Questionnaire (EDE-Q) and various measures of psychosocial functioning at baseline, and again after weeks 3, 6, 9, and 12 of treatment.

Results: Multilevel modeling revealed that, over the 12 weeks, patients with AN-BP and AN-R had slower improvements in global eating disorder pathology, shape concerns, and self-compassion than those with EDNOS and BN. Patients with AN-BP had slower improvements in shame, social safeness (i.e., feelings of warmth in one's relationships), and received social support compared to those with AN-R, BN, and EDNOS.

Conclusions: These findings support the need for more effective and comprehensive clinical interventions for patients with AN and especially AN-BP. Results also highlight not-yet studied processes that might contribute to the poor outcomes AN patients often face during and after treatment.

Keywords: Anorexia nervosa, Transdiagnostic, Treatment process, Treatment outcome, Change trajectories, Self-compassion, Received social support, Shame, Social safeness

Background

Individuals with Anorexia Nervosa (AN) typically fare worse than those with other eating disorders, and it is unclear why [1-3]. Patients with AN are more likely to drop out of treatment prematurely and less likely to experience sustained symptom remission following treatment [4-9]. They also face a risk of mortality that tends to be higher than that of other psychiatric groups [10-12]. Although it is known that AN is a persistent and destructive illness, we know little about why long-term outcomes are poorer for this eating disorder than for others.

In an attempt to understand the dismal outcomes associated with AN, many researchers have sought to identify prognostic factors within AN-only samples. With regards to pre-treatment predictors, certain characteristics of the disorder, such as binge-purge behaviours and a lower BMI, and various psychosocial variables, such as perfectionism, obsessive-compulsive traits, and socially inhibited interpersonal patterns, have emerged as predictors of poorer outcome over time [13-20]. Certain discharge variables have also predicted long-term outcome in AN. Relapse appears more likely among patients who leave treatment with a greater drive to exercise, residual concerns about weight and shape, and a lower readiness to maintain treatment gains [20,21]. Alcohol abuse and poor social adjustment at discharge have also predicted elevated mortality risk at long-term follow-up [12]. Pre-treatment and post-treatment patient factors therefore seem to be important predictors of long-term outcomes in AN.

Next research steps

Although the field has identified numerous pre- and post-treatment predictors of outcome among individuals with AN, there are two gaps in the literature which, if addressed, might help to explain why AN patients fare worse than those with other eating disorders. First, there

* Correspondence: allison.kelly@uwaterloo.ca
[1]Department of Psychology, University of Waterloo, Waterloo, ON N2L 3G1, Canada
Full list of author information is available at the end of the article

is a scarcity of research on the processes that occur for AN patients *during* treatment [16,22,23]. Most treatment studies assess patients at two discrete time points (i.e., pre and post). Associated analytic approaches typically exclude patients for whom an observation is missing, leaving a biased sample. In addition, linear change is assumed, but never confirmed. We therefore suggest that it is important to assess patients' functioning at various time points over the course of treatment to allow for analytical approaches that can more precisely model patterns of change. Identifying the ways in which symptoms and psychosocial functioning change – or remain the same – during treatment might shed light on the poor long-term outcomes AN patients face.

Second, there is little research on the ways in which eating disorder diagnostic groups differ in their experiences over the course of eating disorders treatment. This relative absence of research may stem from practical issues that make between-group comparisons difficult during treatment. First, patients with severe AN often attend different treatment programs from those with other eating disorder patients. Second, weight restoration is generally the most studied outcome variable in AN, but is often not a relevant indicator of progress in other eating disorder groups. We suggest value in designing studies that overcome these barriers and render comparisons between diagnostic groups possible. Such studies may shed light on how individuals with AN differ from those with other eating disorders, not only at the start and end of treatment, but also as treatment unfolds.

The present study

We sought to address the aforementioned gaps in the literature on AN by comparing the change processes of patients with AN-R, AN-BP, BN, and EDNOS during specialized eating disorders treatment. We believed such an approach would help us glean important information about the factors we may be failing to adequately assess and target during treatment. Given the prognostic relevance of eating disorder symptoms and psychosocial factors in predicting long-term outcomes, we sought to compare the trajectories of eating disorder subtypes in both domains. We therefore administered multiple repeated measures of variables that have transdiagnostic relevance to eating disorder patients, rendering between-group comparisons possible. We assessed eating disorder symptoms with the Eating Disorders Examination Questionnaire (EDE-Q) and assessed psychosocial functioning with measures of shame, social safeness, received social support, and self-compassion.

Gilbert's transdiagnostic theory of psychopathology [24,25] inspired our selection of psychosocial variables. Shame is a painful self-conscious feeling that derives from seeing oneself as defective and imagining others share this view. Gilbert proposed that shame contributes to the maintenance of self-destructive behaviours seen in many forms of psychopathology including eating disorders. Feelings of social safeness, however, are considered antidotal to shame. Social safeness is an emotional sense of warmth, belonging, and calmness, and is thought to arise from the soothing system in the brain, which is sensitive to signals of compassion from others and self [26,27]. According to Gilbert, the soothing system is paramount to sustained well-being because it evolved to tone down the threat system, which is highly implicated in shame and psychopathology [28,29]. Gilbert proposed that receiving compassion from others and/or self is the optimal ways to stimulate the soothing system. Therefore, we additionally examined received social support, as an indicator of compassion received from others, and self-compassion, defined as a kind, caring attitude toward personal distress and shortcomings [30].

We hypothesized that, compared to patients with BN and EDNOS, those with AN would have slower improvements over time in eating disorder pathology, shame, social safeness, received social support, and self-compassion. Given past research documenting the poor prognoses associated with AN-BP, we expected that these slower rates of improvement in AN would be especially pronounced among those with the AN-BP subtype of the illness.

Methods

Sample

Participants were 89 patients admitted to the Toronto General Hospital's adult eating disorders program between September 2010 and August 2012. To be admitted into either program, individuals must meet DSM-IV-TR criteria for an eating disorder based on the Eating Disorder Examination [31]. Exclusion criteria for treatment included a diagnosis of binge eating disorder, having an active substance-related disorder, being younger than 18, and being unwilling to comply with the treatment norms. Please see Figure 1 for a flow chart of the recruitment process. The majority (72.2%) of participants was admitted to the eating disorder program's day hospital, and 27.8% was admitted to the program's inpatient unit.

Enough information was collected during intake assessments to classify patients based on revised DSM-5 criteria. We therefore present the DSM-5 diagnostic breakdown of our sample, but for simplicity, we group those with specified and unspecified eating disorders under EDNOS. Twenty-six (29.2%) participants had AN-R, 17 (19.1%) had AN-BP, 26 (29.2%) had BN, and 20 (22.5%) had EDNOS. BMI at admission differed by diagnostic group; means were 15.8 (SD = 1.97) for AN-R,

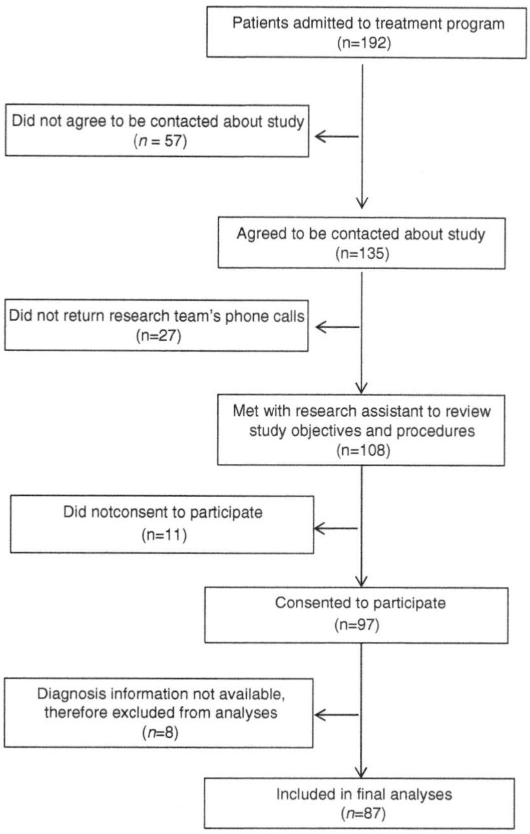

Figure 1 Recruitment and participation flow-chart.

17.08 (SD = 1.54) for AN-BP, 24.52 (SD = 6) for BN, and 23.02 (SD = 4.15) for EDNOS. Of those with EDNOS, three had subthreshold AN-R, four had subthreshold AN-BP, five had subthreshold BN, four had purging disorder, and four had unspecified eating disorders. Eight of those with EDNOS had BMIs between 18 and 20, and the remaining 12 had BMIs of 20 and above. The mean number of previous admissions into the treatment program was 1.29 (SD = .77) and this number did not differ by diagnostic group.

Our sample was predominantly female (97%) and the ethnic breakdown was 79.2% Caucasian, 4.5% East Asian, 1.4% South Asian, 2.8% African-Canadian, 10.8% Latino, and 1.5% mixed race. Participants' mean age was 28 years (SD = 9.6); a minority of patients (17.4%) was between 17 and 19 years of age and the remainder was 20 and older. The diagnostic groups did not differ in any of our demographic variables.

Treatment programs

The day hospital and inpatient eating disorders programs at the Toronto General Hospital are run by multidisciplinary teams, consisting of psychiatrists, psychologists, nurses, dieticians, social workers, and occupational therapists. Treatment consists of group therapy as well as staff-supported meals and snacks. The program focuses on medical stabilization, nutritional rehabilitation and normalized eating, eradication of symptomatic behaviours, and in the case of underweight patients, weight restoration [32]. Patients are admitted to these programs on an ongoing basis whenever a spot becomes available. As such, group make-up fluctuates over time. The duration of treatment also varies by patient. Those admitted to the day hospital commit to eight weeks of intensive treatment, and then go onto a less intensive version of treatment. Those admitted to the inpatient unit remain in the program until they have reached a BMI of 20, and then move into the day hospital for eight weeks. Unless patients choose to leave treatment prematurely or are asked to leave because of non-compliance, patients across programs remain in some version of treatment for at least 12 weeks.

Procedure

Ethics approval was obtained from the University Health Network Research Ethics Board. Participants were asked to complete online questionnaires at the start of their admission, and again after three, six, nine, and 12 weeks of treatment. Questionnaires were emailed to them in the form of a web link, and participants were asked to try and complete them within 48 hours of receiving them. On average, participants completed assessments 4.3 (SD = 1.1) weeks apart from one another.

Measures

Eating disorder symptoms

The 36-item Eating Disorder Examination–Questionnaire (EDE-Q) was used to assess eating disorder symptoms over the previous 28 days [33]. Although questionnaires in this study were administered every 21 days, the fact that the average participant completed surveys late (ever 4.3 weeks) made the assessment windows consistent with the EDE-Q time frame. The EDE-Q generates scores from 0 to 6 on four subscales of Shape Concern, Weight Concern, Eating Concern, and Dietary Restraint. These subscales represent transdiagnostic eating disorder symptoms. A global score of eating disorder pathology is calculated by taking the mean of these four subscale scores. The EDE-Q's test-retest reliability and internal consistency are strong [34]. In the present sample, Cronbach alphas were .96 for the global score, .89 for Shape Concern, .81 for Weight Concern, .88 for Eating Concern, and .83 for Dietary Restraint. Participants had a mean EDE-Q global score of 4.04 (SD = 1.32) at the time of their admission, confirming their clinically severe eating disorder pathology [35].

Shame

Shame was assessed using the 25-item Experience of Shame Scale (ESS) [36]. The ESS generates global shame score, computed by taking the mean of all items, as well as subscale scores representing body shame, character shame, and behaviour shame. A factor analysis of all ESS items in our sample supported a one-factor solution. Sample items from the ESS, rated from 1 (not at all) to 4 (very much) include: "Have you felt ashamed of the sort of person you are?" and "Have you tried to cover up or conceal things you felt ashamed of having done?" The ESS has evidence of high test-retest reliability, good discriminant and construct validity, and high internal consistency, the latter of which was reflected by a Cronbach's alpha of .95 in our sample. Participants had a mean global shame score of 3.15 (SD = .65) at the time of their admission.

Social safeness

We assessed social safeness with the Social Safeness and Pleasure Scale (SSPS) [26]. This 11-item measure uses a 0–4 scale to ask participants to rate the extent to which they experience a sense of warmth, reassurance, and belonging in their social relationships. Sample items include: "I feel easily soothed by those around me," I feel connected to others," and "I feel a sense of warmth in my relationships with people." This measure has been found to have strong internal consistency, which was demonstrated by a Cronbach's alpha of .94 in our sample. Mean social safeness at baseline was 1.4 (SD = .95).

Received social support

We measured received social support (RSS) with the Social Provisions Scale (SPS-short) [37]. The SPS-short is a 6-item measure that can be used to assess perceptions that social support would be available if needed (perceived social support), as well as actual social support received (RSS). We administered the RSS version only. Using a 7-point Likert scale, participants rated the extent to which they received each of six social provisions over the previous three weeks: guidance, assistance, emotional closeness, social integration, reassurance of worth, and opportunity for nurturance. Sample items include: "To what extent did another person(s) come to your assistance," and "To what extent did another person(s) provide you with a sense of emotional security and well-being." The scale's Cronbach's alpha was .80, demonstrating adequate internal consistency. Participants' mean baseline score was 4.6 (SD = 1.36).

Self-compassion

The 12-item Self-Compassion Scale-Short Form (SCS-SF) was used to assess self-compassion [38]. The SCS-SF asks participants to use a 5-point scale to rate their typical reactions at times of personal distress. Sample items include "I try to be kind and patient towards those aspects of my personality I don't like," "I try to see my failings as part of the human condition," and "When something painful happens I try to take a balanced view of the situation." This shortened version of the Self-Compassion Scale correlates near perfectly with the full, 26-item version [30]. In the current study, the SCS-SF had a Cronbach's alpha of .85, demonstrating good internal consistency. Participants' mean self-compassion score at baseline was 2.04 (SD = .68).

Patterns of missing data

At baseline (Time 0), participants completed all questionnaires through a study-specific survey with the exception of the EDE-Q, which was administered as part of the clinical intake process. Time 0 responses on the EDE-Q were available for 80 of the 89 participants; eight patients did not complete their questionnaire, and six patients left treatment before returning their responses. Responses for all other study measures (e.g., shame, self-compassion) at Time 0 were available for all 89 participants. On average, participants completed 3.65 out of 5 assessments over the 12 study weeks, with 58 of the 89 participants completing three or more questionnaires.

Analytic strategy

Our primary analytic approach was multilevel modeling with maximum likelihood estimation. This is the recommended statistical approach when modeling participant trajectories over time [39]. Two notable advantages of multilevel modeling in longitudinal studies are its ability to model change trajectories without fixed data collection schedules, and its ability to retain data from participants for whom observations are missing at random (MAR). MAR means that the observations that are missing are unrelated to the unobserved value(s) but may be related to the unobserved value(s) through other variables in the model for which observations are not missing [40]. We found evidence to support the MAR assumption in the present data set.

We tested our hypotheses using PROC MIXED in SAS 9.3. Dependent variables were EDE-Q eating disorder symptoms, shame, social safeness, received social support, and self-compassion across all available time points between weeks 0 and 12 of treatment inclusive. Because participants commonly completed surveys later than they were asked, we used time stamps to enter the precise time point in their treatment course (i.e., 3 weeks, 4.5 weeks, etc.) at which they completed each of their surveys for greater precision [41].

All multilevel models contained a fixed and random effects portion, and an unstructured error covariance. We included a random effect for intercept and time.

Fixed effects were time, diagnosis (AN-R, AN-BP, BN, EDNOS), Diagnosis x Time, baseline levels of the outcome variable (covariate), and the former's interaction with time. Demographic variables (e.g., age, marital status, living circumstances), treatment program (i.e., inpatient vs. day hospital), BMI, and their interactions with time were initially included as fixed effects, but these terms were dropped from final models because none was significant.

Preliminary analyses revealed that baseline EDE-Q global and subscale scores varied by diagnostic group; therefore, we sought to control for shared variance between eating disorder pathology and diagnosis in our models. We therefore included the relevant baseline EDE-Q score and its interaction with time as fixed effects in our models. In all models, a significant effect for Diagnosis x Time would indicate that the dependent variables changed over a time as a function of participants' eating disorder diagnosis. We then probed significant Diagnosis x Time interactions with simple slope estimates, representing rates of change, for each diagnostic group. Contrasts were then used to compare rates of change across AN-R, AN-BP, EDNOS, and BN. In addition, mean point estimates of the dependent variable were calculated and plotted for each diagnostic group at weeks 0, 3, 6, 9, and 12.

Results

Preliminary analyses

First, Pearson zero-order correlations were computed between study variables at baseline to provide information on the distinguishability of our dependent variables from one another (see Table 1). Inter-correlations between EDE-Q subscales indicate that these variables shared anywhere from 46% to 69% of their variance, whereas the EDE-Q subscales shared anywhere from 74% to 83% of their variance with the EDE-Q global scale. No other pair of variables shared more than half of their variance indicating that the psychosocial variables are related to one another, and to eating disorder pathology, but are distinguishable constructs.

Second, a series of multiple regressions was conducted, using PROC GLM in SAS, to determine whether the four diagnostic groups differed on any of our study variables at baseline. We found that diagnosis predicted baseline EDE-Q global scores, F (3, 76) = 2.93, $p < .05$, eating concerns, F (3, 76) = 3.48, $p < .05$, weight concerns, F (3, 76) = 2.78, $p < .05$, and shape concerns, F (3, 76) 4.38, $p < .01$, but not restraint, F (3, 76) = 1.0, *n.s.* Contrasts revealed that individuals with AN-R reported lower total and subscale scores than the other groups, *p*'s < .01. Controlling for baseline EDE-Q Global, diagnosis also emerged as a significant predictor of baseline social safeness, F (3, 74) = 3.32, $p < .01$. Contrasts revealed that on average, the AN-R and AN-BP groups reported feeling less socially safe at baseline than the EDNOS and BN groups, F (1, 76) = 8.61, $p < .01$. There was no effect of diagnosis on baseline received social support, shame, or self-compassion, indicating that patients across the four diagnostic groups did not differ from one another in these variables at the start of the study.

Does diagnosis predict rate of change in outcome variables?

Eating disorder symptoms

We first examined EDE-Q Global scores as the dependent variable. A significant effect was found for Diagnosis x Time, F (3, 214) = 2.66, $p < .05$. Simple slope estimates revealed that all diagnostic groups had significant decreases in EDE-Q global pathology over time, *p*'s < .001. Simple slope estimates for each diagnostic group are presented in Table 2. Planned contrasts revealed that on average, individuals with AN-R and AN-BP had slower EDE-Q Global decreases over time than those with EDNOS and BN, F (1, 214) = 7.81, $p < .01$. Mean point estimates in EDE-Q Global scores were calculated

Table 1 Zero-order correlations between study variables at baseline

	EDE-Q Global	EDE-Q Restraint	EDE-Q Weight	EDE-Q Shape	EDE-Q Eating	Shame	Safeness	Self-Compassion	RSS
EDE-Q global	–	.86[a]***	.91[a]***	.91[a]***	.90 [a]***	.67[b]***	-.49[c]***	-.45[b]***	-.26[c]*
EDE-Q restraint		–	.68 [a]***	.69 [a]***	.71[a]***	.52[b]***	-.40[c]***	-.29[b]*	-.26[c]*
EDE-Q weight			–	.83[a] ***	.75[a]***	.60[b]***	-.40[c]***	-.43[b]***	-.24[c]*
EDE-Q shape				–	.76[a]***	.62[b]***	-.44[c]***	-.43[b]***	-.21[c]
EDE-Q eating					–	.64[b]***	-.49[c]***	-.47[b] ***	-.22[c]
Shame						–	-.62 [c] ***	-.52[d]***	-.24[c]*
Social safeness							–	.61 [c] ***	.63 [c]***
Self-compassion								–	.34[c]***
RSS									–

[a]$n = 89$; [b]$n = 87$; [c]$n = 76$; [d]$n = 75$.
Note. EDE-Q, eating disorders examination questionnaire. *RSS*, received social support.
*p < .05; ***p < .001.

Table 2 Estimated rates of change (Slopes) in dependent variables by diagnostic group

	AN-R	AN-BP	BN	EDNOS	*Planned Contrasts*
EDE-Q Global	−11 (.03) ***	-.11 (.03) ***	-.18 (.03) ***	-.20 (.03) ***	AN < BN & EDNOS *
EDE-Q Restraint	-.22 (.03) ***	-.16 (.03) ***	-. 21 (.02) ***	-.32 (.03) ***	AN-BP < Others ***
EDE-Q Shape concern	-.00 (.04)	-.04 (.04)	-. 16 (.04) ***	-.15 (.04) ***	AN < BN & EDNOS ***
Shame	-.05 (.02) **	-.01 (.02)	-.07 (.02) ***	-.10 (.02) ***	AN-BP < Others **
Social safeness	.03 (.02) *	-.01 (.02)	.02 (.01)	.07 (.02) *	AN-BP < Others *
					EDNOS > Others *
Received social support	.00 (.04)	-.06 (.03) *	-.01 (.03)	.08 (.03) *	AN-BP < Others *
					EDNOS > Others *
Self-compassion	-.00 (.01)	-.01 (.01)	.05 (.01) ***	.06 (.02) ***	AN < BN & EDNOS ***

Note. EDE-Q, eating disorders examination questionnaire. The last column presents the results of planned contrasts between diagnostic groups for dependent variables where Diagnosis x Time emerged as a significant predictor.
$^{*}p < .05$; $^{**}p < .01$; $^{***}p < .001$.

and graphed for each diagnostic group at weeks 0, 3, 6, 9, and 12 (see Figure 2a).

We then examined each EDE-Q subscale separately as a dependent variable. There was no Diagnosis x Time effect when predicting Eating Concerns, F (3, 214) = .74, *n.s.*, or Weight Concerns, F (3, 214) = 1.38, *n.s.* Diagnosis x Time did, however, predict Restraint, F (3, 214) = 5.2, $p < .01$, and Shape Concerns, F (3, 214) = 4.3, $p < .01$. With regards to Restraint, simple slope estimates revealed that all diagnostic groups showed significant decreases in dietary restraint over time, p's < .001 (see Table 1). Contrasts additionally revealed that the EDNOS group improved at a faster rate than the average of the other three diagnostic groups, F (1, 214) = 12.51, $p < .001$. Furthermore, the AN-BP group improved at a slower rate than the average of the other three groups, F (1, 214) = 8.34, $p < .01$. Those with AN-R and BN were similar in their improvements, F (1, 214) = .28, *n.s.*

With regards to shape concerns, simple slope estimates revealed non-significant improvements over time for those with AN-R and AN-BP and significant decreases over time for those with BN and EDNOS, p's < .001 (see Table 2). Planned contrasts additionally revealed that those with AN-R and AN-BP improved at a significantly slower rate than those with EDNOS and BN, F (1, 214) = 12.12, $p < .001$.

Shame

There was a significant effect of Diagnosis x Time predicting changes in shame, F (3, 185) = 4.03, $p < .01$. As presented in Table 2, simple slope estimates revealed significant decreases in shame over time in the AN-R, BN, and EDNOS groups. The AN-BP group, however, did not improve over time, and this trajectory differed significantly from the average rate of change of the other three diagnostic groups, F (1, 185) = 8.45, $p < .01$ (see Figure 2b).

Social safeness

A significant effect was found for Diagnosis x Time, F (3, 181) = 2.63, $p = .05$ predicting changes in social safeness. As seen in Table 2, simple slope estimates indicated that the AN-R and EDNOS groups had significant increases in social safeness over time; the AN-BP and BN groups, however, reported no changes in social safeness over time. Planned contrasts revealed that the trajectory of the AN-BP group had a significantly slower change trajectory from the average of the other three diagnostic groups, F (1,181) = 5.47, $p < .05$. In addition, the EDNOS group had a significantly faster change trajectory than the average of the other three groups, F (1,181) = 5.24, $p < .05$ (see Figure 2c).

Received social support

We found a significant effect for Diagnosis x Time predicting changes in received social support, F (3, 181) = 2.94, $p < .05$. Simple slope estimates, presented in Table 2, revealed that the AN-R and BN groups had no changes in received social support over time. The AN-BP group, however, had significant decreases in in received support over time, and the EDNOS group had significant increases over time. Once again, the AN-BP group differed significantly in its trajectory compared to the average trajectory shown by the AN-R, BN, and EDNOS groups, F (1,181) = 6.02, $p < .05$. The EDNOS group also differed significantly, showing a faster rate of change than the average of the other three diagnostic groups, F (1,181) = 6.28, $p < .05$. Figure 2d displays a graphic representation.

Self-compassion

Diagnosis x Time predicted changes in self-compassion, F (3, 183) = 5.71, $p < .001$. Simple slope estimates, seen in Table 2, indicated non-significant improvements over time for the AN-R and AN-BP diagnostic groups. The BN and EDNOS groups, however, showed significant increases in self-compassion over time. The average rate

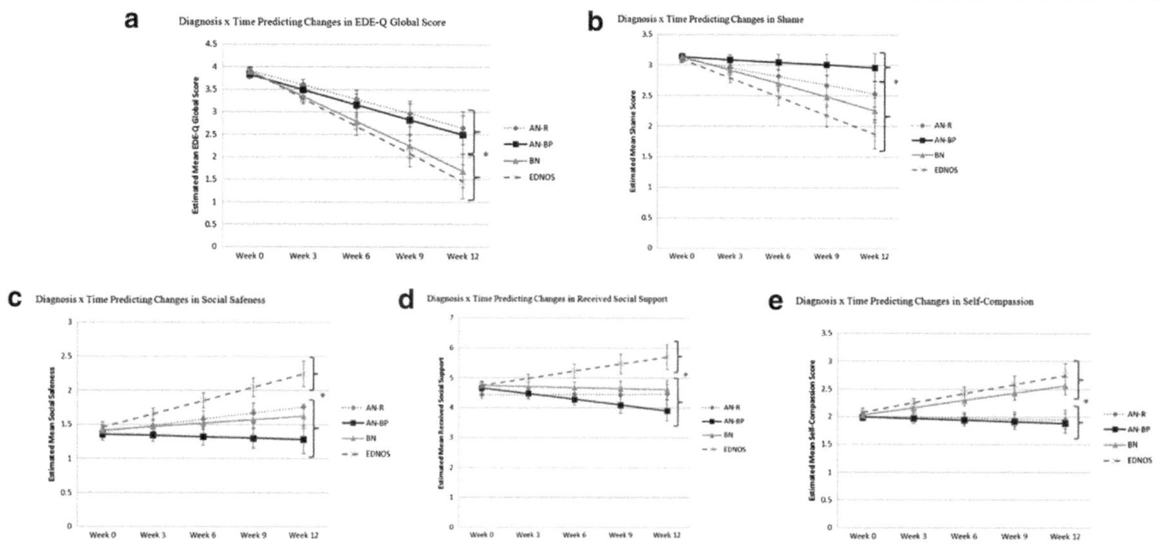

Figure 2 Diagnosis x time predicting changes in eating disorder symptoms and psychosocial functioning. Displays estimated means and standard error bars for **a)** EDE-Q global, **b)** shame, **c)** social safeness, **d)** received social support, and **e)** self-compassion at baseline, week 3, week 6, week 9, and week 12 for each diagnostic group.

of improvement in the BN and EDNOS groups was significantly greater than the average of the AN-R and AN-BP groups, F (1, 183) = 16.45, $p < .001$. See Figure 2e for a graphic representation.

Summary

As presented in Table 2, individuals with AN-BP had slower improvements in dietary restraint, shame, social safeness, and received support compared to those with AN-R, EDNOS, and BN. Individuals with AN-BP and AN-R had comparable trajectories in global eating disorder pathology, shape concerns, and self-compassion, and these rates of change were poorer than those experienced by patients with EDNOS and BN.

Discussion

This was the first study to our knowledge to compare eating disorder diagnostic groups' trajectories of change over multiple time points during treatment. Of note, changes in all outcome variables occurred in a linear manner. We found that compared to patients with BN and EDNOS, patients with AN, and especially those with AN-BP, had the slowest improvements in eating disorder symptoms and psychosocial functioning over 12 weeks of treatment. Both the AN-BP and AN-R groups had slower improvements in global eating disorder pathology, shape concerns, and self-compassion over time compared to those with BN and EDNOS. The AN-BP group had slower and generally non-significant improvements in dietary restraint, shame, social safeness, and received social support compared to those with AN-R, BN, and EDNOS. These results suggest previously unknown ways in which patients with AN, and particularly AN-BP, fare worse than other eating disorders patients over the course of specialized treatment.

Eating disorder pathology

Using the EDE-Q as a transdiagnostic indicator of eating disorder pathology, we found that patients with AN-BP had the slowest improvements in dietary restraint over 12 weeks of treatment. In addition, both AN-BP and AN-R patients had the slowest improvements in global eating disorder pathology and shape concerns. The fact that AN patients generally improved more slowly than other eating disorder patients is perhaps not surprising given what is known about the recalcitrant nature of AN. It is noteworthy, though, that although AN patients had slower improvements in shape concerns over treatment, there was no effect of diagnosis on changes in weight concerns or eating concerns over 12 weeks, suggesting that patients with AN-R and AN-BP only differ from those with BN and EDNOS in their rates of improvement on certain aspects of eating disorder pathology. It is nevertheless important to note that the EDE-Q subscales correlated fairly highly with one another, and with the EDE-Q global score, making it important to replicate this finding in future research.

Shame and social safeness

Over 12 weeks of treatment, individuals with AN-R, BN, and EDNOS experienced significant increases in social safeness and decreases in shame. Individuals with AN-

BP, however, did not show significant improvements in these areas, and their trajectories differed from the average trajectory of the other three groups. These findings suggest that compared to their fellow patients, AN-BP sufferers experienced a more persistent sense of isolation and defectiveness over the course of treatment, with no improvement in feelings of inadequacy and faultiness, or in feelings of social connectedness, warmth, and belongingness. The lack of improvement in shame that AN-BP patients tend to show is particularly concerning in light of growing research documenting the maintaining role that shame plays in the eating disorders [42-44]. Findings are also noteworthy given the group-based nature of our treatment programs, where staff and co-patients are encouraged to be supportive of another. Our results suggest there may something unique about individuals with AN-BP that limits the emotional benefits they are able to derive from group-based therapy.

Received social support

Individuals with AN-BP reported significant decreases in received social support over time, a trajectory that differed significantly from the average of the three other diagnostic groups. EDNOS patients were the only group to show improvements in received support over time, and those with AN-R and BN reported no changes. Because received support was assessed through self-report, it is difficult to know whether the decreases AN-BP patients reported were objective in nature, or whether they primarily reflected patients' emotional sense of insecurity and isolation. The measure of received support also does not allow us to determine whether patients responded to items based on their experiences within the treatment context, outside of treatment, or both. In future research, it would be interesting to examine whether certain interpersonal patterns characteristic of AN-BP, such as being cold/distant, socially inhibited, and vindictive/self-centered [19], may lead these patients to lose favour among co-patients and therapists as treatment progresses.

Self-compassion

Patients with AN-R and AN-BP had slower and non-significant changes in self-compassion over 12 weeks compared to patients with BN and EDNOS. This finding suggests that whereas BN and EDNOS patients come to relate to their distress with more kindness and patience over the course of therapy, individuals with AN do not. Rather, they report no improvements in their self-compassion – that is, their tendency to respond to their feelings of inadequacy with self-kindness rather than self-judgment, mindfulness rather than over-identification, and a perspective that suffering is common to humanity rather than isolating. It would be interesting to know whether these persistently low levels of self-compassion contribute to the poorer outcomes AN patients tend to experience during and after treatment for their eating disorder. Indeed, there is growing evidence that deficits in self-compassion are associated with more severe and prolonged eating disorder pathology in eating disorder patients [45].

Limitations and future research

This study has a number of limitations. First, it was correlational in nature meaning we must be cautious about interpreting the results. Specifically, we cannot conclude that patients' eating disorder diagnosis played a causal role in determining their change trajectories. Second, the sample was quite heterogeneous in nature, and treatment intensity varied across patients. Although these sample and treatment characteristics were partly inevitable due to the nature of our research question, it would be advisable to replicate the present findings in a treatment setting where patients across diagnostic groups undergo the same intensity and duration of treatment. Indeed the present results should be viewed as preliminary. Third, there were no follow-up assessments of patients beyond the 12-week study. In future research, it will be interesting to examine the ways in which patients trajectories change or remain the same after treatment. Fourth, although our sample size was relatively large, it will be important to replicate our results in even larger transdiagnostic samples of eating disorder patients.

Conclusions

The present study provides evidence that patients with AN, and especially those with AN-BP, undergo processes during treatment that differ from those with BN and EDNOS. In particular, their symptoms and psychosocial functioning improve at a slower pace, and often – particularly in the case of AN-BP – at a non-significant pace. Previous research has found that within AN-only samples, poorer psychosocial functioning and more severe illness markers predicted worse outcomes. Our findings extend this research by suggesting that it is not just a subset of AN patients who warrant greater clinical attention. Rather, the trajectories of change AN and especially AN-BP patients showed in our study suggest that compared to patients with BN and EDNOS. Our findings suggest that AN patients may require more comprehensive interventions than those with other eating disorders. It might be important to investigate psychotherapeutic approaches whose integration into current treatments would allow clinicians to better target shame, social safeness, social support, and self-compassion.

Competing interests
The authors declare that they have no competing interests.

Authors' contributions
AK took the lead in devising the study, collecting and analyzing data, and writing up results. JC provided input at all stages. Both authors read and approved the final manuscript.

Acknowledgements
The authors would like to thank the Ontario Mental Health Foundation for their grant support.

Author details
[1]Department of Psychology, University of Waterloo, Waterloo, ON N2L 3G1, Canada. [2]Department of Psychology, Memorial University of Newfoundland, St. John's, NL A1B 3X9, Canada.

References
1. Herzog DB, Dorer DJ, Keel PK, Selwyn SE, Ekeblad ER, Flores AT, Greenwood DN, Burwell RA, Keller MB: **Recovery and relapse in anorexia and bulimia nervosa: a 7.5-year follow-up study.** *J Am Acad Child Psy* 1999, **38:**829–837.
2. Gowers SG, Clark A, Roberts C, Griffiths A, Edwards V, Bryan C, Smethurst N, Byford S, Barrett B: **Clinical effectiveness of treatments for anorexia nervosa in adolescents: randomised controlled trial.** *Brit J Psych* 2007, **191:**427–435.
3. Keel PK, Brown TA: **Update on course and outcome in eating disorders.** *Int J Eat Disorder* 2010, **43:**195–204.
4. DeJong H, Broadbent H, Schmidt U: **A systematic review of dropout from treatment in outpatients with anorexia nervosa.** *Int J Eat Disorder* 2012, **45:**635–647.
5. Halmi KA, Eckert E, Marchi P, Sampugnaro V, Apple R, Cohen J: **Comorbidity of psychiatric diagnoses in anorexia nervosa.** *Arch Gen Psychiat* 1991, **48:**712–718.
6. Wallier J, Vibert S, Berthoz S, Huas C, Hubert T, Godart N: **Dropout from inpatient treatment for anorexia nervosa: critical review of the literature.** *Int J Eat Disorder* 2009, **42:**636–647.
7. Nilsson EW, Gillberg C, Gillberg ICR, Råstam M: **Ten-year follow-up of adolescent-onset anorexia nervosa: personality disorders.** *J Am Acad Child Psy* 1999, **38:**1389–1395.
8. Råstam M, Gillberg C, Wentz E: **Outcome of teenage-onset anorexia nervosa in a Swedish community-based sample.** *Eur Child Adoles Psy* 2003, **12:**i78–i90.
9. Wentz E, Gillberg C, Gillberg IC, Råstam M: **Ten-year follow-up of adolescent-onset anorexia nervosa: psychiatric disorders and overall functioning scales.** *J Child Psychol Psyc* 2001, **42:**613–622.
10. Birmingham CL, Su J, Hlynsky JA, Goldner EM, Gao M: **The mortality rate from anorexia nervosa.** *Int J Eat Disorder* 2005, **38:**143–146.
11. Crow S, Peterson C, Swanson S, Raymond N, Specker S, Eckert E, Mitchell J: **Increased mortality in bulimia nervosa and other eating disorders.** *Am J Psychiat* 2009, **166:**1342–1346.
12. Franko DL, Keshaviah A, Eddy KT, Krishna M, Davis MC, Keel PK, Herzog DB: **A longitudinal investigation of mortality in anorexia nervosa and bulimia nervosa.** *Am J Psychiat* 2013, **170:**917–925.
13. Deter HC, Herzog W: **Anorexia nervosa in a long-term perspective: results of the Heidelberg-Mannheim Study.** *Psychosom Med* 1994, **1994**(56):20–27.
14. Fassino S, Pierò A, Tomba E, Abbate-Daga G: **Factors associated with drop-out from treatment for eating disorders: a comprehensive literature review.** *BMC Psychiatry* 2009, **9:**67.
15. Salbach-Andrae H, Schneider N, Seifert K, Pfeiffer E, Lenz K, Lehmkuhl U, Korte A: **Short-term outcome of anorexia nervosa in adolescents after inpatient treatment: a prospective study.** *Eur Child Adoles Psy* 2009, **18:**701–704.
16. Hjern A, Lindberg L, Lindblad F: **Outcome and prognostic factors for adolescent female in-patients with anorexia nervosa: 9-to 14-year follow-up.** *Brit J Psych* 2006, **189:**428–432.
17. Crane AM, Roberts ME, Treasure J: **Are obsessive-compulsive personality traits associated with a poor outcome in anorexia nervosa? A systematic review of randomized controlled trials and naturalistic outcome studies.** *Int J Eat Disorder* 2007, **40:**581–588.
18. Carter JC, Kelly AC, Norwood SJ: **Interpersonal problems in Anorexia Nervosa: social inhibition as defining and detrimental.** *Pers Indiv Differ* 2012, **53:**169–174.
19. Hartmann A, Zeeck A, Barrett MS: **Interpersonal problems in eating disorders.** *Int J Eat Disorder* 2010, **43:**619–627.
20. Strober M, Freeman R, Morrell W: **The long-term course of severe anorexia nervosa in adolescents: Survival analysis of recovery, relapse, and outcome predictors over 10–15 years in a prospective study.** *Int J Eat Disorders* 1997, **22:**339–360.
21. Carter JC, Blackmore E, Sutandar-Pinnock K, Woodside DB: **Relapse in anorexia nervosa: a survival analysis.** *Psychol Med* 2004, **34:**671–679.
22. Lund BC, Hernandez ER, Yates WR, Mitchell JR, McKee PA, Johnson CL: **Rate of inpatient weight restoration predicts outcome in anorexia nervosa.** *Int J Eat Disorder* 2009, **42:**301–305.
23. Bewell CV, Carter JC: **Motivation to change mediates the impact of eating disorder symptomatology on treatment outcome in anorexia nervosa.** *Int J Eat Disorder* 2008, **41:**368–371.
24. Gilbert P (Ed): *Compassion: Conceptualisations, Research, and Use in Psychotherapy.* London: Routledge; 2005.
25. Gilbert P: *The Compassionate Mind: A New Approach to Life' Challenges.* Oakland: New Harbinger Publications; 2010.
26. Gilbert P, McEwan K, Mitra R, Franks L, Richter A, Rockliff H: **Feeling safe and content: a specific affect regulation system? Relationship to depression, anxiety, stress, and self-criticism.** *J Posit Psychol* 2008, **3:**182–191.
27. Gilbert P, McEwan K, Mitra R, Richter A, Franks L, Mills A, Bellew R, Gale C: **An exploration of different types of positive affect in students and in patients with bipolar disorder.** *Clin Neuropsychiatry* 2009, **6:**135–143.
28. LeDoux J: *The Emotional Brain.* London: Weidenfeld & Nicolson; 1998.
29. Panksepp J: *Affective Neuroscience.* London: Oxford University Press; 1998.
30. Neff KD: **The development and validation of a scale to measure self-compassion.** *Self Identity* 2003, **2:**223–250.
31. Fairburn CG, Cooper Z: **The Eating Disorder Examination.** In *Binge Eating: Nature, Assessment, and Treatment.* 12th edition. Edited by Fairburn CG, Wilson GT. New York: Guilford Press; 1993:317–360.
32. Olmsted MP, McFarlane TL, Carter JC, Trottier K, Woodside DB, Dimitropoulos G: **Inpatient and day hospital treatment for anorexia nervosa.** In *The Treatment of Eating Disorders: A Clinical Handbook.* Edited by Grilo CM, Mitchell JE. New York: Guildford Press; 2010:198–211.
33. Fairburn CG, Beglin SJ: **Assessment of eating disorders: Interview or self-report questionnaire?** *Int J Eat Disorder* 1994, **16:**363–370.
34. Luce KH, Crowther JH: **The reliability of the eating disorder examination—self-report questionnaire version (EDE-Q).** *Int J Eat Disorder* 1999, **25:**349–351.
35. Mond JM, Hay PJ, Rodgers B, Owen C: **Eating disorder examination questionnaire (EDE-Q): norms for young adult women.** *Behav Res Ther* 2006, **44:**53–62.
36. Andrews B, Qian M, Valentine JD: **Predicting depressive symptoms with a new measure of shame: the experience of shame scale.** *Brit J Clin Psychol* 2002, **41:**29–42.
37. Cutrona CE, Russell DW: **The provisions of social relationships and adaptation to stress.** *Adv Pers Rel* 1987, **1:**37–67.
38. Raes F, Pommier E, Neff KD, Van Gucht D: **Construction and factorial validation of a short form of the self-compassion scale.** *Clin Psychol Psychot* 2011, **18:**250–255.
39. Singer JD, Willett JB: *Applied Longitudinal Data Analysis: Modeling Change and Event Occurrence.* New York: Oxford University Press; 2003.
40. Little RJ: **Modeling the drop-out mechanism in repeated-measures studies.** *J Am Stat Assoc* 1995, **90:**1112–1121.
41. Tasca GA, Gallop R: **Multilevel modeling of longitudinal data for psychotherapy research: I.** *Basics Psychother Res* 2009, **19:**429–437.
42. Troop NA, Allan S, Serpell L, Treasure JL: **Shame in women with a history of eating disorders.** *Eur Eat Disord Rev* 2008, **16:**480–488.

43. Kelly AC, Carter JC, Borairi S: **Are improvements in shame and self-compassion early in eating disorders treatment associated with better patient outcomes?** *Int J Eat Disorder.* in press.
44. Goss K, Allan S: **Shame, pride and eating disorders.** *Clin Psychol Psychot* 2009, **16**:303–316.
45. Kelly AC, Carter JC, Zuroff DC, Borairi S: **Self-compassion and fear of self-compassion interact to predict response to eating disorders treatment: a preliminary investigation.** *Psychother Res* 2013, **23**:252–264.

4

Prevalence and characteristics of avoidant/restrictive food intake disorder in a cohort of young patients in day treatment for eating disorders

Terri A Nicely[1], Susan Lane-Loney[2], Emily Masciulli[2], Christopher S Hollenbeak[3] and Rollyn M Ornstein[2*]

Abstract

Background: Avoidant/Restrictive Food Intake Disorder (ARFID) is a "new" diagnosis in the recently published DSM-5, but there is very little literature on patients with ARFID. Our objectives were to determine the prevalence of ARFID in children and adolescents undergoing day treatment for an eating disorder, and to compare ARFID patients to other eating disorder patients in the same cohort.

Methods: A retrospective chart review of 7-17 year olds admitted to a day program for younger patients with eating disorders between 2008 and 2012 was performed. Patients with ARFID were compared to those with anorexia nervosa, bulimia nervosa, and other specified feeding or eating disorder/unspecified feeding or eating disorder with respect to demographics, anthropometrics, clinical symptoms, and psychometric testing, using Chi-square, ANOVA, and post-hoc analysis.

Results: 39/173 (22.5%) patients met ARFID criteria. The ARFID group was younger than the non-ARFID group and had a greater proportion of males. Similar degrees of weight loss and malnutrition were found between groups. Patients with ARFID reported greater fears of vomiting and/or choking and food texture issues than those with other eating disorders, as well as greater dependency on nutritional supplements at intake. Children's Eating Attitudes Test scores were lower for children with than without ARFID. A higher comorbidity of anxiety disorders, pervasive developmental disorder, and learning disorders, and a lower comorbidity of depression, were found in those with ARFID.

Conclusions: This study demonstrates that there are significant demographic and clinical characteristics that differentiate children with ARFID from those with other eating disorders in a day treatment program, and helps substantiate the recognition of ARFID as a distinct eating disorder diagnosis in the DSM-5.

Keywords: Avoidant restrictive food intake disorder, Children and adolescents, Day treatment, DSM-5

Background

Historically, children and adolescents have not been easily diagnosed with eating disorders (EDs) based on past versions of the Diagnostic and Statistical Manual of Mental Disorders (DSM), including the 4th edition. In fact, over 50% of these patients met criteria for Eating Disorder Not Otherwise Specified (EDNOS), likely leading to missed diagnoses and difficulty obtaining appropriate and timely treatment [1-3]. With the preparations for publication of the 5th edition of the DSM (DSM-5), the Eating Disorders Work Group was assigned the tasks of improving clinical utility of the diagnostic categories and reducing the frequency of EDNOS. One of the imperatives was to recognize new disorders and eliminate others by exploring the clinical profiles of patients who fell under the heterogeneous EDNOS category. In

* Correspondence: rornstein@hmc.psu.edu
[2]Division of Adolescent Medicine and Eating Disorders, Penn State Hershey Children's Hospital, 905 West Governor Road, Suite 250, 17033 Hershey, PA, USA
Full list of author information is available at the end of the article

addition, the DSM-5 as a whole has attempted to take a developmental, or life-span, approach to all disorders.

Feeding Disorder of Infancy or Early Childhood, a diagnosis in the DSM-IV, delineated a persistent eating dysfunction leading to weight loss or failure to gain weight, with the requirement that patients be less than six years of age. This was a non-specific diagnostic category that was rarely used in practice and for which there was insufficient literature [4]. A great number of patients are over six years old at the time of initial ED evaluation, even if some have had symptoms from an early age, and have been necessarily given the diagnosis EDNOS in the past. Feeding Disorder of Infancy or Early Childhood also excluded those children with abnormal eating patterns or nutritionally deficient or limited diets, but who were growing normally secondary to sufficient caloric intake, possibly due to the use of nutritional supplements. The inability of DSM-IV to capture such patients was significant, as they often presented with considerable impairment, both physically and functionally [5].

Clinicians and researchers have long recognized specific types of EDs that fall under the umbrella of EDNOS. The Great Ormond Street (GOS) classification system captured a way to describe these types of patients, and was often utilized by clinicians for descriptive purposes. These criteria were actually found to have a higher inter-rater reliability for younger patients than the DSM-IV [1]. The GOS categories include: Food Avoidant Emotional Disorder (FAED), Selective Eating, and Functional Dysphagia, as well as Anorexia Nervosa (AN) and Bulimia Nervosa (BN).

FAED was first described as a combination of inadequate food intake and emotional disturbance; these young people knew that they were underweight and wanted to be heavier, but found this difficult to achieve [6]. The GOS system further clarified this group, and differentiated their presentation by the absence of weight and shape concerns in the presence of significant food restriction. Somatic complaints were frequent as well as more general psychopathology, e.g. generalized anxiety [4,5].

Selective eating, also known as "picky eating", is a common problem of childhood, with anywhere between 13 to 22% of children between 3 and 11 years of age being reported to be picky eaters at any given time [7]. While young children are typically thought to "grow out of" their pickiness, studies have shown that between 18 and 40% of the rigidity concerning food persists into adolescence [8-10]. Patients with selective eating are usually not underweight, as they take in adequate calories from preferred foods, but their diets may be lacking in micronutrients. Some selective eaters have sensory concerns related to the taste, smell, color, or texture of foods, which may limit their intake to such a narrow range of acceptable foods that weight loss, or failure to gain appropriate weight, may occur. Studies have shown a higher prevalence of boys with selective eating, as well as a high degree of co-morbid anxiety [11,12].

Functional dysphagia is a fear of swallowing or an inability to eat or swallow food, especially solid or lumpy foods. There is generally a fear of gagging, choking, or vomiting, often subsequent to actual traumatic episodes or witnessed episodes. Sometimes an illogical connection in the child's mind leads to development of the phobia. Some children present with food refusal specifically out of fears of vomiting, contamination, poisoning, or defecation as well. Many cases of acute food refusal due to specific fears present clinically malnourished and ill, as they often lose weight rapidly. They can easily be mistaken with AN on initial presentation due to the severity of the restriction; however, they are not concerned with weight or shape [4,5].

The DSM-5 has subsumed and expanded Feeding Disorder of Infancy or Early Childhood to capture a greater number of patients who present with avoidant or restrictive eating, but are clearly different from those with AN in that there are no disturbed cognitions about weight and/or shape, or a wish to lose weight. It has been renamed Avoidant/Restrictive Food Intake Disorder (ARFID) and includes those types of patients recognized in the GOS system. Patients with ARFID may present with clinically significant restrictive eating leading to weight loss or lack of weight gain, nutritional deficiencies, reliance on tube feeding or oral nutritional supplements and/or disturbances in psychosocial functioning (see Table 1) [13]. Additionally, they may exhibit similar physical signs and symptoms as patients with AN due to semi-starvation.

Very little has been published on patients with ARFID. Recently, a large multicenter study of children and adolescents presenting as new patients to adolescent medicine ED programs, revealed a 14% prevalence of ARFID, with unique clinical characteristics, including younger age and a greater number of males [14,15]. An 11-year retrospective chart review of adolescent ED patients in Canada reported a 5% prevalence of ARFID [16]. These patients were compared to a matched sample of AN patients, and demonstrated a younger age at presentation, and a higher likelihood of being male. There were specific behaviors and symptoms in the ARFID group, including food avoidance, decreased appetite, abdominal pain, and emetophobia. Both of these studies included all new patients presenting for initial assessments to tertiary care ED programs.

Due to the dearth of literature on ARFID, we sought to determine the prevalence and clinical characteristics of ARFID in young patients admitted to a day treatment program for EDs, and to compare patients with ARFID to those with AN, BN, and Other Specified Feeding or

Table 1 Diagnostic Criteria for Avoidant/Restrictive Food Intake Disorder

WHAT IS ARFID?	WHAT ARFID IS NOT
• A problem with eating or feeding (e.g. seeming disinterest in food or eating; repulsion to certain foods based on their sensory qualities; fears about aversive effects of eating) leading to recurrent inability to take in adequate nutrition and/or energy coupled with one (or more) of the following:	• The eating problems are not due to body image disturbance, and anorexia nervosa or bulimia nervosa cannot be diagnosed instead.
o Major nutritional deficiency.	• Feeding or eating problems are not the result of scarcity of food or a culturally endorsed tradition.
o Substantial weight loss (or lack of weight gain).	• The disordered eating is not due to a concomitant medical problem or another psychiatric disorder, so that if the medical or psychiatric disorder is treated, the eating problems resolves.
o Reliance on nasogastric or gastric tube feeding or oral nutrition supplements.	
o Impaired psychosocial function.	

Adapted from the Diagnostic and Statistical Manual of Mental Disorders, 5th Edition, American Psychiatric Association, 2013.

Eating Disorders/Unspecified Feeding or Eating Disorder (OSFED/UFED) in the same cohort.

Methods

Participants

A retrospective chart review was conducted on 177 patients admitted to a day program for children and adolescents with EDs between August 4th, 2008 and May 1st, 2012. This program treats female and male patients, ages 7 to 17 years, with EDs and co-morbid psychopathology. The majority of patients in the program have restrictive EDs, based mostly on the younger average age. However, patients with purging disorders are treated as well. While we treat some patients with sensory features related to food, who may or may not also have an autism spectrum disorder diagnosis, it is important to clarify that patients with longstanding feeding issues and autism are not typically admitted to our program, and are usually managed in the Feeding Disorders Program at our institution.

Initial ED and co-morbid psychiatric diagnoses were made upon admission to the program based on a comprehensive diagnostic psychiatric evaluation, by both a trained child and adolescent psychiatrist and either an experienced clinical psychologist or a licensed social worker/clinical psychiatric specialist, using DSM-IV-TR criteria. Some of the co-morbid diagnoses were based on history conveyed by the parent to the health care provider. DSM-5 ED diagnoses were determined retrospectively and agreed upon together through careful discussion by two of the psychiatric specialists and an adolescent medicine physician, all of whom were personally involved with the cases, using a checklist based on the proposed DSM-5 diagnostic criteria, which were almost identical to the published criteria. Therefore, these diagnoses were not made in a blinded fashion.

Of the 177 eligible subjects, a total of four participants were excluded from the study. Two were excluded for having medical conditions that were retrospectively determined to fully account for their disordered eating behaviors. Two subjects were excluded for having Binge Eating Disorder and composed too small a distinct group for data analysis.

Measures

Demographics, historical and clinical features

Data collected at intake included age, gender, and ethnicity. Historical information included past history of ED and/or other mental health treatment, other medical disorders and consultations by other medical specialists, presence of weight loss, percentage of body weight lost, length of illness, use of nutritional supplements, presence of purging behaviors, excessive exercise, history of food allergies, fears of choking and/or vomiting, and sensory issues related to food. This information was gathered from the initial evaluations by the adolescent medicine physician, the psychiatrist, and the psychologist or clinical social worker.

Anthropometrics

Weight and height were measured by trained staff at initial presentation. Gowned weights were obtained on a hospital-grade SECA digital scale and recorded to the nearest tenth of a kg. Heights were measured in bare feet using a fixed stadiometer with a right angle headpiece and recorded to the nearest tenth of a cm. BMI was calculated using the standard formula (kg/m^2) and the % Median Body Weight (%MBW) was determined based on the 50th percentile BMI-for-age.

Psychometric measures

The Children's Eating Attitudes Test (ChEAT) [17] The ChEAT is a 26-item scale assessing attitudes and behaviors associated with food and eating, validated in patients as young as 8 years old, adapted from the original EAT-26 [18]. A score of ≥ 20 is considered clinically significant relative to the normative population. The three subscales reflecting varying types of eating pathology include: Dieting, Bulimia/Food Preoccupation, and Oral Control [18].

Children's Depression Inventory (CDI) [19]. The CDI is a 27-item self-report inventory for assessing depression in children between the ages of 7 and 17 years. The measure yields a Total score (M = 50; SD = 10) and five factors: Negative Mood, Interpersonal Problems, Ineffectiveness, Anhedonia, and Negative Self-Esteem (M = 10; SD = 3).

Revised Children's Manifest Anxiety Scale (RCMAS) [20]. The RCMAS is a 37 item self-report instrument designed to measure anxiety for children and adolescents ages 6 to 17 years. The measure yields a Total Anxiety score based upon 28 items, with 9 items comprising the Lie Scale which is designed to detect responses that are socially desirable. The Total Anxiety Score is expressed as a T-score (M = 50, SD = 10) and there are three factor-based subscales, expressed as scaled scores (M = 10, SD = 3): Physiological Anxiety, Worry/Oversensitivity, and Social Concerns/Concentration.

The Child Behavior Checklist (CBCL) [21]. The CBCL provides three global measurements which are expressed as a T- score (M = 50; SD = 10) including Total Score; Internalizing; and Externalizing Scales. In addition, the measure includes 14 Syndrome Scores which reflect clusters of psychiatric symptoms. These scales are also expressed as T-scores (M = 50; SD = 10) and include the following scales: Anxious/Depressed, Withdrawn/Depressed, Somatic Complaints, Social Problems, Thought Problems, Attention Problems, Rule-Breaking Problems, Aggressive Behavior, Affective Problems, Anxiety Problems, Somatic Complaints, ADHD Problems, Oppositional Defiant Problems, and Conduct Problems. It is completed by parents and/or other caregivers.

Statistical analysis

Analysis included descriptive statistics, chi-square, analysis of variance (ANOVA), and Pearson's correlation. Bonferroni correction was used to adjust for Type I error, with thresholds set at $p < 0.01$ for patient characteristics, $p < 0.007$ for ED symptoms and features, and $p < 0.008$ for psychiatric co-morbidities. Post-hoc testing to examine between-groups effects was performed with the Hochberg GT2 test. Data were entered and analyzed using SPSS (version17.0, SPSS Inc., Chicago, Illinois).

This study was approved by the Institutional Review Board of the Penn State Hershey Medical Center/College of Medicine.

Results

Demographics and anthropometrics

Using the proposed DSM-5 criteria, 39 (22.5%) patients met criteria for ARFID, 93 (53.8%) for AN, 20 (11.6%) for BN, and 21 (12.1%) for OSFED/UFED. Notably, all patients diagnosed with ARFID carried a DSM-IV diagnosis of EDNOS. None were diagnosed with DSM-IV Feeding Disorder of Infancy or Early Childhood, as all were over six years old at intake. Of the 173 participants included, 92% were female with a mean age of 13.5 years (SD = 2.03) (range 7.2 -16.9 years). The cohort was predominantly Caucasian (95%), reflecting the ethnic/racial makeup of the geographic area. There was no significant difference in duration of illness between those patients with ARFID and the other ED groups.

Patients with ARFID were found to be younger than those with other EDs (11.1 years, SD = 1.7 vs. 14.2 years, SD = 1.5; $p < 0.0001$) and to have a greater percentage of males (20.5% vs 4.5%; $p = 0.008$). Of the patients who had lost weight as part of their ED, those with AN lost a greater percentage of their premorbid weight than the other ED groups, including those with ARFID (Table 2). There was a significant difference found in %MBW between those with ARFID and BN, but not between ARFID and AN, or OSFED/UFED (Table 2). While the degree of malnutrition was similar to that of patients with AN, those with ARFID were found to have a greater dependence on nutritional supplements, fears of vomiting and/or choking, and texture/sensory issues pertaining to food (all $p < 0.0001$).

Psychometric assessment and psychiatric co-morbidities

Patients with ARFID were less likely to report typical ED symptoms, e.g. purging behaviors and excessive exercise, during intake interview (all $p < 0.0001$). In addition, they had significantly lower total scores on the ChEAT (14.86, SD = 2.10) than those of the remaining patients overall (27.51, SD = 17.28) ($p < 0.0001$) (Figure 1). Post-hoc analysis revealed significant differences among patients with ARFID and all other groups for the total ChEAT score. While patients with ARFID also had significantly lower scores on both the Dieting and Bulimia Nervosa/Food Preoccupation subscales ($p < 0.0001$), there was no significant difference between groups on the Oral Control subscale. An interesting finding on chart review was that while patients with ARFID did not have true body image distortion, as seen in AN, 21% exhibited body preoccupation with somatic concerns. For example, some children were fixated on fears of physical illness due to issues related to shape/weight, e.g. high cholesterol and/or obesity leading to heart disease, either because of personal experiences with relatives or information in their school curriculum. Others who were chronically underweight due to their feeding and eating disturbance had suffered teasing

Table 2 Clinical characteristics of patients by eating disorder diagnosis

	ARFID (N = 39)	AN (N = 93)	BN (N = 20)	OSFED/UFED (N = 21)	*p*-value
Patient Characteristics (mean or %)					
Age (years) (SD)	11.1 (1.7)*	14.0 (1.5)	14.9 (1.1)	14.2 (1.7)	<0.0001
% MBW (SD)	87.1 (13.0)	82.6 (9.2)	108.1 (19.5)*	93.2 (6.8)	<0.0001
% Body Weight Lost (SD)	10.5 (8.4)	18.5 (10.2)*	6.4 (6.5)	14.8 (12.2)	<0.0001
Length of illness (months) (SD)	9.8 (13.2)	8.6 (7.9)	15.9 (11.9)	9.8 (4.9)	N.S.
% Female	79.5	95.7	100	90.5	0.008
% Male	20.5*	4.3	0	9.5	
Symptoms & Features (%)					
Enteral Supplement Use	46*	20	0	0	<0.0001
Purge-vomit	0	6	95*	38	<0.0001
Excessive exercise	15*	68	65	52	<0.0001
Food allergy	20	5	10	5	N.S.
Fear of choking or vomiting	44*	1	0	0	<0.0001
Sensory issues	26*	1	0	0	<0.0001
Recent medical specialist consult	46	19	20	33	N.S.
Psychiatric comorbidities (%)					
Mood disorder	33*	48	80	76	<0.0001
Anxiety disorder	72*	37	25	14	<0.0001
Autism Spectrum Disorder	13*	0	0	0	0.001
Attention Deficit Disorder	4*	0	1	1	N.S.
Learning Disorder	10*	2	2	0	<0.0001
Cognitive impairment	26*	2	10	0	<0.0001

*Significant finding on post-hoc analysis using Hochberg GT2 test.
AN = Anorexia Nervosa ARFID = Avoidant/Restrictive Food Intake Disorder.
BN = Bulimia Nervosa OSFED/UFED = Other Specified Feeding or Eating Disorder/Unspecified Feeding or Eating Disorder % MBW = % Median Body Weight.

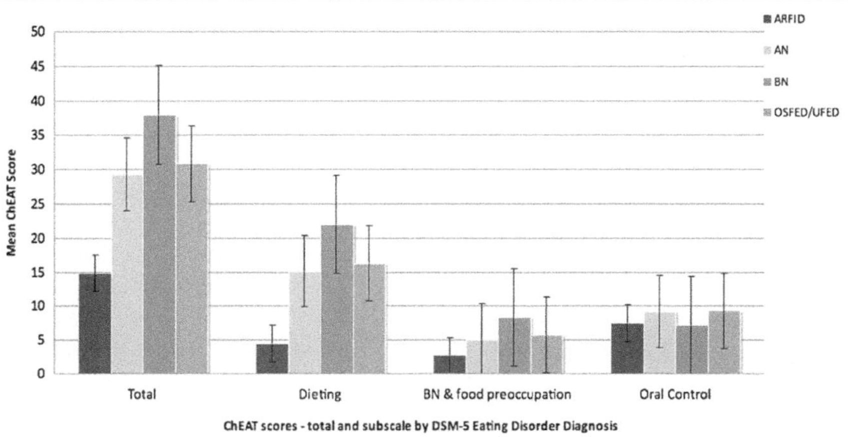

Figure 1 Total and subscale ChEAT scores by DSM-5 Diagnosis. ChEAT = Children's Eating Attitudes Test. All differences between groups significant at p < 0.0001 except Oral Control = N.S.

by their peers because of their low weight, which may have led to body image concerns, although of a different nature than typically seen in AN and BN.

There was a significantly higher comorbidity of anxiety disorders in patients with ARFID (72%) than the other ED groups (31%), as determined by clinician diagnosis ($p < 0.0001$). Furthermore, this was supported by parental report on the CBCL (p =0.005). However, there were no significant differences between groups on the total RCMAS score. Autism spectrum disorder ($p = 0.001$), learning disorders ($p < 0.0001$), and cognitive impairment ($p < 0.0001$) were also seen more frequently in the patients with ARFID, based on past history reported at initial assessment (Table 2). On the CBCL, children with ARFID had significantly more social problems ($p = 0.001$) and attention problems ($p < 0.0001$) than those with AN. There was a lower comorbidity of depression diagnosed in children with ARFID (23%) than the other EDs (57%) ($p < 0.0001$), and total CDI scores were lower in this group as well (54.4 vs. 60.0, $p = 0.05$). Additionally, children with ARFID were found to have significantly lower scores on the CDI subscales Negative Mood (p =0.02) and Negative Self Esteem ($p < 0.0001$). There were no significant differences between the groups on the Interpersonal Problems, Ineffectiveness, or Anhedonia subscales, however.

A smaller percentage of children with ARFID (35%) sought outpatient psychotherapy before coming to the program, compared to patients in the other ED groups (AN = 60.22%, EDNOS = 75%, BN = 80%; $p = 0.002$). However, there were no differences in the past history of higher levels of psychiatric care, e.g. inpatient, residential, or day treatment. In contrast, more children with ARFID (46.2%) had seen other medical specialists for consultation (e.g. gastroenterology, endocrinology) before coming to program than those with other EDs (26.1%), although this did not reach statistical significance with the Bonferroni correction ($p = 0.02$).

Discussion

This study adds to the literature on ARFID by comparing a cohort of children and adolescents undergoing day treatment for EDs, including patients with this "new" diagnosis. Notably, almost a quarter of our patients were diagnosed with ARFID, which illustrates the significant prevalence of this disorder amongst children and adolescents requiring an intensive level of ED treatment in a tertiary care setting. This was a higher prevalence than that found in the multicenter studies [14,15], which might be accounted for by the fact that our patients were encountered over four years in a day treatment setting, as opposed to all ED patients presenting for initial evaluation over a one-year period. The prevalence rate was in even starker contrast to the 11-year retrospective review from Canada, where the prevalence was only found to be 5% [16]. There is no mention of age range in that study, only that the patients were adolescent ED patients assessed in a pediatric tertiary care hospital program. Our study included children and adolescents between 7 and 17 years, which may have been a slightly lower range than the Canadian study; this might also justify the higher prevalence of ARFID found in our cohort. Another possible explanation for the discrepancy in prevalence rates across studies is that younger patients with atypical EDs, like ARFID, may be increasingly referred to adolescent medicine ED programs in more recent years, as there has been greater recognition of these presentations as true EDs. The Canadian study reviewed records starting in 2000 and it would be interesting to know whether the prevalence increased annually over the 11 years. In our experience, referrals from primary care providers tend to generate more referrals once they are successfully managed. Lastly, the higher prevalence in our cohort may reflect the fact that many children and adolescents with ARFID present acutely and significantly malnourished, requiring a higher level of care, such as day treatment.

Similar to the multicenter and Canadian studies [15,16], our results demonstrate that there are significant demographic and diagnostic characteristics that differentiate children with ARFID from those with other EDs. First, while female patients remain the majority, there was a higher preponderance of male patients in the ARFID group than in the other ED groups. Children and adolescents with ARFID were more likely to present at a younger age with significant weight loss or failure to gain appropriate weight, were more dependent on oral or enteral nutritional supplementation, and had significantly more fears of choking and/or vomiting, and texture and/or sensitivity issues regarding food. These findings are consistent with those in studies of early-onset EDs [2,22,23], as well as in the recent multicenter study [15], and many are relevant and important features in making the diagnosis of ARFID [24].

Based on DSM-5 criteria, a patient cannot have body image distortion and be diagnosed with ARFID. However, our data revealed that 21% of patients diagnosed with ARFID had body preoccupation with somatic concerns. It is important to reiterate that none of the patients with ARFID had been diagnosed with AN using DSM-IV criteria, which underscores the absence of true body image distortion. During evaluation of a young patient with possible ARFID versus AN, it is critical to probe about body concerns that need to be distinguished from body image distortion. For example, if a patient has worries about becoming fat, this may have something to do with events in the family's medical history, e.g. an overweight parent or grandparent with a recent myocardial infarction or diabetes diagnosis. Children and adolescents are often privy to this information, but may make illogical associations based on their cognitive developmental stage. This knowledge may then trigger restrictive eating behaviors. Thorough history-taking can often elicit this information.

As has been documented in other studies of patients with acute food avoidance without weight/shape concerns [2,15,22,25,26], there were no significant differences in our study between % MBW in patients with ARFID and AN; however, patients with AN lost a significantly greater percentage of their premorbid body weight. This may be explained by the fact that our patients with ARFID, notably those with the acute food refusal seen in functional dysphagia, may have presented sooner after the onset of illness than those with AN. The data may not fully bear this out due to the heterogeneity of the ARFID category (e.g. more chronic selective eaters vs more acute food refusal), which might balance out the length of illness data. Furthermore, young patients may present relatively early in the course of their illness, based on their age alone.

Based on both clinician and parental report, patients with ARFID had significantly more anxiety and less depression than patients with other EDs, which is similar to findings in the large multicenter study on ARFID [15]. However, our study is the first of patients with ARFID to use standardized measures obtained from parents to aid in evaluation. There were no self-reported significant differences found between children with ARFID and those with other EDs on the RCMAS or any of its subscales, which could be due to the generally high comorbidity of anxiety symptoms in EDs. Alternatively, younger patients (those more likely to be diagnosed with ARFID) may have had a harder time filling out the questionnaire than older subjects, perhaps in understanding the questions or acknowledging symptoms of anxiety, due to cognitive developmental stage. It is important to clarify that ARFID is not simply a type of anxiety disorder, as the severity of the eating disturbance exceeds that which might be seen in an anxiety disorder and necessitates further clinical attention (see Table 1) [13].

Other than the use of outpatient psychotherapy, there were no significant differences between the groups in terms of prior mental health treatment, including hospitalizations for EDs or other mental health issues, admissions to day treatment programs, intensive outpatient programs, or residential treatment facilities. It should be taken into consideration, however, that ours is a young, relatively treatment-naïve population, and that the rate of past mental health admissions would be very different when looking at an older population of patients. Additionally, children with ARFID may be more likely seen as medically ill initially, and the early referrals may tend to gravitate toward the medical as opposed to mental health arena, as a trend in our data revealed, although it was not significant.

There were several strengths to this study, including the large sample size and the use of both clinical and standardized psychometric measures for patient assessment. Additionally, the use of multiple informants (patients, parents, and clinicians) adds to the validity of the findings. Furthermore, experienced clinicians completed all assessments and the adolescent medicine physician involved in deciding on the retrospective DSM-5 diagnoses was integrally involved in the efforts leading up to the inclusion of ARFID in the DSM-5. As ARFID is still a relatively "new" diagnosis, there are no formalized assessment tools available yet. However, instruments will likely be developed, capturing the clinical features and diagnostic criteria which will help standardize diagnosis. There are some available resources to help guide the clinician in evaluation [24,27].

However, there are several limitations that deserve mention. The retrospective nature of this study, and the fact that diagnoses were made on DSM-5 criteria that had not yet been formalized by the time of its completion, need to be taken into consideration. However, as previously mentioned, the published DSM-5 criteria were essentially the same as the proposed criteria used for this study. Careful discussion amongst experienced clinicians very familiar with all of the cases was undertaken to decide upon the appropriate DSM-5 diagnosis for each patient; this did not allow for direct assessment of inter-rater reliability. The absence of blinding of the clinicians may have introduced bias to the outcome of the study, possibly leading to a higher prevalence of ARFID than previously seen in other studies. Lastly, our patients were undergoing day treatment, which implies a certain severity of illness, and may limit the generalizability to patients in other settings, or non-clinical populations. Despite these limitations, this study provides support for ARFID as a separate diagnostic category.

Conclusions

This is the first study to examine patients with the diagnosis of ARFID in a cohort of patients undergoing day treatment and adds to the limited literature available on this new diagnosis. The inclusion of psychometric measures from both patients and parents has not been documented to date. Children and adolescents with ARFID are clearly distinct from those with other EDs and can now be identified and labeled more specifically and accurately. Ideally, this will enable more timely recognition and access to care. The degree of both physical and psychosocial dysfunction with which these patients present indicates the need for prompt and appropriate treatment. The relatively high prevalence of patients with

ARFID in this treatment setting may indicate the need for an intensive level of care for many of these children and adolescents, depending on their initial presentation. Future research on ARFID, with respect to course, prognosis and treatment is warranted.

Competing interests
None of the authors have any competing interests relative to the publication of this manuscript.

Authors' contributions
TN was involved with the study design, revised the database, carried out all data analysis, and was involved with drafting the manuscript. SLL was involved with the study design, was part of the group of providers determining the DSM-5 diagnoses, reviewed the data analysis, and was involved with drafting of the manuscript. EM was involved with the study design, was part of the group of providers determining the DSM-5 diagnoses, reviewed the data analysis, and reviewed the manuscript. CH supervised the statistical analysis, reviewed the data analysis, created the tables, and reviewed the manuscript. RO conceived of the study, was involved with the study design, was part of the group of providers determining the DSM-5 diagnoses, reviewed the data analysis, and drafted and reviewed the manuscript. All authors read and approved the final manuscript.

Author information
SL is a clinical psychologist who has specialized in the care of patients with eating disorders for almost 20 years. She is the Program Director for the day program described in the manuscript.
RO is an Adolescent Medicine physician with clinical and research expertise in the area of eating disorders for 16 years. She was a Special Interest Group leader at both the Society for Adolescent Health and Medicine Annual Meeting and the International Conference on Eating Disorders. She just completed her tenure on the Scientific Program Committee for the 2014 ICED. She serves as the Adolescent Medicine Director for the day program described in the manuscript.

Acknowledgements
No funding sources.
The authors would like to acknowledge Debra K. Katzman, MD for her careful and critical review of the manuscript.

Author details
[1]Penn State College of Medicine, 500 University Drive, 17033 Hershey, PA, USA. [2]Division of Adolescent Medicine and Eating Disorders, Penn State Hershey Children's Hospital, 905 West Governor Road, Suite 250, 17033 Hershey, PA, USA. [3]Departments of Surgery and Public Health Sciences, Penn State College of Medicine, 500 University Drive, 17033 Hershey, PA, USA.

References

1. Nicholls D, Chater R, Lask B: **Children into DSM don't go: a comparison of classification systems for eating disorders in childhood and early adolescence.** *Int J Eat Disord* 2000, **28**(3):317–324.
2. Madden S, Morris A, Zurynski YA, Kohn M, Elliot EJ: **Burden of eating disorders in 5-13-year-old children in Australia.** *Med J Aust* 2009, **190**(8):410–414.
3. Peebles R, Hardy KK, Wilson JL, Lock JD: **Are diagnostic criteria for eating disorders markers of medical severity?** *Pediatrics* 2010, **125**(5):e1193–e1201.
4. Bryant-Waugh R, Markham L, Kreipe RE, Walsh BT: **Feeding and eating disorders in childhood.** *Int J Eat Disord* 2010, **43**(2):98–111.
5. Nicholls D, Bryant-Waugh R: **Eating disorders of infancy and childhood: definition, symptomatology, epidemiology, and comorbidity.** *Child Adolesc Psychiatr Clin N Am* 2009, **18**(1):17–30.
6. Higgs JF, Goodyer IM, Birch J: **Anorexia nervosa and food avoidance emotional disorder.** *Arch Dis Child* 1989, **64**(3):346–351.
7. Chatoor I: **Feeding disorders in infants and toddlers: diagnosis and treatment.** *Child Adolesc Psychiatr Clin N Am* 2002, **11**(2):163–183.
8. Mascola AJ, Bryson SW, Agras WS: **Picky eating during childhood: a longitudinal study to age 11 years.** *Eat Behav* 2010, **11**(4):253–257.
9. Nicklaus S: **Development of food variety in children.** *Appetite* 2009, **52**(1):253–255.
10. Jacobi C, Schmitz G, Agras WS: **Is picky eating an eating disorder?** *Int J Eat Disord* 2008, **41**(7):626–634.
11. Timimi S, Douglas J, Tsiftsopoulou K: **Selective eaters: a retrospective case note study.** *Child Care Health Dev* 1997, **23**(3):265–278.
12. Nicholls D, Christie D, Randall L, Lask B: **Selective eating: symptom, disorder or normal variant.** *Clin Child Psychol Psychiatry* 2001, **6**(2):257–270.
13. APA: *Diagnostic and Statistical Manual of Mental Disorders.* 5th edition. Washington, DC: American Psychiatric Association; 2013.
14. Ornstein RM, Rosen DS, Mammel KA, Callahan ST, Forman S, Jay MS, Fisher M, Rome E, Walsh BT: **Distribution of eating disorders in children and adolescents using the proposed DSM-5 criteria for feeding and eating disorders.** *J Adolesc Health* 2013, **53**(2):303–305.
15. Fisher MM, Rosen DS, Ornstein RM, Mammel KA, Katzman DK, Rome ES, Callahan ST, Malizio J, Kearney S, Walsh BT: **Characteristics of avoidant/restrictive food intake disorder in children and adolescents: a "new disorder" in DSM-5.** *J Adolesc Health* 2014, **55**(1):49–52.
16. Norris ML, Robinson A, Obeid N, Harrison M, Spettigue W, Henderson K: **Exploring avoidant/restrictive food intake disorder in eating disordered patients: a descriptive study.** *Int J Eat Disord* 2013, **47**(5):495–499.
17. Maloney MJ, McGuire JB, Daniels SR: **Reliability testing of a children's version of the eating attitude test.** *J Am Acad Child Adolesc Psychiatry* 1988, **27**(5):541–543.
18. Garner DM, Olmsted MP, Bohr Y, Garfinkel PE: **The eating attitudes test: psychometric features and clinical correlates.** *Psychol Med* 1982, **12**(4):871–878.
19. Kovacs M: *Children's Depression Inventory (CDI).* New York, NY: Multi Health Systems, Inc.; 1992.
20. Reynolds CR: *Manual, Revised Children's Manifest Anxiety Scale.* Los Angeles, CA: Pro-Ed, Inc. 1985.
21. Achenbach TM: *Manual for the Child Behavior Checklist/4-18 and 1991 Profile.* Burlington, Vermont: University of Vermont Department of Psychiatry; 1991.
22. Pinhas L, Morris A, Crosby RD, Katzman DK: **Incidence and age-specific presentation of restrictive eating disorders in children: a Canadian paediatric surveillance program study.** *Arch Pediatr Adolesc Med* 2011, **165**(10):895–899.
23. Peebles R, Wilson JL, Lock JD: **How do children with eating disorders differ from adolescents with eating disorders at initial evaluation?** *J Adolesc Health* 2006, **39**(6):800–805.
24. Bryant-Waugh R: **Avoidant restrictive food intake disorder: an illustrative case example.** *Int J Eat Disord* 2013, **46**(5):420–423.
25. Rhodes P, Prunty M, Madden S: **Life-threatening food refusal in two nine-year-old girls: re-thinking the Maudsley model.** *Clin Child Psychol Psychiatry* 2009, **14**(1):63–70.
26. Nicholls DE, Lynn R, Viner RM: **Childhood eating disorders: British national surveillance study.** *Br J Psychiatry* 2011, **198**(4):295–301.
27. Bryant-Waugh R, Kreipe RE: **Avoidant/restrictive food intake disorder.** *Psychiatr Ann* 2012, **42**(11):402–405.

5

Restrained eating and self-esteem in premenopausal and postmenopausal women

Suzana Drobnjak[1], Semra Atsiz[1], Beate Ditzen[1,3], Brunna Tuschen-Caffier[2] and Ulrike Ehlert[1*]

Abstract

Background: There has been limited research about disordered eating in middle-aged women, and to date, few data exist about restrained eating behavior in postmenopausal women. Therefore, the aim of this study was to examine eating behavior with a specific focus on menopause as an associated factor in restrained eating. Beyond this, we were interested in how postmenopausal status and self-esteem would interact to determine eating patterns in women in middle age.

Methods: We conducted an online survey in women aged between 40 and 66. Eating behavior was assessed with the Eating Disorder Examination-Questionnaire (EDE-Q) in premenopausal ($N = 318$) and postmenopausal women ($N = 250$). All participants rated their self-esteem using the Rosenberg Self-Esteem Scale (RSE) and reported their weight, height, waist circumference, and hip circumference.

Results: 15.7% of all participants showed clinically meaningful scores on restrained eating. Postmenopausal women showed significantly higher scores on the EDE-Q subscale of restrained eating as compared to premenopausal women, but when controlling for body mass index, however, this finding was no longer significant. Further exploratory analyses suggest that particularly low or high self-esteem levels are associated with restrained eating. Self-esteem might serve as a mediator between menopausal status and restrained eating, however results of these additional analyses were inconsistent.

Conclusions: Restrained eating may appear in middle-aged women. Particularly in postmenopausal women, restrained eating might be associated with lower and higher self-esteem.

Keywords: Menopause, Middle age, Restrained eating, Self-esteem, Eating behavior

Background

An increasing number of middle-aged women from highly industrialized countries are practicing disordered eating behaviors [1]. Eating disorders often show a chronic course, functional impairment, and seem to increase the risk of several health problems such as future obesity, depressive disorders, suicide attempts, anxiety disorders, and substance abuse [2]. Besides clinically diagnosed eating disorders such as anorexia nervosa and bulimia nervosa [3], disordered eating includes a wide range of eating-related problems [4]. Such behavior occurs relatively frequently but does not meet full criteria for the diagnosis of an eating disorder [4,5]. In general, disordered eating is a well-researched phenomenon, which is mainly assessed in adolescent and young adult women [3]. So far, few studies have investigated disordered eating in women between the ages of 40 and around 65 years [6], although health professionals have recently begun to focus their attention on disordered eating among this age group [7]. Admissions of middle-aged women to eating disorder inpatient treatment has increased over the last ten years [8,9].

Although in several studies, restrained eating has been identified as a main risk factor for young women to develop an eating disorder [10], as yet, specific trajectories of eating disorders in middle-aged women remain unknown. In general, restrained eating is defined as an intentional restriction of energy intake with the aim of losing or controlling weight [11]. Despite this definition, several studies indicate that restrained eating predicts

* Correspondence: u.ehlert@psychologie.uzh.ch
[1]Department of Psychology, Division of Clinical Psychology & Psychotherapy, University of Zurich, Binzmuehlestrasse 14/26, Zurich 8050, Switzerland
Full list of author information is available at the end of the article

weight gain and might be a risk factor for future onset of obesity [12,13].

Several studies found biological (e.g. body mass index), psychological (e.g. self-esteem), and sociocultural influences (e.g. weight-related teasing) [1] to predict disordered eating patterns – and these seem to be independent of age. However, a specific factor associated with eating behavior in middle-aged women might be menopause status. Menopause is defined as the permanent cessation of the primary functions of the human ovaries [14]. Menopause can be determined retrospectively, once 12 months have elapsed with no menstrual cycle, and this time frame distinguishes menopause from other related terms such as premenopause, perimenopause and postmenopause [14]. Premenopause describes a period of time with regular menstrual cycles. Perimenopause is a period of time when menstrual cycles begin to become irregular. Finally, postmenopause starts after the final menstrual period. After 12 months of amenorrhea, it can be determined that a woman has entered postmenopause [14].

Menopausal transition is a complex psychophysiological process [14]. During the menopausal transition, women could gain an average of 2 to 2.5 kg in weight over 3 years, which is often regarded as the major contributing factor to midlife body weight gain in women [15]. Besides this, it has been shown that a shift to an abdominal fat redistribution occurs [16]. Since slimness is an important criterion of female attractiveness in many societies [17,18], it can be assumed that middle-aged women may experience a loss of attractiveness due to the age-related naturally occurring weight gain [19]. However, the data regarding body image in this age group are contradictory. Although researchers found that the perception of attractiveness is not influenced by age or menopausal status [19], postmenopausal women reported less positive attitudes about their appearance than premenopausal women [20].

Overall, body weight and female self-experienced attractiveness are closely connected, as are self-rated attractiveness and self-esteem [21]. Additionally, as supported by meta-analyses, self-esteem seems to be associated with disordered eating [22]. Lower self-esteem, which means a reduced sense of contentment, self-acceptance, and a reduced appraisal of one's own worth, predicts higher rates of eating disorders in young women [22-25] and body dissatisfaction or symptoms of bulimia nervosa in middle-aged women [7,26,27].

Our study was designed with two aims: first, to examine the association between menopausal status and disordered eating, with a particular focus on restrained eating in middle-aged women. Our hypothesis was that postmenopausal women will show increased scores in disordered eating than premenopausal women. Our second aim was to examine the role of self-esteem in disordered eating in this age group. We hypothesized that low self-esteem will be positively associated with disordered eating in postmenopausal women.

Methods

Data collection and participants

Potential participants were contacted by email using mailing lists and websites from women's organizations (e.g. www.frauenlandsgemeinde.ch) in Switzerland. The information of the advertisement in the internet in order to inform and recruit the women contained a brief explanation about the study: We introduced the background of the study with the fact that little has been known about eating behavior and related factors in middle-aged women. After this short introduction we informed potential study participants that the online questionnaire would contain questions about demographics, their eating behavior, psychological variables, and menstrual cycle status. Email recipients were also informed that the online survey would take about 15 minutes. The inclusion criteria was age over 40 and female gender. At the end of our information letter, we referred to the link, which had to be opened in order to get to the questionnaire. The survey was programmed using the software *Unipark* (http://www.unipark.info/1-0-online-befragungssoftware-fuer-studenten-und-universitaeten-unipark-home.htm). Overall, we sent about 5'000 Email invitations and 1101 potential participants started to fill out our questionnaire. The drop-out rate (participants who did not fill out the questionnaire completely) in our study was 40.2%.

Participation in the study was voluntary and all women gave their informed consent. Only participants who agreed with the informed consent were able to fill out the questionnaire. Upon completion of the questionnaire, the participants were thanked for their filling in the questionnaire and informed that their anonymity would be guaranteed. Participants who were interested in a follow-up study or who wished to receive further information on the study results could leave their e-mail addresses. Additionally, contact information was provided for the unlikely event that responding to stress or symptom-related questions caused acute psychological problems. This study was conducted in accordance with rules and regulations of the appropriate ethics committee (The Faculty of Arts and Humanities of the University of Zurich, Switzerland).

We excluded participants with the following criteria: age under 40 or over 66, pregnancy, self-reported Affective Disorder, Eating Disorder or Anxiety Disorder, last menstruation more than 15 years ago and participants who did not complete all questions. After the completion of the study, menopausal status was defined as follows: premenopausal women (N = 318) reported to have a regular or irregular menstrual cycle in the past 12 months, which means that participants with a possible perimenopausal status were in the group premenopausal women included, too. Postmenopausal women (N = 250) had not had a menstrual cycle during the past 12 months. The women were asked to provide the date (day, month, year) of their last menstruation. The detailed process of recruitment and the selection of the two groups from a large sample are shown in Figure 1.

Assessment measures

The online survey consisted of 58 items. The first section of questions comprised items addressing sociodemographic, general health-related, and menstrual cycle-related variables. The second section of the survey consisted of questions about eating behavior and self-esteem, presented in a randomized order.

Body Mass Index and Waist-to-Hip Ratio

Participants were asked to indicate their weight and height, and BMI was calculated as weight divided by the square of height in cm. Besides this, participants were asked to measure their waist (at the midpoint between the lower margin of the last palpable rib and the top of the iliac crest) and hip circumference (widest portion of the buttocks) [28]. Waist-to-hip ratio (WHR) was calculated by dividing the waist by the hip circumference [28]. In addition, we illustrated the definition of the WHR measurement with a picture. WHO norms [28] define obesity for females as a WHR above 0.85, or a BMI above 30). BMI and WHR were used as control variables in this study.

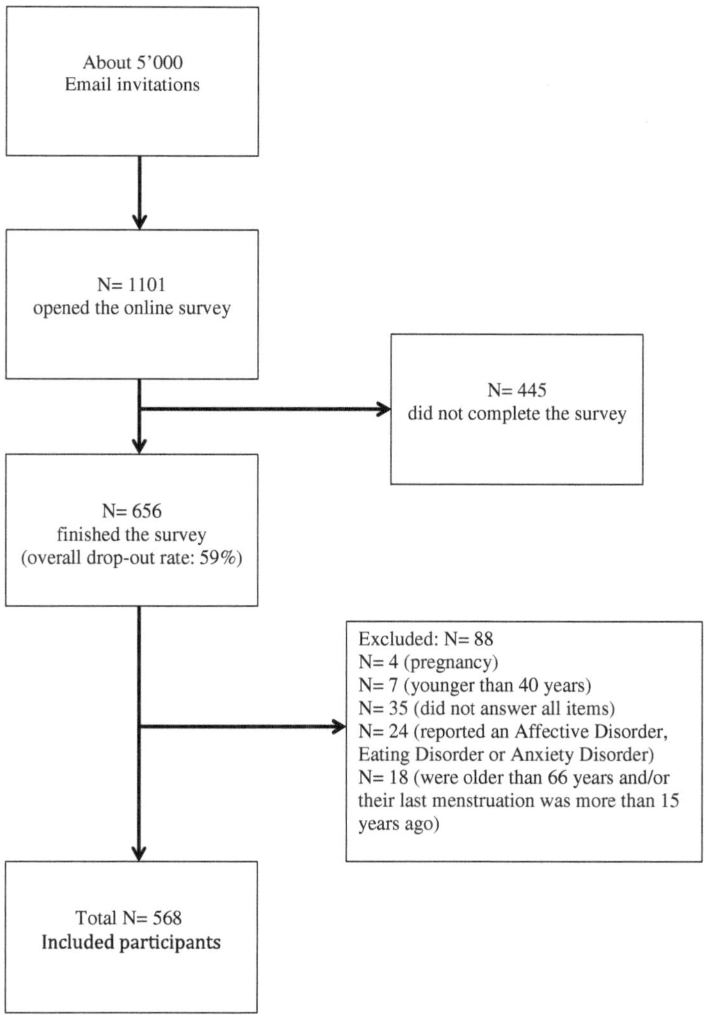

Figure 1 Process of data selection.

Eating behavior

Eating behavior was assessed with the German version of the Eating Disorder Examination-Questionnaire (EDE-Q) [29,30]. The EDE-Q is a self-report instrument with 36 items covering the previous 28 days. It contains four subscales measuring restrained eating, shape concern, weight concern, and eating concern, to be summarized with a global score. The items can be answered on a 7-point scale, with higher scores reflecting greater eating-related pathology. Frequencies of disordered eating behaviors including binge eating and various compensatory behaviors are also assessed. Based on this questionnaire, "extreme dietary restraint" was defined with reference to the EDE-Q "food avoidance" item, namely "going without food for a period of eight or more waking hours on average three or more times per week in order to influence weight or shape" [31,32]. For the EDE-Q, norms for anorexia nervosa, bulimia nervosa, and eating disorders not otherwise specified are available for young women [29,30,33]. The scores of the subscale "restrained eating" range from 0.1 to 2.6 among women without diagnosed eating disorders, while means of restrained eating between 2.7 and 6 are found in women with eating disorders. Women with clinically meaningful scores show values ranging between 3.7 and 6.0 for "shape concern", between 3.09 and 6.0 for "weight concern", and between 1.85 and 6 for "eating concern" [30].

Additional six items measure diagnostically relevant information, e.g. symptoms of binge eating. In our study, we analyzed the item 13 "Over the past 28 days, how many times have you eaten what other people would regard as an unusually large amount of food (given the circumstances)?" and item 14 "On how many of these times did you have a sense of having lost control over your eating (at the time you were eating)?". These key behavioral items were dichotomized for any occurrence (≥1 episode versus 0 episodes over the past 28 days) and regular occurrence (≥4 or < 4 episodes in the last 28 days) [31].

In this study, the Cronbach's alpha for each subscale was acceptable (restrained eating = .78; shape concern = .89; weight concern = .77; eating concern = .82).

Self-esteem

Self-esteem was assessed with the German version [34] of the self-esteem scale (RSE) [35], which is a widely used self-esteem inventory in social science research. The scale contains 10 items to be scored from 1 = "totally disagree" to 4 = "totally agree". Negatively coded items were recoded in order to calculate the sum score. In the present study, the Cronbach's alpha for SES was .74, which is acceptable.

Data analysis

Following overall descriptive data analysis and the analysis of frequencies and intensities of disordered eating behavior, and the key behavioral factors for binge eating, premenopausal women and postmenopausal women were compared with regard to eating behavior, such as restrained eating, shape concern, eating concern and weight concern, using multivariate ANOVAs. Furthermore, BMI, age and WHR were included as covariates, and univariate ANOVAs with menopause status as factor and restrained eating or self-esteem as dependent variables were conducted. An additional univariate ANOVA was performed with menopause status as factor and "extreme dietary restraint" as dependent variable including the control variables BMI, age and WHR.

Results

Participants' characteristics

Table 1 provides descriptive data of the total study sample (N = 568 women, aged from 40 to 66 years).

Frequencies and intensities of disordered eating behavior

80.8% (N = 459) of all participants show a score higher than 0 on restrained eating. 15.7% (N = 116) of the participants show clinically relevant scores on restrained eating. 10.7% (N = 61) participants reported "Extreme dietary restraint", defined as going without food for a period of eight or more waking hours on average three or more times per week. Of these 61 participants, one participant reported a BMI < 18.5, 42 a BMI between 18.5 and 25, and 18 women reported a BMI over 25.

Comparable scores were found in the subscales eating concern, weight concern and shape concern, with 56.9% to 82% of all participants reporting low to moderate manifestations of disordered eating. 6% to 12.5% reported clinically meaningful scores on these subscales. Figure 2 displays the distributions of eating patterns.

In addition, results of the key behavioral features showed the following results: 69.7% (N = 396) showed no occurrence of eating large amounts of food (EDE-Q item 13), whereas 30.3% (N = 172) scored higher than 1. 86.7% (N = 493) reported no regular occurrence of this behavior whereas 13.3% (N = 75) showed scores higher than 4. 77.5% (N = 440) showed no occurrence of lost control during eating (EDE-Q item 14), whereas 22.5% (N = 128) scored higher than 1. 89.2% (N = 507) reported no regular occurrence of this behavior whereas 10.8% (N = 61) showed a score over 4.

Correlations between eating behavior and associated variables

Most correlations were significant at the .001 level, except for WHR and menstrual status, where the associations with the other variables were mostly insignificant (see Table 2).

Table 1 Characteristics of study population

Characteristics	Premenopausal (N = 318)	Postmenopausal (N = 250)	Group difference t-test/Chi-square
Age	M = 46.40, SD = 3.96	M = 54.98, SD = 5.19	T = −22.499, p = .000
Education			
Any type of college and higher	N = 228 (71.7%)	N = 139 (49.6%)	χ^2 = 6.698, p = .153
Marital status			
Married/in a relationship	N = 200 (62.9%)	N = 190 (76.0%)	χ^2 = 0.536, p = .464
Single/separated/divorced	N = 118 (37.1%)	N = 60 (24.0%)	χ^2 = 1.002, p = .317
Employment	76-100%	N = 152 (47.8%)	N = 95 (38.0%)
unemployed/up to 75%	N = 166 (52.2%)	N = 155 (62.0%)	χ^2 = 3.003, p = .391
Children	M = 1.4, SD = .49	M = 1.26, SD = .44	T = −1.144, p = .253
Months after beginning of the last menstruation	M = 1.00, SD = 1.79	M = 97.81, SD = 68.36	T = 24.497, p = .000
BMI	M = 23.34, SD = 3.86	M = 23.74, SD = 4.53	T = −1.133, p = .258
WHR	M = 0.812, SD = 0.07	M = 0.828, SD = 0.09	T = −1.758, p = .080
EDE-Q$_{_restrained}$	M = 1.23, SD = 1.32	M = 1.45, SD = 1.35	T = −1.983, p = .048
EDE-Q$_{_eating}$	M = 0.46, SD = 0.87	M = 0.48, SD = 0.82	T = − 0.295, p = .768
EDE-Q$_{_weight}$	M = 1.28, SD = 1.29	M = 1.29, SD = 1.27	T = − 0.080, p = .936
EDE-Q$_{_shape}$	M = 1.63, SD = 1.45	M = 1.67, SD = 1.47	T = − 0.305, p = .761
RES	M = 39.77, SD = 4.64	M = 38.86, SD = 4.82	T = 2.288, p = .023

Note: EDE-Q $_{restrained}$ = subscale restrained eating of the EDE-Q; EDE-Q $_{eating}$ = subscale eating concern of the EDE-Q; EDE-Q $_{weight}$ = subscale weight concern of EDE-Q; EDE-Q $_{shape}$ = subscale shape concern of the EDE-Q; BMI = body mass index; RSE = Rosenberg Self-Esteem Scale.

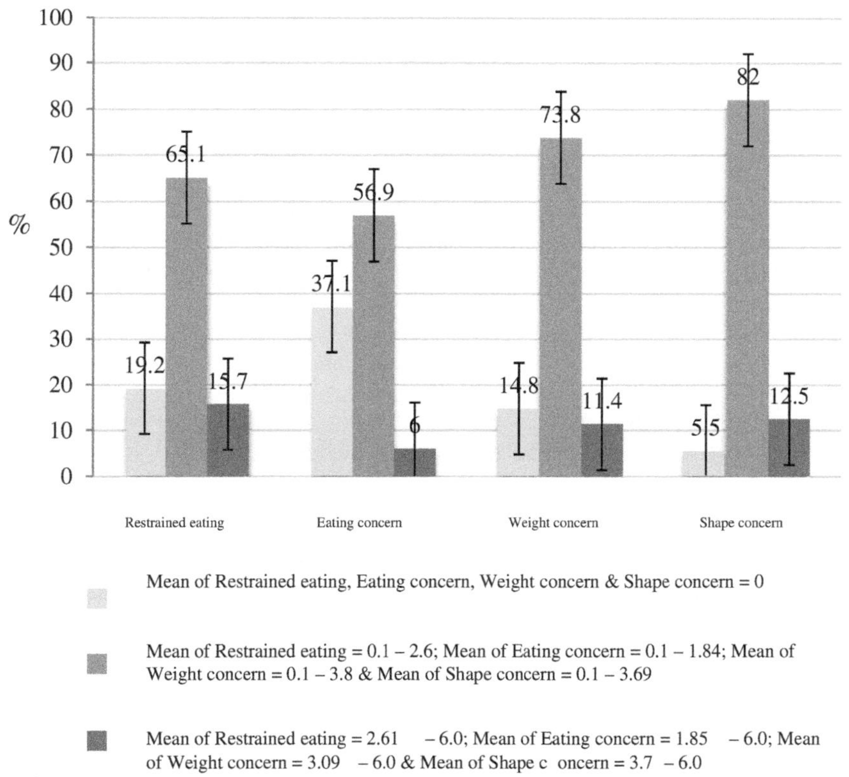

Figure 2 Manifestations of disordered eating behavior.

Table 2 Correlations between all variables in the study

		1	2	3	4	5	6	7	M	SD	Range
1	m.status	-							-.087	.997	−1, +1
2	RSE	-.096[a]	-						39.351	4.717	17-50
3	EDE-Q $_{restraint}$	.088[a]	-.213						1.340	1.345	0-6
4	EDE-Q $_{eating}$	.005[b]	-.396	.555					. 467	.843	0-6
5	EDE-Q $_{weight}$	.000[b]	-.333	.642	.716	-.333			1.281	1.280	0-6
6	EDE-Q $_{shape}$	.012[b]	-.322	.638	.701	.910			1.651	1.451	0-6
7	BMI	.039[b]	-.043[b]	.200	.267	.456	.427	-	23.495	4.144	14-46
8	WHR	.096[b]	-.027[b]	.032[b]	.063[b]	.142[a]	.186	.283	.8182	0.081	.45-1.27

Note: Unless otherwise noted, all coefficients were significant at the p = .001 level; [a]: significant at p < .05; [b]: non-significant; m.status = menopausal status; RSE = Rosenberg Self-Esteem Scale; EDE-Q $_{restraint}$ = subscale restrained eating of the EDE-Q; EDE-Q $_{eating}$ = subscale eating concern of the EDE-Q; EDE-Q $_{weight}$ = subscale weight concern of EDE-Q; EDE-Q $_{shape}$ = subscale shape concern of the EDE-Q; BMI = body mass index; WHR = Waist-to-Hip Ratio.

Group differences

The overall multivariate analyses (Hoteling-Spur) with menopause status as factor and the subscales of EDE-Q and RSE as dependent variables revealed a main effect of menopause status change [F(5, 562) = 2.584, p = .025, partial $\eta^2 = .022$]. Results obtained by multivariate ANOVAs indicate that restrained eating in postmenopausal women is increased compared to premenopausal women (F[1, 566] = 3.931, $p = 0.048$, partial $\eta^2 = .007$), and self-esteem is decreased in postmenopausal women (F[1, 566] = 5.234, $p = 0.023$, partial $\eta^2 = .009$). No significant differences in other eating behavior variables, such as eating concern (F[1, 566] = 0.087, $p = 0.768$, partial $\eta^2 = .000$), weight concern (F[1, 566] = 0.006, $p = 0.936$, partial $\eta^2 = .000$), and shape concern (F[1, 566] = 0.093, $p = 0.761$, partial $\eta^2 = .000$), were observed between pre- and postmenopausal women (see Table 1). No covariates were included in this multivariate analysis.

Results obtained by univariate ANOVAs with menopause status as factor and BMI as dependent variable indicate that Body mass index (BMI) did not differ between the groups (F[1, 566] = 1.284, $p = 0.258$, partial $\eta^2 = .002$). Additionally, WHR did not differ between the groups (F[1, 330] = 3.091, $p = 0.080$, partial $\eta^2 = .009$).

Results obtained by univariate ANOVAs with menopause status as factor and restrained eating as dependent variable show that when controlling for BMI, WHR and age, BMI was a significant covariate (F[1, 327] = 18.038, $p = 0.000$, partial $\eta^2 = .052$).

The results with the subgroup of women who reported "Extreme dietary restraint" showed a different pattern of findings: The univariate ANOVAs with menopause status as factor and restrained eating as dependent variable show that when controlling for BMI, WHR and age, menopause status (F[1,24] = 4.615, $p = 0.042$, partial $\eta^2 = .161$) and WHR (F[1,24] = 5.406, $p = 0.029$, partial $\eta^2 = .184$) were significant predictors of restrained eating.

Results obtained by univariate ANOVAs with menopause status as factor and self-esteem as dependent variable show that when controlling for BMI, WHR and age, menopause status (F[1, 327] = 5.789, $p = 0.017$, partial $\eta^2 = .017$) is a significant predictor of self-esteem.

Associations between self-esteem and restrained eating

U-shaped association between self-esteem and restrained eating

Results from the multiple regression analysis with self-esteem and self-esteem squared as independent variables and restrained eating as dependent variable are shown in Table 3 and suggest a U-shaped relationship (see Figure 3). Overall, self-esteem explained 6.1% of the variance in restrained eating.

A mediation analysis with menopause status as an independent, restrained eating as a dependent variable and self-esteem as potential mediator based on the Baron & Kenny [36] and Sobel method [37] suggested that self-esteem mediated the relationship between menopause status and restrained eating. However, the bootstrapping approach by Preacher and Hayes ([38], and as available as an SPSS-syntax on their homepage, http://www.afhayes.com/spss-sas-and-mplus-macros-and-code.html) did not provide significant results. We, thus, do not further interpret the results from the aforementioned mediation analyses.

Discussion

This study focused on the role of menopausal status and self-esteem in terms of their relationship with eating behavior in normal-weight middle-aged women. Overall,

Table 3 Multiple regression analysis with restrained eating as dependent variable

	Unstandardized coefficients, *B*	SE	Standardized coefficients, *β*	Level of significance, *p*
Constant	9.566	1.946		.000
RSE	-.382	105	−1.340	.000
RSE^2	.004	.001	1.134	.002

Note: RSE = Rosenberg Self-Esteem Scale.

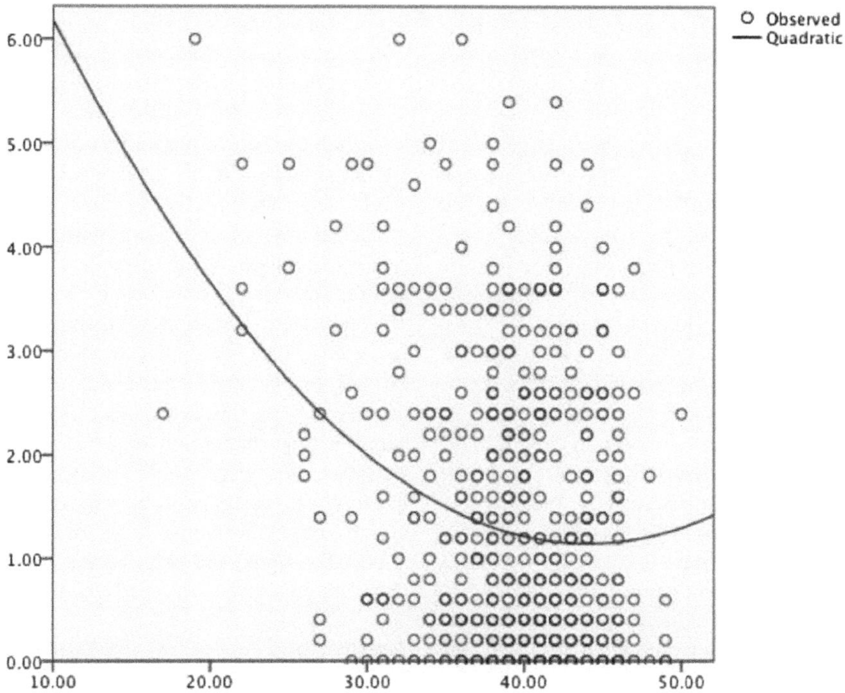

Figure 3 U-shaped relationship between self-esteem and restrained eating.

the results suggest that restrained eating is a relavitely frequent behavior among middle-aged women: 15.7% of all participants report restrained eating scores in a clinically meaningful range. In addition, 10.8% - 13.3% of all participants showed a regularly occurrence of binge eating symptoms. Compared to premenopausal women, postmenopausal women report a decreased self-esteem and higher levels of restrained eating, whereas this effect disappears when BMI and age are controlled for. However, even when controlling for BMI, WHR and age, both menopause status and WHR seem to be in a relationship with extreme dietary restraint. Self-esteem was associated with restrained eating, showing a U-shaped curve. Based on these data, it might be followed that self-esteem mediates the relationship between menopausal status and restrained eating, however the results of the additional mediation analyses were inconsistent.

The assessed mean scores of the subscales of the EDE-Q indicate that middle-aged women's eating concerns are comparable with those of young adult women [31]. However, to date, no normative data for this older age group are available. In the present study, a subsample of 6–15.7% women showed subscale scores in a clinically meaningful range, thus suggesting that negative body image and eating disorders may appear in older women [39,40].

Even tough a recent study examined overweight middle-aged participants and showed increased restrained eating in postmenopausal women, our finding that normal-weight postmenopausal women show increased restrained eating when not controlling for BMI could be seen in a similar line [41]; we have also found an associtation between menopausal status and restrained eating.

The authors described that postmenopausal women (M = 51.7 years) reported higher levels of dietary restraint than premenopausal women (M = 35.7 years). However, in that study, postmenopausal women still had a significantly higher BMI than premenopausal women. To the best of our knowledge, this is the first study in this field, examining participants with normal weight. Although restrained eating and BMI are modestly positively correlated, it is highly surprising that restrained eating differs between the average normal-weighted pre- and postmenopausal women. This finding might have interesting implications for further studies.

Furthermore, menopause-related changes in body fat distribution or increasing BMI in middle-aged women are seen as having a negative impact on appearance [42-44,25]. Beyond this, the physiological changes after menopause could be associated with increased feelings of body dissatisfaction and lower psychological well-being than in the years before menopause [45,46]. When internalized ideals of appearance no longer seem achievable [45], this may affect body image and eating behaviors. This effect seems to be even greater the more physical appearance is seen as an integral part of the self-concept [46].

It is difficult to distinguish the association between menopause and restrained eating or BMI from age or age-related factors, such as sedentary lifestyle, slowed metabolism, or less sleep. All of these factors have independently been associated with weight gain [47]. Indeed, our data suggest that postmenopausal women showed higher restrained eating and, when controlling for BMI, WHR and age, only BMI seems to be in a modest positive relationship with restrained eating in middle-aged women. Previous research suggests positive [48], negative [49], or no relationships between BMI and restrained eating. However, in normal-weight groups, restrained eating and BMI seem to be positively associated [48,50,51]. It might therefore follow that in normal-weight populations, restrained eating may serve as a marker for the tendency to overeat – which could then call for constant counter-regulation.

In younger women, several studies have shown that decreased self-esteem is a risk factor for developing disordered eating behavior [22]. However, results regarding this relationship in middle-aged women have been inconsistent, with some suggesting a positive and some a negative relationship [26,52]. The U-shaped relationship found in the present study now suggests that low as well as high self-esteem might be associated with restrained eating, although the findings are more robust for the former. This finding seems to integrate the previous and seemingly contradictory results. Many women seem to link their self-esteem to their appearance. The realization that one is no longer able to fulfill societal ideals of appearance was found to have a negative impact on self-esteem [46]. Given that restrained eating is intended to maintain or decrease a particular weight [22], and weight loss was found to improve self-esteem [53], increased restrained eating could be regarded as a measure to raise self-esteem [54].

However, the results should also be interpreted in light of the study's strengths and limitations. Online-based data collection allows access to a broad sample of participants as well as the assessment of data in a short period of time [55]. Nevertheless, this is a cross-sectional study and the results should be interpreted with caution because our results show only associations without causal meanings; only longitudinal study might provide more conclusive answers to the question of whether menopausal status and self-esteem might cause disordered eating in middle-aged women. Furthermore, potential problems with online recruitment may occur. Online studies are based on self-reported data, which leads to the inability to verify the inclusion and exclusion criteria. In addition, individuals with high BMI or circumferences might not want to share this information, even if it is anonymous. For example, even tough we tried to provide a clear definition of the WHR measurement, it might be subjective what the "widest portion of the buttocks" is, and therefore cause biased results. Overall, the recruited participants might be a biased selective population. It could also explain why the BMI is in a normal weight range. In addition, mixing potential perimenopausal and postmenopausal women may have biased the results – a limitation which is due to our online assessment lacking an endocrine validation of menopausal status. We acknowledge that future and methodological more rigorous studies in this field might use endocrine assessments. However, with this initial investigation in this relatively large sample, endocrine analyses would not have been feasible.

Moreover, participants in this online study may have reported specific eating behaviors as a consequence of their educational and professional background.

Conclusions

In conclusion, this study focused on menopausal status, self-esteem and eating patterns in middle-aged women, and in so doing, might shed light on this relatively understudied topic. It shows that not only women with diagnosed eating disorders may show eating-related changes, but also non-diagnosed, healthy, middle-aged and normal-weighted women may have increased scores, especially in restrained eating. It remains to be analyzed whether it is specifically menopausal status or other age-related factors, which influence self-esteem in middle-aged women. As described in a recent study, it can be hypothesized that menopausal transition could represent a window of vulnerability to eating-related changes [56]. In Western societies, menopausal transition is often perceived as a time of emotional and physical health impairment [43]. Independently, disordered eating is influenced by a multitude of bio-psycho-social factors [24,57]. Thus, while not every woman is necessarily predisposed to developing restrained eating patterns during her menopausal transition, her experienced self-esteem might influence this relationship. According to recent data, over 70% of women aged over 50 years report dissatisfaction with their current weight and shape, being compared to when they have younger [58], likely, being vulnerable to develop disordered eating. This suggests that women in midlife might be particularly vulnerable to developing disordered eating behavior. Further studies could help identify specific risk groups for disordered eating in this age group, in order to develop prevention and treatment options for the most vulnerable. With increased ageing in our societies and stable youth-related norms of attractiveness, the demand for such interventions might well increase over the coming years.

Competing interests
The authors declare that they have no competing interests.

Authors' contributions
SD designed the study, recruited the participants, analyzed the data and wrote the manuscirpt. SA helped to recruite the participants and analyze the data. BD supervized the data analysis and edited the manuscript. BTC was involved in the discussion of the data analysis and its implications. UE designed the study with SD, supervised it and edited the manuscript. She was the chief supervisor of the study and manuscript. All authors read and approved the final manuscript.

Acknowledgements
The authors would like to thank all the women who participated in this study. There were no funding sources for this project.

Author details
[1]Department of Psychology, Division of Clinical Psychology & Psychotherapy, University of Zurich, Binzmuehlestrasse 14/26, Zurich 8050, Switzerland. [2]Department of Psychology, Division of Clinical Psychology & Psychotherapy, Albert-Ludwigs University, Engelbergerstrasse 41, Freiburg 79106, Germany. [3]Institute of Medical Psychology in the Center for Psychosocial Medicine, University Hospital Heidelberg, Bergheimer Str. 20, Heidelberg 69115, Germany.

References
1. Slevec JH, Tiggemann M: **Predictors of body dissatisfaction and disordered eating in middle-aged women.** *Clin Psychol Rev* 2011, **31**:515–524. doi: 10.1016/j.cpr.2010.12.002.
2. Wilson GT, Becker CB, Heffernan K: **Eating disorders.** In *Child Psychopathology.* 2nd edition. Edited by Mash EJ, Barkley RA. New York: Guilford Press; 2003:687–715.
3. Association AP: *Diagnostic and Statistical Manual of Mental Disorders (4th ed. TR).* Washington DC: Author; 2000.
4. Pereira RF, Alvarenga M: **Disordered eating: identifying, treating, preventing, and differentiating it from eating disorders.** *Diabetes Spectrum* 2007, **20**:141–148.
5. Machado PPP, Machado BC, Gonçales S, Hoek HW: **The prevalence of eating disorders not otherwise specified.** *Int J Eat Disord* 2007, **40**:212–217.
6. Zerbe K, Domnitei D: **Eating disorders at middle age, part 1.** *Eat Disord Rev* 2004, **15**:1–3.
7. Procopio CA, Holm-Denoma JM, Gordon KH, Joiner TE: **Two-three-year stability and interrelations of bulimotypic indicators and depressive and anxious symptoms in middle-aged women.** *Int J Eat Disord* 2006, **39**:312–319.
8. Cumella EJ, Kally Z: **Comparison of middle-age and young women inpatients with eating disorders.** *Eat Weight Disord* 2008, **13**:183–190.
9. Cumella EJ, Kally Z: **Profile of 50 women with midlife-onset eating disorders.** *Eat Disord* 2008, **16**:193–203. doi: 10.1080/10640260802016670.
10. Stice E, Ng J, Shaw H: **Risk factors and prodromal eating pathology.** *J Child Psychol Psychiatry* 2010, **51**:518–525. doi: 10.1111/j.1469-7610.2010.02212.x.
11. Burger KS, Stice E: **Relation of dietary restraint scores to activation of reward-related brain regions in response to food intake, anticipated intake, and food pictures.** *Neuroimage* 2011, **55**:233–239. doi: 10.1016/j.neuroimage.2010.12.009.
12. Field AE, Austin SB, Taylor CB, Malspeis S, Rosner B, Rockett HR, Gillman MW: **Relation between dieting and weight change among preadolescents and adolescents.** *Pediatrics* 2003, **112**:900–906.
13. Stice E, Presnell K, Shaw H, Rohde P: **Psychological and behavioral risk factors for onset of obesity in adolescent girls: a prospective study.** *J Consult Clin Psychol* 2005, **73**:195–202.
14. Nelson HD: **Menopause.** *Lancet* 2010, **371**:760–770. doi: 10.1016/S0140-6736(08)60346-3.
15. Wing RR, Matthews KA, Kuller LH, Meilahn EN, Plantinga PL: **Weight gain at the time of menopause.** *Arch Intern Med* 1991, **151**:97–102.
16. Polotsky HN, Polotsky AJ: **Metabolic implications of menopause.** *Semin Reprod Med* 2010, **5**:426–434. doi: 10.1055/s-0030-1262902.
17. Swami V, Frederick DA, Aavik T, Alcalay L, Allik J, Anderson D: **The attractive female body weight and female body dissatisfaction in 26 countries across 10 world regions: results of the international body project I.** *Pers Soc Psychol Bull* 2010, **36**:309–325. doi: 10.1177/0146167209359702.
18. Tunaley JR, Walsh S, Nicolson P: **'I'm not bad for my age': the meaning of body size and eating in the lives of older women.** *Ageing Society* 1999, **19**:741–759.
19. Koch PB, Mansfield PK, Thurau D, Carey M: **"Feeling Frumpy": the relationship between body image and sexual response changes in midlife women.** *J Sex Res* 2005, **42**:215–223.
20. McCabe MP, Ricciardelli LA, James T: **A longitudinal study of body change strategies of fitness center attendees.** *Eat Behav* 2007, **8**:492–496.
21. Thornton B, Moore S: **Physical attractiveness contrast effect: implications for self-esteem and evaluations of the social self.** *Pers Soc Psychol Bull* 1993, **19**:474–480.
22. Stice E: **Risk and maintenance factors for eating pathology: a meta-analytic review.** *Psychol Bull* 2002, **28**:825–848.
23. Leary MR, Baumeister RF: **The nature and function of self-esteem: sociometer theory.** *Soc Psychol* 2000, **32**:1–62.
24. LePage ML, Crowther JH, Harrington EF, Engler P: **Psychological correlates of fasting and vigorous exercise as compensatory strategies in undergraduate women.** *Eat Behav* 2008, **9**:423–429. doi: 10.1016/j.eatbeh.2008.06.002.
25. Tylka TL, Sabik NJ: **Integrating social comparison theory and self-esteem within objectification theory to predict women's disordered eating.** *Sex Roles* 2010, **63**:18–31.
26. Green SP, Pitchard ME: **Predictors of body image dissatisfaction in adult men and women.** *Soc Behav Pers* 2003, **31**:215–222.
27. Webster J, Tiggemann M: **The relationship between women's body satisfaction and self-image across the life span: The role of cognitive control.** *J Genet Psychol* 2003, **162**:241–252.
28. WHO: *Waist Circumference and Waist-Hip Ratio, Report of a WHO Expert Consultation.* Geneva: World Health Organization (WHO); 2012.
29. Fairburn CG, Beglin SJ: **Assessment of eating disorders: interview or self-report questionnaire?** *Int J Eat Disord* 1994, **16**:363–370.
30. Hilbert A, Tuschen-Caffier B, Karwautz A, Niederhofer H, Munsch S: **Eating disorder examination-questionnaire.** *Evaluation der deutschsprachigen Übersetzung Diagnostica* 2007, **53**:144–154.
31. Mond JM, Hay PJ, Rodgers B, Owen C: **Eating Disorder Examination Questionnaire (EDE-Q): norms for young adult women.** *Behav Res Ther* 2006, **44**:53–62.
32. Cooper Z, Fairburn CG: **Refining the definition of binge eating disorder and nonpurging bulimia nervosa.** *Int J Eat Disord* 2003, **34**:S89–S95.
33. Carter JC, Stewart DA, Fairburn CG: **Eating disorder examination questionnaire: norms for young adolescent girls.** *Behav Res Ther* 2001, **39**:625–632.
34. Janich H, Boll T: *Übersetzung des Self-Esteem Fragebogens von Rosenberg (1965).* Trier: Universität Trier, Fachbereich I – Psychologie; 1982. unpublished manuscript.
35. Rosenberg M: *Society and the Adolescent Self-Image.* Princeton, N.J.: Princeton University Press; 1965.
36. Baron RM, Kenny DA: **The moderator-mediator variable distinction in social psychological research: conceptual, strategic, and statistical considerations.** *J Pers Soc Psychol* 1986, **51**:1173–1182.
37. Sobel ME: **Asymptotic confidence intervals for indirect effects in structural equation models.** In *Sociological Methodology.* Edited by Leinhardt S. Washington, DC: American Sociological Association; 1982:290–312.
38. Preacher KJ, Hayes AF: **SPSS and SAS procedures for estimating indirect effects in simple mediation models.** *Behav Res Method Ins Comp* 2004, **36**:727–731.
39. Gadalla TM: **Eating disorders and associated psychiatric comorbidity in elderly Canadian women.** *Arch Womens Ment Health* 2008, **11**:357–362. doi: 10.1007/s00737-008-0031-8.
40. Mangweth-Matzek B, Rupp CI, Hausmann A, Assmayr K, Mariacher E, Kemmler G, Whitworth AB, Biebl W: **Never too old for eating disorders or body dissatisfaction: A community study of elderly women.** *Int J Eat Disord* 2006, **39**:583–586.
41. Copeland AL, Martin PD, Geiselman PJ, Rash CJ, Kendzor DE: **Predictors of pretreatment attrition from smoking cessation among pre- and postmenopausal, weight-concerned women.** *Eat Behav* 2006, **7**:243–251.
42. McKinley NM: **The developmental and cultural contexts of objectified body consciousness: a longitudinal analysis of two cohorts of women.** *Dev Psychol* 2006, **42**:679–687.

43. Mcquaide S: **Women at midlife.** *Soc Work* 1998, **43:**21–31.
44. McLean SA, Paxton SJ, Wertheim EH: **Factors associated with body dissatisfaction and disordered eating in women in midlife.** *Int J Eat Disord* 2010, **43:**527–536. doi: 10.1002/eat.20737.
45. Cash TF, Melnyk SE, Hrabosky JI: **The assessment of body image investment: an extensive revision of the appearance schemas inventory.** *Int J Eat Disord* 2004, **35:**305–316.
46. McKinley NM, Lyon LA: **Menopausal attitudes, objectified body consciousness, aging anxiety, and body esteem: European American women's body experiences in midlife.** *Body Image* 2008, **5:**375–380. doi: 10.1016/j.bodyim.2008.07.001.
47. Filozof C, Gonzalez C: **Predictors of weight gain: the biological Behavioral debate.** *Obes Rev* 2000, **1:**21–26.
48. de Lauzon-Guillain B, Basdevant A, Romon M, Karlsson J, Borys JM, Charles MA: **Is restrained eating a risk factor for weight gain in a general population?** *Am J Clin Nutr* 2006, **83:**132–138.
49. Boschi V, Iorio D, Margiotta N, D'Orsi P, Falconi C: **The three- factor eating questionnaire in the evaluation of eating behaviour in subjects seeking participation in a dietotherapy programme.** *Ann Nutr Metab* 2001, **45:**72–77.
50. Williamson DA, Lawson OJ, Brooks ER, Wozniak PJ, Ryan DH, Bray GA, Duchmann EG: **Association of body mass with dietary restraint and disinhibition.** *Appetite* 1995, **25:**31–41.
51. Bellisle F, Clement K, Le Barzic M, Le Gall A, Guy-Grand B, Basdevant A: **The eating inventory and body adiposity from leanness to massive obesity: a study of 2509 adults.** *Obes Res* 2004, **12:**2023–2030.
52. Johnson F, Pratt M, Wardle J: **Dietary restraint and self-regulation in eating behavior.** *Int J Obes* 2012, **36:**665–674. doi: 10.1038/ijo.2011.156.
53. Vasiljevic N, Ralevic S, Kolotkin RL, Marinkovic J, Jorga J: **The relationship between weight loss and health-related quality of life in a Serbian population.** *Eur Eat Disord Rev* 2012, **20:**162–168. doi: 10.1002/erv.1114.
54. Crocker J, Park LE: **Seeking self esteem: Construction, maintenance and protection of self-worth.** In *Handbook of Self and Identity.* Edited by Leary MR, Tangney JP. New York: The Guilford Press; 2003:291–313.
55. Reips UD: **Standards for Internet-based experimenting.** *Exp Psychol* 2002, **49:**243–256.
56. Mangweth-Matzek B, Hoek HW, Rupp CI, Kemmler G, Pope HG Jr, Kinzl J: **The menopausal transition-a possible window of vulnerability for eating pathology.** *Int J Eat Disord* 2013, **46:**609–616. doi: 10.1002/eat.22157.
57. Hunter M, Rendall M: **Bio-psycho-socio-cultural perspectives on menopause.** *Best Pract Res Clin Obstet Gynaecol* 2007, **21:**261–274.
58. Gagne DA, Von Holle A, Brownley KA, Runfola CD, Hofmeier S, Branch KE, Bulik CM: **Eating disorder symptoms and weight and shape concerns in a large web-based convenience sample of women ages 50 and above: results of the gender and body image (GABI) study.** *Int J Eat Disord* 2012, **45:**832–844. doi: 10.1002/eat.22030. Unipark [http://www.unipark.info/1-0-online-befragungssoftware-fuer-studenten-und-universitaeten-unipark-home.htm] SPSS Syntax [http://www.afhayes.com/spss-sas-and-mplus-macros-and-code.html]

6

Weight-control behaviour and weight-concerns in young elite athletes – a systematic review

Anne Werner[1*], Ansgar Thiel[2], Sven Schneider[3], Jochen Mayer[2], Katrin E Giel[1] and Stephan Zipfel[1]

Abstract

Weight-control behaviour is commonly observed in a wide range of elite sports, especially leanness sports, where control over body weight is crucial for high peak performance. Nonetheless, there is only a fine line between purely functional behaviour and clinically relevant eating disorders. Especially the rapid form of weight manipulation seems to foster later eating disorders. So far, most studies have focussed on adult athletes and concentrated on manifest eating disorders. In contrast, our review concentrates on young athletes and weight-control behaviour as a risk factor for eating disorders.

An electronic search according to PRISMA (Preferred Reporting Items for Systematic Reviews and Meta-Analyses) Statement was performed using Pubmed, PsychInfo and Spolit. The following search terms were used: *weight-control, weight-control behaviour, weight gain, weight loss, pathogenic weight-control behaviour* and *weight-concerns*, each of them combined with *elite athlete, young elite athlete, adolescent elite athlete* and *elite sports*.

Overall, data are inconsistent. In general, athletes do not seem to be at a higher risk for pathogenic weight concerns and weight-control behaviour. It does seem to be more prevalent in leanness sports, though. There is evidence for pathogenic weight-control behaviour in both genders; male athletes mostly trying to gain weight whereas females emphasise weight reduction. There is not enough data to make predictions about connections with age of onset.

Young elite athletes do show weight-control behaviour with varying degrees of frequency and severity. In particular, leanness sports seem to be a risk factor for weight manipulation. Further research is needed for more details and possible connections.

Keywords: Young elite athlete, Weight-control behaviour, Weight concern, Leanness sports

Review

Introduction

Weight-control behaviour is accepted in a wide range of elite sports [1,2]. Many sports require "low body weight and/or low fat/muscle ratio (leanness)" to achieve good results ([1] page 5, [3]). Quite often, this causes problems in terms of pathogenic weight-control behaviour or eating disorders. Research into adult elite athletes so far has suggested that pathogenic weight-control behaviour, disordered eating or clinically relevant eating disorders are common in elite sports [2,4-12]. However, there is much less evidence on these aspects in young elite sports.

* Correspondence: anne.werner@med.uni-tuebingen.de
[1]Department of Psychosomatic Medicine and Psychotherapy, University Hospital Tübingen, Osianderstr, 5, 72076, Tübingen, Germany
Full list of author information is available at the end of the article

For many athletes across various sport disciplines there is a direct causal connection between success and low body weight [13], with weight regulation playing a decisive role. Thus, Dosil classified so-called "high risk sports in connection with pathogenic weight-control behaviour" [2]. These are: 1. aesthetic sports, e.g. rhythmic and artistic gymnastics, ice-skating or dancing; 2. weight division sports, e.g. judo or rowing; 3. gym sports, e.g. aerobics; 4. endurance sports and 5. low-weight performance sports, e.g. distance running. In general athletes in these high-risk sports emphasize their slim appearance [2,3,13].

Weight-control behaviour can be pathogenic or non-pathogenic. Pathogenic weight-control behaviour is used to "manage emotions, weight and body size" [14] hence introduces a second dimension, namely feelings. This clearly distinguishes it from the non-pathogenic weight-control, which is purely functional and targeted in line with sport specific demands. Pathogenic refers to all unhealthy ways of controlling weight and can be carried out in two ways: gradual and rapid [10,15]. Gradual weight-control behaviour is a method of reducing or gaining weight in a more careful, continuous way, for example through restraint, selective eating or exercising over a longer period of time. Nonetheless, it can get out of control and might lead to sub-clinical eating disorders, with excessive exercising or long lasting dieting being risk factors for eating disorders [8,16,17]. On the other hand, rapid weight-control is characterized by a fast change of body weight through compensatory behaviour over a shorter time period (e.g. vomiting, obsessive sweating through sauna in plastic suits or using medication like laxatives). It might also – in connection with the pressure to be thin for a better athletic performance – increase the risk of developing an eating disorder [4,7,8,10,15,18-21]. In general, it is well recognized that dissatisfaction with either shape or weight of the body and a resulting dieting behaviour are risk factors for the development of eating disorders [22,23].

Elite athletes form a special population, as they participate in a highly competitive system, in which the main evaluation criterion is "victory or defeat" in sport competitions and sporting events [24]. Therefore, the main orientation is towards peak performances and outstanding bodily achievements. In order to attain this, elite athletes from almost all sport disciplines must focus on their body in some way [8]. This clearly distinguishes them from non-athletes and, consequently, has to be taken into account when evaluating the effect of amount of training, weight loss methods, eating patterns or psychological "profile" [8,20]. Sport specific weight-control behaviour can be purely functional and necessary for performance improvement, particularly in leanness-sports [25], making it a non-pathogenic form of weight-control. This means that the very same behaviour (e.g. restriction in eating) might be pathological in one context and non-pathological in another. However, the line between functional, non-pathogenic and sub-clinical pathogenic behaviour might be thin. Additionally, young athletes might be under double pressure, as they are not only under the normal strain from society, but the sport-specific demands on top [18].

Over the last decades, several studies and reviews have shown a higher prevalence of eating disorders among athletes compared to non-athletes. In contrast, this review will focus on pathogenic weight-control behaviour (e.g. restricted/disordered eating, abuse of medication) and weight-concerns (e.g. body dissatisfaction) rather than manifest eating disorders in elite athletes. We defined "elite athletes" as those actively competing at minimum in the national teams of their respective home country and/or being part of the national squad team. Additionally, we decided to focus on young elite athletes aged 12 to 25, as there is a substantial gap of knowledge on eating and weight-management behaviour in young and adolescent elite athletes. It has been reported that athletes start to manipulate their weight as early as aged 9 to 14 [26,27]. Empirical evidence suggests that the onset of eating and weight problems in the general population often happens during adolescence leaving young athletes potentially at double risk [28]. As young elite athletes often still attend college and educational systems vary in different countries, we decided to set the upper age limit to 25.

Therefore, the aim of this review is to have a closer look at weight-control behaviour in young elite athletes, providing a comprehensive overview of the data published to answer the following questions:

1. Are young elite athletes more at risk for pathogenic weight-control behaviour than non-athletes? Is there some kind of functionality for (pathogenic) weight-control behaviour in young elite sports?
2. Are young elite athletes competing in leanness-sports more at risk for pathogenic weight-control behaviour than athletes competing in non-leanness sports?
3. Are young elite female athletes more at risk for pathogenic weight-control behaviour than young male athletes?

Answers could be used to develop special guidelines for dealing with the occurring weight-control behaviour in young elite athletes, similar to those already shown for adults [12].

Methods

The systematic procedure of this literature review follows the PRISMA-Statement (Preferred Reporting Items for Systematic Reviews and Meta-Analyses) [29]. An electronic search was performed using Pubmed, PsychInfo and Spolit. Additionally, references from retrieved articles were examined for cross-references. The final database search was carried out on February 27, 2012. We applied no language or year restrictions. As one study eligible for our review only had a Norwegian full text, a bilingual research assistant translated the article.

Search strategy was performed by using search terms based on the Medical Subject Heading (MeSH) with 24 combinations performed in each database. The terms *weight-control, weight-control behaviour, weight gain, weight loss, pathogenic weight-control behaviour* and *weight-concerns* were each combined with *elite athlete, young elite athlete, adolescent elite athlete* and *elite sports.*

Inclusion criteria for the search procedure were that our search terms appeared either in title or abstract.

Additionally, studies had to focus on (a) "elite" athletes (defined as athletes competing at minimum in the national teams of their respective home country and/or being part of a national selection squad), (b) athletes still actively competing at time of assessment, (c) young or adolescent athletes (defined as younger than 25 years on average including the standard deviation of the sample) and (d) the terms "weight concerns" or "weight-control behaviour" as primary outcome variable. Reviews and meta-analyses were also included. We excluded dissertations and essays.

Two blinded reviewers assessed the abstracts and full texts independently for inclusion and exclusion criteria. The inter-rater-reliability was κ =0.80 and 0.82, respectively, reflecting a good to very good agreement. In cases of disagreement, a common conclusion based on consent could be found.

Results

After excluding duplicates, we found a total of 568 articles of which 15 were eligible for our review (see flow chart, Figure 1). Thirteen articles looked at "weight-control behaviour" or "pathogenic weight-control behaviour" as the primary outcome variable; only two articles looked at weight-control behaviour alone [4,19]. Another two studies focused on "weight-concerns" as the primary outcome variable [30,31], with one additionally looking at weight-control behaviour [31]. All studies eligible for inclusion were either in English or German. Table 1 gives an overview of all articles included in the review (see additional files). All results presented are significant unless stated otherwise.

Weight-control behaviour in young athletes and non-athletes

According to cross-sectional cohort studies using questionnaires (e.g. Rapid Weight Loss Questionnaire, Eating Disorder Inventory) or standardized clinical interviews, young elite athletes are not more at risk for developing or showing pathogenic weight concerns or weight-control behaviour than non-athletes [13,30,32-35].

Two studies found no difference between controls and athletes [30,35]. Arroyo et al. [30] examined 56 elite

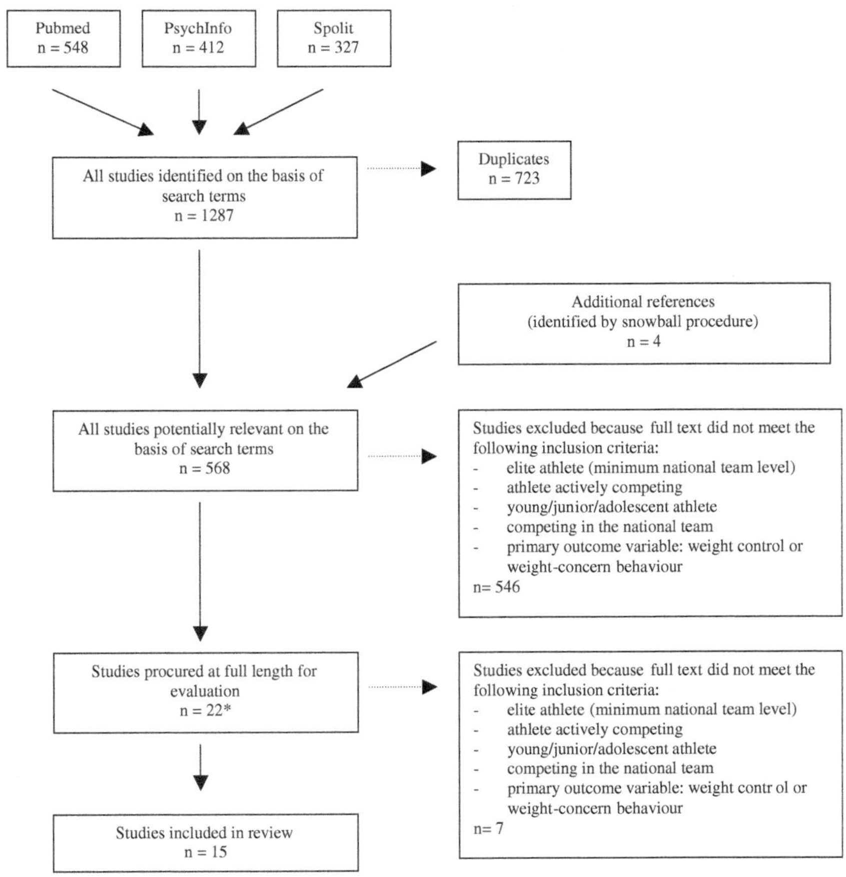

Figure 1 Flow-chart overview of literature search process.

Table 1 Overview of all studies included in the review

Author	Age in years (mean, SD)	Gender	Sample size total	Sample size athletes	Sample size controls	Sports type	Competition level	Controls	Outcome	Instruments	Results
Anderson et al., 2011 [18]	19.14 +/− 1.86	females only	414	414	0	gymnastics, swimming/ diving	NCAA Division-I	n/a	WC, WCB	Body Parts Satisfaction Scale, Dietary Intent Scale	No significant difference between athletes competing in leanness and non-leanness sports.
Arroyo et al., 2008 [30]	19.6 +/− 1.3	males only	56	28	28	soccer	Professional soccer team	age- and BMI-matched students; engagement in recreational sports <3hrs/week	WC	Somatomorphic matrix test	No significant difference between athletes and controls
Artioli et al., 2010 [4]	19.3 +/− 5.3 not specified according to gender	607 male, 215 female	822	822	0	judo	national and international	n/a	WCB	Rapid Weight Loss Questionnaire	Athletes were engaged in several forms of pathogenic weight control behaviour. No gender differences could be found. An earlier start of using weight-control methods leads to more aggressive variants.
Ferrand et al., 2005 [32]	athletes: 15.4 +/− 1.2 (swimmers) and 16.5 +/− 0.93 (rest) controls: 16.3 +/− 1.1	not specified; only the swimmers included males	132	82	50	synchron. swimming, non-leanness sports (basketball, handball, soccer, volleyball)	national	non-athlete college students; no further elaboration about their sports activities	WC, WCB	Canadian-French version of Body-Esteem Scale, French version of Eating Attitudes Test	Athletes showed more weight concerns but not more weight-control behaviour than controls. No significant difference between athletes competing in leanness and non-leanness sports.
Galli et al., 2009 [47]	23 +/− 0.68	males only	10	10	0	baseball, diving, football, golf, lacrosse, skiing, swimming	national and international	n/a	WC, WCB	Qualitative study using semi-structured interviews	Athletes did show some weight concerns.
Greenleaf et al., 2009 [19]	20.16 +/− 1.31	females only	204	204	0	basketball, cheerleading cross-country, field hockey, golf, gymnastics, rowing, skiing, soccer, softb., swimming, synchron. swimming, tennis, track&field, volleyball	NCAA Division-I	n/a	WCB	Adapted version of Questionnaire of Eating Disorder Diagnosis, Bulimia Test-Revised	No significant difference between athletes competing in leanness and non-leanness sports.

Table 1 Overview of all studies included in the review *(Continued)*

Johnson et al., 1999 [44]	19.9 20.1 (male), 19.6 (female); no SD given	883 male, 562 female	1445	1445	0	basketball, tennis, cross-country, football, gymnastics, nordic skiing, swimming, volleyball, wrestling	NCAA Division-I	n/a	WC, WCB	Self-created questionnaire including subscales from EDI-2, Rosenberg Self-Esteem Scale and Body Cathexis Scale	No significant difference between athletes competing in leanness and non-leanness sports. Female athletes have more pathogenic weight concerns and weight-control behaviour than male ones.
Marshall et al., 1996 [31]	20.8 +/– 3.8 (juniors 17.1 +/– 0.9 and seniors 22.5 +/– 3.2)	not specified	111	111	0	field hockey	national and international	n/a	WC, WCB	EDI	Athletes did show weight concerns. No difference in pathogenic weight concerns and weight-control behaviour in connection with age.
Martinsen et al., 2010 [13]	15-16 (range) no mean given not specified according to gender	athletes: 389 male, 217 female controls: 197 male, 158 female	961	606	355	50 different sports types, classified into leanness and non-leanness sports	students at elite sport schools, no further elaboration of competition level	age-matched 1st year high school students; no further elaboration about their sports activities	WC, WCB	EDI-2	Controls used pathogenic weight-control behaviour significantly more often than athletes. Different reasons for weight control. No significant difference between athletes competing in leanness and non-leanness sports. Female athletes have more pathogenic weight concerns and weight-control behaviour than male
Parks and Read, 1997 [42]	14-18 (range) no mean given	males only	74	74	0	cross-country running, football	national	n/a	WC, WCB	Body Esteem Scale, Body Size Drawings, Eating Attitudes Test, Reason for Exercising Inventory	Athletes competing in leanness sports showed more pathogenic weight concerns and weight-control behaviour than athletes competing in non-leanness sports.

Table 1 Overview of all studies included in the review *(Continued)*

Pietrowsky and Straub, 2008 [41]	rowers: 22.00 +/− 2.00 (heavyweight) and 22.06 +/− 2.89 (lightweight) handball: 28.25 +/− 3.91 non-athletes: 25.56 +/−4.47 (restraint eating group) and 28.00 +/− 4.29 (unrestraint eating group)	males only	164	132	32	rowing	national and international	non-athletes; engagement in recreational sports less than once a month; handball players from national team	WC, WCB	Silhouettes similar to the Body Image Assessment, Three-Factor Eating Questionnaire	Controls and athletes lightweight rowers had a more weight concerns if hungry, whereas heavyweight rowers and handball players showed more weight concerns in satiety. All athletes showed weight-control behaviour.
Reinking and Alexander, 2005 [33]	athletes: 19.7 +/− 1.1 controls: 20.2 +/− 1.2	females only	146	84	62	swimming, cross-country, basketball, volleyball, soccer, softball, field hockey	NCAA Division-I	undergraduate students; no further elaboration about their sports activities other than "not athletes in collegiate sports"	WC, WCB	EDI-2	Controls showed more weight concerns and weight-control behaviour than athletes. Athletes competing in leanness sports showed more pathogenic weight concerns and weight-control behaviour.
Rosendahl et al., 2009 [34]	14-18 (range) no mean given not specified according to gender	athletes: 366 male, 210 female controls: 122 male, 169 female	867	576	291	26 different sports: technical, endurance, aesthetic, weight class, ball game, power, antigrav. sports	national and international	students from non-Elite Sports Schools; no further elaboration about their sports activities	WC, WCB	Eating Attitude Test, Silhouettes	Controls more often showed a history of weight-control behaviour than athletes, only significant in females. Athletes competing in leanness sports scored higher for weight control than athletes competing in non-leanness sports. Gender differences in intention.
Rouveix et al., 2007 [35]	athletes: 16.5 +/− 0.5 (male) and 17.2 +/− 1.1 (female) controls: 21.8 +/− 1.8 (male) and 20.2 +/− 3.0 (female)	athletes: 12 male, 12 female controls: 17 male, 14 female	55	24	31	judo	national	random sample with participants not training more than 3hrs/week	WC, WCB	Self-administered questionnaire, French version of Eating Attitudes Test, Body Esteem Scale	No significant difference between athletes and controls concerning weight concerns. Significant difference in weight-control behaviour. There was a gender difference in used methods and ideal body.
Thiel et al., 1993 [45]	21.1 +/− 2.4	males only	84	84	0	rowing, wrestling	national	n/a	WC, WCB	Self-created questionnaire, EDI-2	Athletes did not show pathogenic weight-control behaviour.

WC = weight concerns, *WCB* = weight-control behaviour.

soccer players and 28 age- and BMI-matched non-elite athlete controls with regard to body perception and satisfaction. In both groups around one fifth desired a higher weight and a more muscular appearance. The only difference, though not significant, in perceived body image between athletes and controls was that the soccer players perceived their body sizes smaller than the control group. Rouveix at al [35] compared judo athletes with non-athletic controls. Overall, there were some differences between athletes and controls with regard to weight concerns. Female athletes were less satisfied with their actual weight and wanted to have a lower body weight than their respective controls. Additionally, female athletes had more and higher fluctuations in their weight. However, all differences in satisfaction and perception were not significant. Nonetheless, the authors could show a significant difference in weight-control behaviour. They found, that one-quarter of the examined judo athletes but none of the controls showed a higher risk for pathogenic weight-control measured with the Eating Attitudes Test [36].

Three other studies found a higher prevalence of weight concerns and/or weight-control behaviour in controls than in athletes [13,33,34]. Martinsen et al. [13] examined 606 elite athletes from 50 different sports types (categorized into leanness and non-leanness sports) and compared them with an age-matched control group of 355 high school students. They found pathogenic weight-control behaviour (defined as use of diuretics, laxatives, vomiting and diet pills) more frequently in controls than in athletes. Additionally, there was a different reason for weight-control in male subjects: whereas male controls wanted to improve their appearance, male athletes tried to improve their performance. Rosendahl et al. [34] looked at weight concerns in 567 athletes of elite sports schools compared to 291 non-athlete high school pupils using the Eating Attitude Test [37] and silhouettes for body perception [38]. When looking at disordered eating and dietary experience as prior weight-control behaviour, athletes scored significantly lower than non-athletes with only the difference between female participants being significant. Reinking and Alexander (30) examined 84 female NCAA Division I athletes (16 competing in leanness and 68 in non-leanness sports) and compared them to 62 non-athletes using the Eating Disorder Inventory 2 [39]. All females had a lower mean desired body weight with athletes scoring significantly lower on the Body Dissatisfaction subscale than non-athletes. When assessing the risk for disordered eating, again non-athletes scored significantly higher than athletes.

One study came partly to the conclusion that athletes are more at risk for weight concerns but not weight-control behaviour [32]: Ferrand et al. compared 42 synchronized swimmers and 40 other athletes competing in "non-weight dependant" sports types with a control group of 50 students using the Canadian-French version of Body-Esteem Scale [40] and the French version of the Eating Attitudes Test [36]. Synchronized swimming athletes had more weight concerns than the female control subjects but showed no difference on weight-control behaviour subscales.

Finally, a study by Pietrowsky et al. [41] with male light- and heavy-weight rowers from the German national team examined the body dissatisfaction in connection with leanness and muscularity under hunger and satiety conditions and compared them to handball players and non-athletes using male body silhouettes. Their findings are heterogeneous: As a result, the examined athletes struggle with weight problems, control of eating behaviour and body dissatisfaction, especially those competing in the lightweight group. This result varied between the groups as lightweight rowers and non-athletes had greater body dissatisfaction when hungry, whereas it was the other way round with heavyweight rowers and handball players.

When looking at the data found, several points have to be considered. All studies included used self-reported measures, which are prone to distortion. Two studies [30,34] complemented questionnaires with silhouettes to determine athletes' weight concerns in order to strengthen their statement. However, the study of Rosendahl et al. raises major concerns [34]. The authors did not clarify at which level their "elite" athletes compete, in particular there were 101 athletes described as currently not belonging to a specific team. Additionally, there was no definition of the sports activities in the comparison group, so that any comparative conclusions must be drawn with care. Most worryingly, the two groups (athletes versus non-athletes) were already significantly different in their basic demographic characteristics. A lack of clear definitions appeared in two more studies, with neither elaborating what the control groups' sports activities were [13,32].

In contrast, the study by Reinking et al. did not clearly distinguish between their athletes and controls [33]: 43.6% of the control group participated in sports activities 4 times per week and more, which makes the distinctive feature of the athlete group questionable. Furthermore, only athletes from one year at one university have been examined, and these were a "convenience sample", with athletes voluntarily joining after an information session, which may have prevented students with severe weight-control behaviours or disturbed body images from participating. It remains unclear, therefore, how generalizable the results are.

Although the non-athletes in Pietrowsky et al.'s study were well controlled with regard to their sport activity (less than once a month) their results must also be interpreted with care [41]. Only the light- and heavyweight rowers were within our category of "young athlete" whereas the other participants all belonged to older age groups. This makes comparisons beyond the different rower groups unreliable. A very specific problem resulted from the sample composition of Ferrand et al.'s study [32]: One of their subgroups, swimmers, consisted of female and male athletes whereas the two other groups were female samples only. Any result found could thus be due to gender characteristics rather than sports type specific or control group related.

A further weakness of many of the studies was sample size. For example, both Arroyo et al. and Martinsen et al. had a substantial difference in group sizes between athletes and controls, which might distort the results [13,30]. Two other studies [35,41] only examined very smalls groups so that it is hard to determine how valid results are even if relatively specific instruments were used [35].

Summarizing these data, larger studies in particular seem to suggest that young elite athletes are not more at risk for pathogenic weight concerns and weight-control behaviour than non-athletic controls. Participating in elite sports might even be a protective factor. However, due to the overall limited number of studies, with simultaneously dozens of different sport types to be examined there is not enough data in total. Additionally, several methodological problems across the different studies make a clear final conclusion impossible.

Weight-control behaviour in connection with type of sport

Three studies suggest that restrict weight-control is particularly prevalent in leanness-sports defined as sports emphasising leanness or low body weight (such as aesthetic or endurance sports) [33,34,42]. Reinking and Alexander [33] could show that within their NCAA Division I athletes, those competing in leanness sports scored significantly higher on the sub score for Body Dissatisfaction than those competing in non-leanness sports. Equally, athletes from leanness sports had a lower mean desired body weight than athletes from non-leanness sports. Parks et al. [42] compared 30 male cross-country runners with 44 male football players. They could show a significant difference between these two groups, with runners expressing more weight concerns and aiming for less weight than footballers who wanted to if anything gain weight. Rosendahl at al [34] could show in addition to the comparisons with controls mentioned above that athletes competing in leanness sports scored higher for weight-control behaviour than those competing in non-leanness sports.

In contrast, four other studies did not find any differences between leanness- and non-leanness sports weight-control behaviour [13,18,19,32]. Greenleaf et al. [19] were looking at 204 NCAA Division I athletes of various sports types from 3 different universities using the Questionnaire for Eating Disorder Diagnosis [43]. As a result, over half of the athletes (54.4%) were dissatisfied with their weight. The majority of them wanted to lose weight, on average around 5.9 kg. Additionally, there was a weight fluctuation of more than 10% within a year in $1/5^{th}$ (in season) to $1/3^{rd}$ (out of season) of the athletes. 25.5% admitted to exercise at least 2 hours a day specifically to reduce their weight, 15.7% were fasting or on a strict diet for the very same reason. However, only a small minority indicated purging behaviour: 2.9% reported vomiting 2–3 times/month, another 1.5% taking diuretic medication 2–3 times/month and 1% using laxatives 1–2 times/week. For all weight concerns and weight-control behaviours, no difference could be found between the various types of sports. Ferrand at al compared weight-concerns in 42 synchronized swimmers and 40 other "non-weight dependant sports types" (e.g. basketball, volleyball, soccer), finding no difference [32]. Martinsen et al. [13] in their study with 606 elite athletes from 50 different sports types showed similar frequencies of pathogenic weight-control methods such as vomiting, laxatives, diuretics and diet pills. 11.1% of the female and 2.1% of the male athletes used pathogenic weight-control methods. When looking at weight concerns and the feeling of being "too fat", 24% of the female athletes and 7.5% of the male ones were dieting now and/or have been on a diet at least three times before due to this reason. Johnson at al [44] could show some differences between different types of sports. However, this was only true in two instances and with no particular connection to the categories of leanness and non-leanness sports: In female athletes gymnasts scored higher on the Drive for Thinness Scale than swimmers and basketball players. Male football players showed greater body dissatisfaction than gymnasts and cross-country athletes.

In their study about psychosocial correlates of bulimic symptoms, Anderson et al. used structural equation modelling to test pathways and constructs in 280 NCAA Division I female gymnasts and 134 NCAA Division I female swimmers/divers from 26 universities [18]. They could show that the level of body dissatisfaction as well as restrictive eating was related to the amount of experienced pressure from teammates and coaches. There was no relation between the two components themselves. No difference with regard to type of sport could be shown.

Looking at weight-dependent sports only, two studies described methods of rapid weight-control amongst judo athletes [4,35]. A large survey by Artioli et al. [4] exploring prevalence and patterns of rapid weight loss among male and female judo competitors shows that most elite judo athletes (86%) have reduced weight rapidly before competition. Most of them regained this lost weight at least partially within one week after competition. The average magnitude of weight reduction was around 2-5% of their body-weight, with some athletes loosing up to 10% ten times or more in their careers. The fluctuation of weight was confirmed by a study from Rouveix et al. showing that rapid weight reduction is an inherent part of the lives of judo athletes [35]. In their study, they could show that during a season 70% of the athletes lost more than 2.8 kg, primarily by increasing exercises or limiting the intake of food and fluids. Nearly two thirds limited their choice of food on a constant basis.

Other studies examined only selected sports types [31,45] describing the prevalence of weight concerns and weight-control behaviour in a particular field. Thiel et al. [45] deliberately chose male athletes of lower weight categories to match them to female athletes from ballet and dancing previously identified as high-risk groups for subclinical eating disorders. The majority of athletes did not score pathologically for weight concerns and weigh-control behaviour. In particular, there was no difference between the male rowers and wrestlers. Only if they formed a subgroup of athletes with the diagnosis of a subclinical eating disorder based on the EDI-2 [39] Drive for Thinness subscale scores, did they find a difference on Body Dissatisfaction scale in comparison to the rest of the subjects. Marshall at al examined 120 female Canadian elite field hockey players [31]. In general, only a very low number of athletes (3.65%) scored pathological on the Drive for Thinness scale of the Eating Disorder Inventory, thus indicating a preoccupation with weight. However, they did find a fivefold higher frequency of athletes scoring at risk for the Body Dissatisfaction (BD) scale, which made the authors conclude a higher prevalence of weight concerns. Interestingly, athletes with high BD scores could be shown to be indeed heavier and with more body fat than their colleagues so there might be some truth in the athletes' perceptions.

Rouveix et al. included a comparably small sample size of only 24 athletes [35]. Reinking et al. on the other hand had a substantial difference in group sizes with only 16 athletes competing in leanness sports as opposed to 68 athletes competing in non-leanness sports [33]. Thiel et al. also showed a significant difference in the group sizes of athletes with only 25 wrestlers but 59 rowers, which further reduce the generalizability of results found [45]. This study raises additional concern because they found differences only after creating a subgroup scoring pathologically for subclinical eating disorders, which makes their conclusions questionable [45].

In contrast, two studies used large, balanced samples [4,44]. A specific problem of the study by Johnson et al. was that large parts of their results were based on a self-created, unvalidated questionnaire that had its main focus on eating disorders [44]. Anderson et al. tried to make their results more generalizable by using a variety of universities to get their sample from which clearly reduces local biases [18]. Again, a lack of clear definitions made interpretation difficult: Two studies did not state clearly at which level their athletes competed [32,34]. In the study of Ferrand et al. [32] only the swimmers were classified as "elite" whereas the other athletes only were referred to as "national" ones without any further specification of the competing level. Additionally, the sample of swimmers consisted of female and male athletes whereas the two other groups were female samples only. Two studies did not state clearly how the sample of athletes was collected so it is hard to judge the quality of each study [35,42,45].

Summed up, the evidence seems to point towards no higher prevalence of pathogenic weight concerns or weight-control behaviour in athletes competing in leanness sports. However, this behaviour does seem to be particularly present in weight-class sports where success is often dependent on the class an athlete is competing in.

Weight-control in connection with gender and age

Although it is suggested that female athletes are more susceptible to developing eating disorders or at higher risk for pathogenic weight-control behaviour than male athletes, one study by Artioli et al. did not find any gender differences [4]. They examined active judo competitors with the Rapid Weight Loss Questionnaire [46]. Their results showed that athletes lose up to 5% of their weight, mostly in connection with an upcoming competition. Increased exercises and restricted fluid intake were the favourite methods to lose weight. They did not find any differences between gender – neither in prevalence nor manifestation of pathogenic weight-control.

Looking at male athletes only, Galli and Reel [47] explored the body image and body enhancing behaviour of male athletes from various sports types in qualitative interviews. The findings show that male athletes want to reduce fat and gain muscle mass, desiring a more muscular, stronger body. An extreme version is the so-called "muscle dysmorphia". Patients who suffer from it perceive their body as too slim or not muscular enough, even if there is no objective evidence [48]. It is a form of body dysmorphic disorder and it is referred to as "reverse anorexia" [49]. As a result of their perception, patients withdraw from social activities out of shame or stick to extensive workouts or usage of anabolic drugs [50]. In Galli's study there was an interesting finding: Although 80% expressed some dissatisfaction regarding their physique and admitted to regularly use body-enhancing strategies (e.g. dieting, efforts to gain weight), 70% had some positive feelings about their bodies at the same time. This was mostly expressed as a confidence in their bodies' abilities [47]. Clear strength of the study by

Galli et al. is clearly the insight gained through qualitative data. However, this also leaves the potential risk of interviewer's bias.

The majority of studies included in this review did find a higher frequency of pathogenic weight concerns and weight-control behaviour in female athletes than in male ones. Martinsen at al [13] could show in their study that female athletes have more concerns about their weight and a higher urge to improve their appearance than male athletes. Additionally, they used more pathogenic weight-control methods than their male counterparts. Johnson et al. [44] examined NCAA Division I athletes from 11 universities all over the States showing a higher frequency of some pathogenic weight-control behaviour in female athletes than in male ones independent of the type of sport. This was true for vomiting and use of laxatives as well as diet pills over a lifetime. However, no statistically significant difference could be shown for use of diuretics or steroids. Male athletes, on the other hand, were using the sauna or steam bath more often than females to lose weight, although this didn't become significant. In general, female athletes wanted to reduce their body fat down to a percentage where they would stop menstruating risking osteoporosis within one year. Rouveix [35] at al examined 24 judo athletes and came to mixed conclusions. Nearly two thirds of the athletes lost more than 2.8 kg over the course of a season with no gender differences. Most common methods were intensification of exercising and reduction of fluid intake. There was a gender difference in methods to reduce weight, though: female athletes fasted significantly more. Interestingly, athletes reported their parents and society as equally important sources for the pressure to lose weight as their own drive to do so. Additionally, there was a clear gender difference for the ideal body with female athletes desiring a much lower body weight than male athletes. A definite strength of this study is its clear definition of the athlete level and a good control of the comparison group, who did not engage in sports activities more than three times a week.

Another interesting finding with regard to gender differences was found in the study of Rosendahl at al [34]: 50% of the examined female but just 10.1% of the male athletes wanted to reduce their weight and 19.6% of the male but just 3.4% of the female athletes wanted to gain weight. This confirms different mindsets and intentions behind weight-control behaviour in female and male athletes.

Only two studies also draw conclusions about the role of age in pathological weight concerns and weight-control behaviour. One study by Artioli et al. suggests that the earlier in life athletes started reducing weight before competition, the more aggressive they were with respect to their methods [4]. Another study from Marshall et al. [31] showed no significant difference in pathological weight concerns and weight-control behaviour between junior and senior field hockey players. However, both studies have their limitations: Whereas Artioli only asked athletes retrospectively where memories could be distorted; Marshall compared two different age groups in a cross-sectional study. Both did not examine athletes longitudinally to follow up the same cohort and their development.

In summary, a number of studies provide evidence for pathogenic weight-control behaviour in both genders. The form of pathogenic weight-control behaviour is different in male and female athletes. Whereas female athletes mostly want to reduce weight and focus on a slim appearance, male athletes mostly want to gain weight through muscle mass.

Concerning weight-control behaviour in connection with age, no uniform conclusion can be drawn, as only two studies looked at it at all. Results are heterogeneous, with one giving evidence that the age of an athlete starting with pathogenic weight-control behaviour might play a decisive role for the prognosis [4] whereas the other does not seem to see any connection with age [31].

Discussion

To our best knowledge, this is the first systematic review on weight-concerns and weight-control behaviour in young elite athletes. It appears that young elite athletes are engaged in pathogenic weight-control behaviour despite long-term health being very important for the development of their sports career and achievement of peak performance.

Comparing athletes with non-athletes or controls, the majority of studies, several of which were large scale, found either no difference or an even lower risk of athletes for pathogenic weight concerns or weight-control behaviour [13,30,33-35,45]. Only one study could show a higher prevalence of pathogenic weight concerns but not weight-control behaviour in athletes [32].

Because of different demands associated with different sports types, we further analysed the studies found according to clusters. We decided to use the classification into leanness and non-leanness sports for the sub-analysis of different sports types, as this is a very common distinction first introduced by Sundgot-Borgen [51] in connection with eating disorders in elite athletes. Several of the studies included in our review used this particular classification. However, we are aware that there might be additional ways of clustering different types of sports that were not considered in this review. Focusing on leanness-sports, three studies give evidence of a higher prevalence of weight-control problems in leanness-sports [33,34,42]. However, four other studies did not find any differences in the prevalence between these two categories [13,18,19,32], and there was no study in which a higher prevalence of pathogenic weight-control behaviour in non-leanness sports could be shown. Whether leanness-sports are a risk factor for pathogenic weight-control or whether the higher prevalence is merely due to a selection bias has to be further investigated.

It was suggested that gender plays an important role for the prevalence of pathogenic weight-control behaviour. In total, only two studies made a clear statement about gender with contradictory results: whereas one study showed no difference between female and male athletes [4], the other one clearly supported the theory that female athletes are more engaged in pathogenic weight concerns and weight-control behaviour [13]. Two other studies showed mixed results within their different outcome variables [35,44]. Additional studies focus on female or male athletes alone, making gender comparison hard. However, they help to get a deeper understanding of gender specific ways to worry about body shape or weight-control.

Our review had to encounter several problems. In general, difficulties seem to arise when looking at the topic of pathogenic weight concerns and weight-control behaviour. Specifically, there does not seem to be a clear common definition of what weight concerns and weight-control behaviour are. As a result, a variety of different measuring instruments are used. This heterogeneity makes consistent conclusions difficult. In our review, we included all studies that used these two terms. However, further research should clarify what these terms comprise exactly to get a better idea of what appropriate measures might be. Another problem arises with choosing appropriate screening instruments. This is due to the fact that in some sports types the very same behaviours can be pathogenic or non-pathogenic depending on circumstances. Normally, screening instruments used are not specifically designed for or even adapted to athletes and their specific demands which might incorrectly classify non-pathogenic, functional behaviour as part of a pathogenic one [25]. Furthermore, the next difficult distinction is the thin line between pathogenic weight-control behaviour and eating disorders in elite sports. This is especially supported by the fact that in leanness-sports a very thin look is considered normal, and more radical forms of weight-control are often accepted by coaches and athletes [2,6,8,52]. Sundgot-Borgen even described a sport-specific variant of anorexia nervosa referred to as "anorexia athletica". According to her, female athletes suffering from it show an intensive fear of gaining weight or even becoming obese, although the athlete is not overweight at all. To achieve their individually set ideal weight, these athletes use a variety of pathogenic weight-control techniques [8]. On the other hand, it is impossible to deny that for some sport disciplines a change of body weight is a necessary part of training and competition. Here, it is most crucial to support athletes in losing or gaining weight in a healthy way. Several organizations and associations have acknowledged this fact and now provide specific guidelines for healthy weight management in elite athletes [9,53]. However, particularly in elite sports, trainers' experience and anecdotal knowledge plays an important role when it comes to the management of athletes' concerns. Therefore it seems crucial to combine the two sources by providing trainers with additional information about the topic of weight concerns and weight-control behaviour in young elite athletes.

Another challenge for this review was the broad heterogeneity of studies. Their sample sizes ranged from 10 to 1445 participants. Some examined groups only consisted of athletes from a special type of sport, and some had no control-groups to give evidence of the differences between athletes and non-athletes Furthermore, results are mostly based on self-rating questionnaires and no expert interviews. This may have affected the validity, because many athletes might not answer truthfully or withhold their pathogenic concerns or weight-control behaviour. When some studies cooperated with the respective sports association or college, it cannot be excluded that athletes held back some information, as they might have been scared to lose privileges within their system. In any case, this would have only lead to an underestimation of the results found. Additionally, the methods differ strongly between cross-sectional studies with big cohorts and qualitative interview studies with small samples. Whereas, for example, Johnson et al. examined nearly 1500 athletes from 11 different universities [44], Galli and Reel examined 10 male athletes over ten in-depth semi-structured interviews regarding body image in male athletes [47]. Both methods are respectable forms of research but make a comparison difficult if not impossible. Finally, we can't exclude publication bias.

Conclusions

Taken together, the examined papers show that there is some prevalence of pathogenic weight concerns and weight-control behaviour in elite athletes. However, there is no certainty that the prevalence is higher than in control groups. Only in leanness-sports, where athletes are encouraged to be thin for either appearance or performance, the prevalence of pathogenic weight-control behaviour is higher in frequency than in non-athletes. The pressure of competitive sports seems therefore to be a risk factor for both genders.

Thus, special attention should be paid to athletes in leanness sports who have experiences with dieting and who show body- or weight-dissatisfaction.

Further research is necessary to get a better understanding of the connection between elite sports and pathogenic weight-control behaviour. This is why our research group examined pathogenic weight-control behaviour, body- and weight-dissatisfaction and subjective eating concepts in young elite athletes in the "GOAL-study" ("The German Young Olympic Athletes' Lifestyle and Health Management Study") [54] It consisted of a quantitative and a qualitative part and collected data from young squad athletes from all Olympic Disciplines allowing us to perform sub-analysis according to each single discipline. First results show that this combined approach provides comprehensive data [55-58]. In addition, long-term studies are needed to see what happens if young athletes stop competing as adults.

Competing interests
The authors declare to have no competing interests.

Authors' contributions
AW and SZ carried out the literature search and drafted the manuscript. AT, JM and KEG have made substantial contributions to conception and design, and interpretation of data. All three have revised the article critically for important intellectual content. SS has made substantial contributions to interpretation of data. He has revised the article critically for important intellectual content. All authors have given final approval of the manuscript version to be published.

Acknowledgments
We would like to thank Franziska Kocher (Postgraduate Student) for her initial input and her support in retrieving the articles as well as Clare Blythe (Research Assistant) for proofreading the manuscript.

Author details
[1]Department of Psychosomatic Medicine and Psychotherapy, University Hospital Tübingen, Osianderstr, 5, 72076, Tübingen, Germany. [2]Institute of Sports Science, Tübingen University, Tübingen, Germany. [3]Mannheim Institute of Public Health, Social and Preventive Medicine, Medical Faculty Mannheim, Heidelberg University, Mannheim, Germany.

References

1. Hagmar M, Hirschberg AL, Berglund L, Berglund B: **Special attention to the weight-control strategies employed by Olympic athletes striving for leanness is required.** *Clin J Sport Med* 2008, **18:**5–9.
2. Dosil J, González-Oya J: **Eating disorders and the Athlete's environment.** In *Eating disorders in athletes.* Chichester, West Sussex, England: John Wiley & Sons, Ltd; 2008:41–63.
3. Platen P: **Essstörungen und Leistungssport.** In *Handbuch essstörungen und adipositas.* Edited by Herpertz S, de Zwaan M, Zipfel S. Heidelberg: Springer Medizin Verlag; 2008:334–340.
4. Artioli GG, Gualano B, Franchini E, Scagliusi FB, Takesian M, Fuchs M, Lancha AH Jr: **Prevalence, magnitude, and methods of rapid weight loss among judo competitors.** *Med Sci Sports Exerc* 2010, **42:**436–442.
5. Brownell KD, Steen SN, Wilmore JH: **Weight regulation practices in athletes: analysis of metabolic and health effects.** *Med Sci Sports Exerc* 1987, **19:**546–556.
6. Sundgot-Borgen J: **Risk and trigger factors for the development of eating disorders in female elite athletes.** *Med Sci Sports Exerc* 1994, **26:**414–419.
7. Sundgot-Borgen J, Garthe I: **Elite athletes in aesthetic and Olympic weight-class sports and the challenge of body weight and body compositions.** *J Sports Sci* 2011, **29**(Suppl 1):101–114.
8. Sundgot-Borgen J, Torstveit MK: **Prevalence of eating disorders in elite athletes is higher than in the general population.** *Clin J Sport Med* 2004, **14:**25–32.
9. American Academy of Pediatrics: **Promotion of healthy weight-control practices in young athletes.** *Pediatrics* 2005, **116:**1557–1564.
10. Sundgot-Borgen J, Larsen S: **Pathogenic weight-control methods and self-reported eating disorders in female elite athletes and controls.** *Scand J Med Sci Sports* 1993, **3:**150–155.
11. Rosen LWMD, Hough DO, Curley V: **Pathogenic weight-control behavior in female athletes.** *Physician Sportsmed* 1986, **14:**79–86.
12. Rosen LWHD: **Pathogenic weight-control behaviors of female college gymnasts.** *Physician Sportsmed* 1988, **16:**141–144.
13. Martinsen M, Bratland-Sanda S, Eriksson AK, Sundgot-Borgen J: **Dieting to win or to be thin? A study of dieting and disordered eating among adolescent elite athletes and non-athlete controls.** *Br J Sports Med* 2010, **44:**70–76.
14. American Psychiatric Association: *Diagnostic and statistical manual of mental disorders.* 4th edition. Washington (DC): American Psychiatric Press; 1994.
15. Fogelholm M, Hiilloskorpi H: **Weight and diet concerns in finnish female and male athletes.** *Med Sci Sports Exerc* 1999, **31:**229–235.
16. Patton GC, Selzer R, Coffey C, Carlin JB, Wolfe R: **Onset of adolescent eating disorders: population based cohort study over 3 years.** *BMJ* 1999, **318:**765–768.
17. Stice E, Davis K, Miller NP, Marti CN: **Fasting increases risk for onset of binge eating and bulimic pathology: a 5-year prospective study.** *J Abnorm Psychol* 2008, **117:**941–946.
18. Anderson CM, Petrie TA, Neumann CS: **Psychosocial correlates of bulimic symptoms among NCAA division-I female collegiate gymnasts and swimmers/divers.** *J Sport Exerc Psychol* 2011, **33:**483–505.
19. Greenleaf C, Petrie TA, Carter J, Reel JJ: **Female collegiate athletes: prevalence of eating disorders and disordered eating behaviors.** *J Am Coll Health* 2009, **57:**489–495.
20. Sundgot-Borgen J, Torstveit MK, Skarderud F: **[Eating disorders among athletes].** *Tidsskr Nor Laegeforen* 2004, **124:**2126–2129.
21. Torstveit MK, Sundgot-Borgen J: **The female athlete triad: are elite athletes at increased risk?** *Med Sci Sports Exerc* 2005, **37:**184–193.
22. Jacobi C, Abascal L, Taylor CB: **Screening for eating disorders and high-risk behavior: caution.** *Int J Eat Disord* 2004, **36:**280–295.
23. Stice E, Shaw HE: **Role of body dissatisfaction in the onset and maintenance of eating pathology: a synthesis of research findings.** *J Psychosom Res* 2002, **53:**985–993.
24. Thiel A, Mayer J, Digel H: *Gesundheit und Spitzensport. Eine sozialwissenschaftliche Analyse.* Schorndorf, Germany: Hofmann; 2010.
25. Torstveit MK, Rosenvinge JH, Sundgot-Borgen J: **Prevalence of eating disorders and the predictive power of risk models in female elite athletes: a controlled study.** *Scand J Med Sci Sports* 2008, **18:**108–118.
26. Alderman BL, Landers DM, Carlson J, Scott JR: **Factors related to rapid weight loss practices among international-style wrestlers.** *Med Sci Sports Exerc* 2004, **36:**249–252.
27. Steen SN, Brownell KD: **Patterns of weight loss and regain in wrestlers: has the tradition changed?** *Med Sci Sports Exerc* 1990, **22:**762–768.
28. Herpertz-Dahlmann B, Wille N, Holling H, Vloet TD, Ravens-Sieberer U: **Disordered eating behaviour and attitudes, associated psychopathology and health-related quality of life: results of the BELLA study.** *Eur Child Adolesc Psychiatry* 2008, **17**(Suppl 1):82–91.
29. Moher D, Liberati A, Tetzlaff J, Altman DG: **Preferred reporting items for systematic reviews and meta-analyses: the PRISMA statement.** *PLoS Med* 2009, **6:**e1000097.
30. Arroyo M, Gonzalez-de-Suso JM, Sanchez C, Ansotegui L, Rocandio AM: **Body image and body composition: comparisons of young male elite soccer players and controls.** *Int J Sport Nutr Exerc Metab* 2008, **18:**628–638.
31. Marshall JD, Harber VJ: **Body dissatisfaction and drive for thinness in high performance field hockey athletes.** *Int J Sports Med* 1996, **17:**541–544.
32. Ferrand C, Magnan C, Philippe RA: **Body-esteem, body mass index, and risk for disordered eating among adolescents in synchronized swimming.** *Percept Mot Skills* 2005, **101:**877–884.
33. Reinking MF, Alexander LE: **Prevalence of disordered-eating behaviors in undergraduate female collegiate athletes and nonathletes.** *J Athl Train* 2005, **40:**47–51.
34. Rosendahl J, Bormann B, Aschenbrenner K, Aschenbrenner F, Strauss B: **Dieting and disordered eating in German high school athletes and non-athletes.** *Scand J Med Sci Sports* 2009, **19:**731–739.
35. Rouveix M, Bouget M, Pannafieux C, Champely S, Filaire E: **Eating attitudes, body esteem, perfectionism and anxiety of judo athletes and nonathletes.** *Int J Sports Med* 2007, **28:**340–345.

36. Leichner P, Steiger H, Puentes-Neuman G, Perreault M, Gottheil N: **[Validation of an eating attitude scale in a French-speaking Quebec population].** *Can J Psychiatry* 1994, **39**:49–54.
37. Garner DM, Olmsted MP, Bohr Y, Garfinkel PE: **The eating attitudes test: psychometric features and clinical correlates.** *Psychol Med* 1982, **12**:871–878.
38. Gutezeit G, Marake J, Wagner J: **[Effect of ideal body image on self assessment of the true body image in childhood and adolescence].** *Prax Kinderpsychol Kinderpsychiatr* 1986, **35**:207–214.
39. Gardner D: *Eating disorder inventory 2: professional manual.* Odessa: Psychol Assess Res; 1983.
40. Beaudoin CS-MD, Bottamini G: **Traduction et validation canadienne-francaise d'une echelle portant sur l'estime de son corps.** *Avante* 2011, **9**:15–20.
41. Pietrowsky R, Straub K: **Body dissatisfaction and restrained eating in male juvenile and adult athletes.** *Eat Weight Disord* 2008, **13**:14–21.
42. Parks PS, Read MH: **Adolescent male athletes: body image, diet, and exercise.** *Adolescence* 1997, **32**:593–602.
43. Mintz LB, OHalloran MS, Mulholland AM, Schneider PA: **Questionnaire for eating disorder diagnoses: reliability and validity of operationalizing DSM-IV criteria into a self-report format.** *J Couns Psychol* 1997, **44**:132–132.
44. Johnson C, Powers PS, Dick R: **Athletes and eating disorders: the National Collegiate Athletic Association study.** *Int J Eat Disord* 1999, **26**:179–188.
45. Thiel A, Gottfried H, Hesse FW: **Subclinical eating disorders in male athletes. A study of the low weight category in rowers and wrestlers.** *Acta Psychiatr Scand* 1993, **88**:259–265.
46. Artioli GG, Scagliusi F, Kashiwagura D, Franchini E, Gualano B, Junior AL: **Development, validity and reliability of a questionnaire designed to evaluate rapid weight loss patterns in judo players.** *Scand J Med Sci Sports* 2010, **20**:e177–e187.
47. Galli N, Reel JJ: **Adonis or Hephaestus? Exploring body image in male athletes.** *Psychology of Men & Masculinity* 2009, **10**:95–108.
48. Pope HG Jr, Gruber AJ, Choi P, Olivardia R, Phillips KA: **Muscle dysmorphia. An underrecognized form of body dysmorphic disorder.** *Psychosomatics* 1997, **38**:548–557.
49. Pope HG Jr, Katz DL, Hudson JI: **Anorexia nervosa and "reverse anorexia" among 108 male bodybuilders.** *Compr Psychiatry* 1993, **34**:406–409.
50. Pope CG, Pope HG, Menard W, Fay C, Olivardia R, Philips KA: **Clinical features of muscle dysmorphia among males with body dysmorphic disorder.** *Body Image* 2005, **2**:395–400.
51. Sundgot-Borgen J: **Prevalence of eating disorders in elite female athletes.** *Int J Sport Nutr* 1993, **3**:29–40.
52. Smolak L, Murnen SK, Ruble AE: **Female athletes and eating problems: a meta-analysis.** *Int J Eat Disord* 2000, **27**:371–380.
53. Turocy PS, DePalma BF, Horswill CA, Laquale KM, Martin TJ, Perry AC, Somova MJ, Utter AC: **National Athletic Trainers' Association position statement: safe weight loss and maintenance practices in sport and exercise.** *J Athl Train* 2011, **46**:322–336.
54. Thiel A, Diehl K, Giel KE, Schnell A, Schubring AM, Mayer J, Zipfel S, Schneider S: **The German Young Olympic Athletes' lifestyle and health management study (GOAL study): design of a mixed-method study.** *BMC Public Health* 2011, **11**:410.
55. Schneider S, Weiss M, Thiel A, Werner A, Mayer J, Hoffmann H, Diehl K: **Body dissatisfaction in female adolescents: extent and correlates.** *Eur J Pediatr* 2013, **172**(3):373–384.
56. Diehl K, Thiel A, Zipfel S, Mayer J, Schnell A, Schneider S: **Elite adolescent athletes and Use of dietary supplements: characteristics, opinions, and sources of supply and information.** *Int J Sport Nutr Exerc Metab* 2012, **22**(3):165–174.
57. Schneider S, Diehl K, Bruhmann B: **[Do boys suffer injury more often than girls in sport?].** *Gesundheitswesen* 2012, **74**:234–235.
58. Diehl K, Thiel A, Zipfel S, Mayer J, Schneider S: **Substance use among elite adolescent athletes: Findings from the GOAL Study.** *Scand J Med Sci Sports* 2012. doi:10.1111/j.1600-0838.2012.01472.x. Epub ahead of print.

The efficacy of Bioelectrical Impedance Analysis (BIA) in monitoring body composition changes during treatment of restrictive eating disorder patients

Charles F Saladino

Abstract

Reviews: Treating restrictive eating disorder patients is metabolically and psychologically complex. Determining body composition is an important diagnostic and treatment option for these patients, because it ascertains whether the acquisition of body mass during refeeding is metabolically appropriate - ideally an approximate 20/80% - 25/75% fat/lean body mass ratio. The purpose of this paper is to evaluate the efficacy of Bioelectrical Impedance Analysis (BIA) during the treatment period of patients with restrictive eating disorders. The search engines PubMed, Medline, and MSN were utilized using combinations of key words, "Bioimpedance Analysis", "body composition determination", "eating disorders", and "anorexia".

Conclusions: The literature indicates that the use of Bioelectrical Impedance Analysis (BIA) in eating disorder patients to be efficacious in determining body composition during the treatment period, and that only assessing weight changes does not necessarily reflect specific changes in various body compartments. Also, utilizing BIA has the advantage of using each patient as his/her own "control", potentially allowing for a more individualized nutrition regimen according to the body composition changes observed during treatment.

Keywords: Bioelectrical Impedance Analysis (BIA), Anorexia, Bulimia, Body composition

Reviews

In the United States, where over 2 trillion dollars yearly is spent on health care, approximately 24 million people of all ages suffer from some form of eating disorder, which collectively forms the highest mortality rate of any mental illness; and the mortality rate associated with anorexia nervosa is 12 times higher than the death rate associated with all causes of death for females 15–24 years old. In addition, almost 50% of people with eating disorders meet the criteria for depression, and only 35% of those receiving any treatment are treated at a facility that specializes in such afflictions [1]. Clearly, treatments for eating disorder patients must include as a goal appropriate restoration of the patients' overall mental and physical health, including the acquisition of proper body composition.

This paper evaluates the efficacy of utilizing BIA as a potential technique to evaluate body composition during the weight gain process in restrictive-eating disorder patients undergoing treatment. In view of the fact that improper dietary intake can have profound metabolic effects [2-4], using BIA during patient treatment can alert the clinician as to whether or not their treatment diet is appropriate.

The literature on determining body composition is extensive, and various other methods (such as anthropometric measurements and dual x-ray absorptiometry - DXA) are available for this purpose. The following discussion will include comparisons as to the efficacy of BIA vs. some of the other methodologies; but this review focuses on BIA to determine body composition in patients being treated for restrictive eating disorders, such as anorexia nervosa and bulimia nervosa.

Correspondence: csaladin@misericordia.edu
Department of Chemistry and Biochemistry, Misericordia University, Dallas, PA 18612, USA

For this literature review, three search engines were utilized: PubMed, Medline, and MSN. An assessment of a cross-section of the literature was conducted using combinations of key words that included "Bioimpedance Analysis," "body composition determination", "eating disorders", and "anorexia". Among the three search engines, in which there was paper overlap, approximately fifty articles were evaluated for relevance to the subject, with 34 chosen to review the use of BIA for measuring body composition - whether or not it applied to patients with restrictive eating disorders.

BIA is an inexpensive and relatively simple method for measuring body composition, first being applied by Hoffer et al. [5] in 1969 to measure total body water and then by Luskaski et al. [6] to determine nutritional status. The instrument uses electrodes to send a harmless very-low level of electric current through the body. Whereas fatty tissue is low in water content and does not conduct electricity well, lean body mass (muscle tissue) is more than 70% water and does conduct an electric current relatively efficiently. BIA measures body fat (FM) (which optimally ranges up to about 25% in women and 20% in men), as well as lean body mass (body cell mass –BCM - plus extracellular mass - ECM) [7,8]. Lean body mass is also referred to as fat free mass (FFM). In addition, the instrument also measures body mass index (BMI) and intracellular and extracellular water.

It is widely accepted that changes in weight and body composition occur with age, health status, and physiological function. In general, aging is associated with a loss of lean body mass and strength; and the elderly can sometimes experience replacement of some muscle mass with fat, but with a stable body weight [9,10], even though weight gain in the young adult into the mid-life years shows an increase in both fat and muscle mass. In addition, intra-abdominal visceral fat and waist circumference often increase with age at a faster rate than total body weight [11-13]; and BMI does not take fat distribution into account [14,15].

Age-related changes in body composition have important correlations to health status later in life. BIA data could theoretically serve as a guideline for good health; and the technique can be used to assess actual body composition and thus overall metabolic well-being. Body composition can correlate to a continuum of health - from longevity and a high level of function on the one hand to morbidity and mortality on the other. Thus, just as early detection of body composition changes resulting from certain diseases allows for early intervention treatments, the restrictive-eating disorder patient could benefit from the clinician having knowledge as to body composition alterations prior to and during therapy.

Mika et al. [16] utilized BIA technology, to evaluated 21 female adolescents with anorexia nervosa (AN) with an initial BMI of 15.5 (15.5 ± 1.1 kg/m^2) and 19 normal-weight, age-matched female controls, each four times between week 3–15 of refeeding with a hyperenergetic diet. They concluded that changes they observed in extracellular mass (ECM)/body cell mass (BCM) index were due to an increase in BCM, and that multi-frequency phase-sensitive BIA would be a promising tool for assessment of nutritional status and body composition in AN patients.

Mattar et al. [17] compared BIA and Dual x-ray absorptiometry (DXA) to measure FFM and FM in 50 female, underweight patients with anorexia nervosa. For the BIA modality, five equations (Sun, Kushner, Sun, Deurenberg, and Roubenoff - validated in healthy populations) were used for the calculations. Comparisons between BIA and DXA used the sum of the squares of differences and Bland-Altman plots. It was concluded that the best estimates of FFM and FM in the anorexic study group was when the Deurenberg equation was used with BIA, because it took into account height, weight, and age, and it was applicable in adults and adolescents ages 13.4 up to 36.9 and for BMI values of 12.8 - 21.

In order to consider being able to obtain body composition at the bedside, Ghosh et al. [18] evaluated an inexpensive hand-held BIA instrument to measure lean body mass, as compared against DXA in potentially malnourished patients. In this study, body composition analysis was obtained from 17 patients with eating disorders, 7 with chronic alcoholic pancreatitis, and 18 with inflammatory bowel disease The results indicated that in thin and non-obese adults, an accurate two compartment (lean body mass and fat mass) measurement could be made in ten minutes using this hand-held BIA instrument.

In a study utilizing BIA, anthropometry, and DXA to assess body composition, plus a basal endocrine profile was obtained, Bruni et al. [19] sought to identify diagnostic criteria that could distinguish 59 patients with functional hypothalamic amenorrhea mostly related to minimal energy deficiency vs. 59 where a failure in adaptive response to stress was prevalent Subjects with eating disorders had a lower BMI and fat mass (measured with both techniques). Leptin levels were positively associated with fat mass and also with body cell mass indexed to height and BIA phase angle parameters. (This parameter is an indicator of the active lean body compartment and cellular health, and will be further explained below). This study demonstrated the value of BIA, which was corroborated with DXA. Further, in a separate report using the same subjects, Bruni et al. [19] demonstrated that a multivariate analysis model confirmed the utility of integrating endocrine data with the study of body composition; and they reported that BIA proved to be a useful clinical alternative to DXA, especially when considering body cell mass and phase angle.

The parameter of phase angle in BIA is based on total body reactance and total body resistance, independent of weight, height, body fat. Lower phase angles appear to be consistent with either cell membrane degeneration or cell death, whereas higher phase angles are consistent with large quantities of healthy cell membranes and body cell mass. This is because phase angle is positively correlated with capacitance and negatively associated with resistance [20].

Of course, the use of phase angle is not limited to anorexic patients, as seen in a report by Schwenk et al. [21] who found that low phase angle remains an independent adverse prognostic marker of clinical progression and survival in HIV-AIDS patients provided with an antiretroviral therapy that was designed to reduce the risk of wasting. Similarly, Gupta et al. [22] evaluated a case series of 52 patients with histologically-confirmed stage IV colorectal cancer. BIA was conducted on all patients and their respective phase angles were calculated. It was concluded that phase angle would be a prognostic indicator in patients with advanced colorectal cancer. Thus, the phase angle parameter of BIA can be an indicator of overall patient health.

In further considering the efficacy of BIA compared to other modalities of body composition analysis, a study by Beshyah [23] compared fat-free mass (FFM) and% body fat mass (BFM) values derived from total body potassium (TBK), BIA, and DXA in hypopituitary adults before and after a six month treatment with growth hormone (GH). The authors reported that before the GH treatment, there was a strong correlation between the three evaluation modalities, and by the end of the study, they concluded that changes in FFM and BFM values derived by DXA in patients receiving growth hormone vs. placebo were not significantly different from those derived by using TBK or BIA.

A recent study by Krachler et el. [24] was designed to determine whether categories of obesity based upon anthropometric-based estimate of the% fat mass (FM%) had a similar discriminative ability for markers of cardiovascular risk evaluated for FM% by DXA or BIA. The study included 205 males and 388 females ranging in age from 40 – 79 years.

Risk factors including weight, blood pressure, triaglycerols, HDL, cholesterol and fasting glucose were also ascertained. The results showed that for grade 1 hypertension, dyslipidemia and impaired fasting glucose and obesity (defined by FM% and BMI equation) had a higher discriminative power than DXA. However, for grade 2 hypertension, FM% discriminated 1.2% lower ($p = 0.05$) than DXA and 2.8% ($p < 0.01$) lower than BIA. They concluded that receiver operation characteristics confirmed BIA as the best predictor of grade 2 hypertension and FM% for grade 1 hypertension.

Moon et el. [25] compared single estimations of fat-free mass (FFM) and tracked FFM in 34 men and 38 women in a control vs. exercise group assessing body composition using BIA equations, DXA, and a 4-C model during weeks 1, 12, and 24 of the study using BIA and DXA compared to a four compartment (4-C) model. Single estimates for DXA and BIA produced high r values (0.79 – 0.95) and low standard errors. Both BIA and DXA equations showed the same significance when comparing groups and times with the 4-C model. Further, individual accuracy for tracking changes were again similar when comparing the two methodologies with the 4-C model in the evaluation of FFM and suggest that the two modalities could be used interchangeably.

Pathophysiological conditions can confound estimates of body composition. For example, Kang et el. [26] conducted a study wherein changes in the difference between BIA and DXA body composition determinations according to edema became an important parameter in peritoneal dialysis patients (PD) patients. After reviewing the data from 409 patients whose body composition was measured by both techniques one or more times, the measurements were divided into four quartiles on the basis of edema index. Significant correlations and intraclass correlations were found for lean body mass (LM), fat mass (FM), and mineral bone content. The authors concluded from the data that when LM is measured by DXA, it is overestimated in PD patients with edema, compared to measurements derived from BIA. However, FM and bone mineral density measured by BIA are overestimated in PD patients, compared to measurements with DXA, especially in patients afflicted with worsening edema; and that the difference between the two modalities grows as the edema worsens. Thus, the authors conclude that a combination of the two methods will allow clinicians to ascertain more accurate body composition evaluations for PD patients with edema.

An interesting study was conducted by Vaz et al. [27] where body composition was analyzed in a group of patients fulfilling DSM-IV criteria for bulimia nervosa (BN). Thus, 43 patients with prior AN (BN-AN group) and 61 without this history (BN-nonAN) were evaluated for height and weight, abdominal diameter, body circumferences, skinfold thickness, and BIA parameters. The results demonstrated that more than 40% of the bulimic patients with an AN history showed a BMI of <20, as well as lower muscle mass and a higher percent of extracellular water. However, these differences were not evident in the second part of the analysis, when only patients with a normal weight range were compared. This indicated that a large number of AN patients tend to retain some clinical traits of the previous condition, remaining in a "subclinical status". In other words, they were thinner and appeared to have less of a challenge in maintaining a lower weight more than without having had prior AN. Importantly, however, these differences no longer existed in the patients who had achieved a normal weight. This raised interesting questions regarding the boundaries between BN and AN.

In a report by Piccoli et al. [28], 74 AN women with a BMI =10 - 17.5 were evaluated for the frequency of disagreement between BIA and anthropometric estimates of FM and FFM. The results showed a correlation coefficient of 0.8 - 0.9 between the two methods; but the calculations revealed that there was a progressive disagreement between the two techniques when the BMI was <15 kg/m^2) The authors concluded that although BIA data could be useful in monitoring the patients during refeeding, neither anthropometric methods nor BIA should be used in patients with a BMI of <15.

However, this conclusion appears to conflict with that of Hannan et al. [29] who pointed out that many methods of measuring body composition are time-consuming and require equipment that is often unavailable; but that BIA is simple and inexpensive and can differentiate between lean and fat tissues. Studying 38 anorexic females with highly variable BMI, the authors concluded from the data that the BIA technique compared favorably with other established methods, even in AN patients with a very low BMI.

A negative conclusion about standard BIA was reported by Haas et al. [30] recently who studied 57 AN women with BIA and Bioimpedance vector analysis (BIVA). The authors suggested that because 47% of the patients showed "implausible" results, BIA had "little utility" in these patients, whereas BIVA could be an alternative modality reflecting ECW volume changes and later real tissue mass increases.

Although many of the various body composition studies that have thus far been presented here focus on anorexia, an interesting and recent report by Marra et al. [31] presented data regarding body composition in underweight ballet dancers and constitutionally lean females. The study utilized phase angle measurements to ascertain whether this parameter differed regarding the type of underweight female adolescents and younger women. Thirty AN patients, 10 constitutionally lean individuals, and 15 classic dancers were evaluated by skin fold thickness and BIA. The results indicated that the BIA-derived phase angle discriminated between different forms of underweight, being an effective marker to detect qualitative changes in body composition. Also, in an earlier study by Marra et al. [32], which evaluated the relationship between BMR and BIA in 86 female anorexic patients, multiple regression analysis indicated that phase angle was a predictor of BMR both when solely BIA variables were considered and when combined with either weight and age or fat-free mass.

In a study by Saladino and Dieffenbach [data unpublished, The Use of Bioelectrical Impedance to Monitor Metabolic/Body Composition Changes Resulting from Dietary Treatment in Restrictive Eating Disorder Patients], which assessed 79 restrictive eating disorder patients within an impatient setting and receiving a modified Mediterranean-style diet, it was observed that 37% gained body cell mass interpreted from BIA as lean body mass, and an additional 39% gained lean body mass and fat mass from this diet ($p \leq 0.05$). Importantly, the BIA data showed that the fat mass acquired by this second group of patients still allowed them to achieve a lean body mass to fat ratio of 80/20 - 75/25. The remaining study group lost lean body mass.

It is well-recognized that the issues which lay at the heart of restrictive eating disorder patients are complex. This is exemplified by the work of Van Wymbeleke et al. [33] who studied 87 female AN patients and included BIA to assess body composition. During the treatment period, it was observed that by day eight, resting energy expenditure (REE) increased significantly (13.4%, $p < 0.01$), based upon an increase in fat-free mass, and that the ratio of REE/FFM remained high thereafter.

However by multivariate analysis, they concluded that the rise in this ratio observed during refeeding was significantly related to energy intake, anxiety, abdominal pain, and depressive mood; and they also noted a significant rise in the REE/FFM ratio with physical activity and cigarette smoking. This rise in REE leveled off after recovery from AN. Thus, many variables can affect the results and interpretation of even efficacious BIA data, and that analysis of such data must be careful, thorough, and with as much knowledge about the patient as possible.

Conclusions

The studies presented in this review demonstrate the metabolic and psychological complexity of understanding and treating restrictive eating disorder patients. However, assessing body mass composition in these patients would be an important component of diagnosis and treatment options; and it is suggested here that such an evaluation would ascertain whether or not the acquisition of body mass during refeeding is metabolically appropriate - ideally achieving an approximate 20/80% - 25/75% fat/lean body mass ratio. In addition, and based upon sometimes conflicting science, it is reasonable to suggest that utilizing BIA techniques to achieve this assessment could be advantageous in patients with eating disorders, such as anorexia nervosa and bulimia nervosa. In addition to the results of the varied studies reviewed here, assessing body composition is also important, because weight changes do not necessarily reflect specific changes in body compartments (including fat free mass and fat mass).

Of course, there are always eating disorder patients with co-morbid disorders that can confound data obtained for a research study or a treatment regimen. However, by utilizing a technique like BIA, clinicians and researchers would have the advantage of using each patient as their own "control" which could potentially allow for a more effective, individualized nutrition regimen according to the body composition changes observed during their treatment period. In addition, BIA might provide information on BMR in anorexic patients and should be explored in evaluating other forms of protein malnutrition. Therefore, in the hands of a qualified clinician who understands the instrumentation as well as human metabolism, it appears that BIA could be a very useful modality in the treatment of patients afflicted with restrictive eating disorders.

Abbreviations

BIA: Bioimpedance analysis; DXA: Dual-energy X-ray absorptiometry; AN: Anorexia nervosa; BN: Bulimia nervosa; BMI: Body mass index; ECM: Extracellular mass; BCM: Body cell mass; FFM: Fat-free mass; FM: Fat mass; ECW: Extracellular water; GH: Growth hormone; PD: Peritoneal dialysis; REE: Resting energy expenditure.

Competing interests

The author declares that he has no competing interests.

Acknowledgements

Thanks to Misericordia University for support in writing this paper.

References

1. ANAD. (n.d.): **Eating Disorders Statistics.** In Retrieved September 17, 2014, from http://www.anad.org/get-information/about-eating-disorders/eating-disorders-statistics/.
2. Nicholls D, Wells DJ, Singhal A, Stanhope R: **Validation of the Dutch Eating Behaviour Questionnaire parent version (DEBQ-P) in the Italian population: a screening tool to detect differences in eating behaviour among obese, overweight and normal-weight preadolescents.** *European Journal of Clinical Nutrition* 2004, **58:**1217–1222.
3. Noordenbox G: **Characteristics and treatment of patients with chronic eating disorders.** *International Journal of Eating Disorders* 2002, **10:**15–29.
4. Dixon JB, Boyd JB, Strauss JG, Laurie C, O'Brien PE: **Changes in body composition with weight loss: obese subjects randomized to surgical and medical programs.** *Obesity* 2007, **15:**1187–1198.
5. Hoffer EC, Meador CK, Simpson DC: **Correlation of whole-body impedance with total body water volume.** *J Appl Physiol* 1969, **27:**531.
6. Lukaski HC, Johnson PE, Bolonchuk WW, Lykken GI: **Assessment of fat-free mass using bioelectrical impedance measurements of the human body.** *Am J Clin Nut* 1985, **41:**810–817.
7. Ellis KJ: **Selected body composition methods can be used in field studies.** *J Nutrition* 2001, **131:**1589S–1595S.
8. Kyle UG, Bosaeus I, De Lorenzo AD, Durenberg P, Elia M, Gomez JM, Heitmann BL, Kent-Smith L, Melchior JC, Pirlich M, Scharfetter H, Schols AM, Pichard C: **Bioelectrical impedance analysis-part 1: review of principles and methods.** *Clin Nutr* 2004, **23:**1226–1243.
9. Gallagher D, Ruts E, Visser M, Heshka M, Baumgartner R, Wang J, Pierson R, Pi-Sunyer F, Heymsfield S: **Weight stability masks sarcopenia in elderly men and women.** *Am J Physiol Endocinol Metab* 2000, **279:**E366–E375.
10. Song MY, Ruts E, Kim J, Janumala I, Heymsfield S, Gallagher D: **Sarcopenia and increased adipose tissue infiltration of muscle in elderly African American women.** *Am J Clin Nutrition* 2004, **79:**874–880.
11. Hughes VA, Roubenoff R, Wood M, Frontera WR, Evans WJ, Fiatarone Singh MA: **Anthropometric assessment of 10-y changes in body composition in the elderly.** *Am J Clinical Nutrition* 2004, **80:**475–482.
12. Fantin F, Francesco VD, Fontana G, Zivelonghi A, Bissoli L, Zoico E, Rossi A, Micciolo R, Bosello O, Zamboni M: **Longitudinal body compositional changes in old men and women: interrelationships with worsening disability.** *J Gerontol A Biol Sci Med* 2007, **62:**1375–1381.
13. Snijder MB, van Dam RM, Visser M, Seidell JC: **What aspects of body fat are particularly hazardous and how do we measure them?** *Int J Epidemiology* 2006, **35:**83–92.
14. Goodpaster BH, Krishnaswami S, Harris TB, Katsiaras A, Kritchevsky S, Simonsick E, Nevitt M, Holvoet P, Newman A: **Obesity, regional body fat distribution, and the metabolic syndrome in older men and women.** *Arch Intrn Med* 2005, **165:**777–783.
15. Ramsay SE, Whincup PH, Shaper AG, Wannamethee SG: **The relations of body composiiton and adiposity measures to ill health and physical diability in elderly men.** *Am J Epidemiol* 2006, **164:**459–469.
16. Mika C, Herpetz-Dahlmann B, Heer M, Holtzkamp K: **Improvement of nutritional status as assessed by multifrequency BIA during 15 weeks of refeeding in adolescent girls with anorexia nervosa.** *J Nutrition* 2004, **134:**3026–3030.
17. Mattar L, Godart N, Melchior JC, Falissard B, Kolta S, Ringuenet D, Vindreau C, Nordon C, Blanchet C, Pichard C: **Underweight patients with anorexia nervosa: comparison of bioelectrical impedance analysis using five equations to dual X-ray absorptiometry.** *Clinical Nutrition* 2011, **30:**746–752.
18. Gosh S, Meister D, Cowen S, Hannan WJ, Gerguson A: **Body composition at the bedside.** *Europ J Gastroent Hepatol* 1997, **9:**783–788.
19. Bruni V, Dei M, Morelli C, Schettino M, Balzi D, Balzi D, Nuvolone D: **Body composition variables and leptin levels in functional hypothalamic amenorrhea and ammenorreah related eating disorders.** *J Ped Adolesc Gynecol* 2011, **24:**347–352.
20. Liedtke RR: *Principles of Bioelectrical Impedance*; http://rjlsystems.com.
21. Schwenk A, Beisenherz A, Römer K, Kremer G, Salzberger B, Marinos E: **Phase angle from bioelectrical impedance analysis remains an independent predictive marker in HIV-infected patients in the era of highly active antiretroviral treatment.** *Am J Clin Nutr* 2000, **72:**496–501.
22. Gupta D, Lammersfeld CA, Burrows JL, Dahlk SL, Vashi PG, Grutsch JF, Hoffman S, Lis CG: **Bioelectrical impedance phase angle in clinical practice: implications for prognosis in advanced colo-rectal cancer.** *Am J Clin Nutr* 2004, **80:**1634–1638.
23. Beshyah SA: **Comparison of measurement of body composition by total body potassium, bioimpedance analysis, and dual energy x-ray absorptiometry in hypopituitary adults before during growth hormone treatment.** *Am. J. Clin. Nutr* 1995, **61:**1186–1194.
24. Krachler B, Volgyi E, Saconen K, Tylavsky FA, Alen M, Cheng S: **BMI and an athropometry-based estimate of fat mass percentage are both valid discriminators of cardiometabolic risk: a comparison with DXA and bioimpedance.** *J Obes* 2013, 14 pages. EPub 2013 Dec.
25. Moon JR, Stout JR, Smith-Ryan AE, Kendall KL, Fukuda DH, Cramer JT, Moon SE: **Tracking fat-free mass changes in elderly men and women using single-frequency bioimpedance analysis and dual-energy x-ray absorptiometry: a four compartment model comparison.** *Eur J Clin Nutr* 2013, **67:**S40–S46.
26. Kang SH, Cho KH, Park JW, Do JY: **Comparison of bioimpedance analysis and dual-energy x-ray absorptiometry body composition measurements in peritoneal dialysis patients according to edema.** *Clin Nephrol* 2013, **79:**261–268.
27. Vaz FJ, Guisado JA, Penas-Lledo EM: **History of anorexia nervosa in bulimic patients: its influence on body composition.** *Int J Eat Disord* 2003, **34:**148–155.
28. Piccoli A, Codognotto M, Di Pascoli L, Boffo G, Caregaro L: **Body mass index and agreement between bioimpedance and anthropometry of body composition compartments in anorexia nervosa.** *J Parental Enteral Nutr* 2005, **29:**148–156.
29. Hannan WJ, Cowen S, Freemen CP, Shapiro CM: **Evaluation of bioeletrical impedance analysis for body composition measurements in anorexia nervosa.** *Clin Phys Physiol Meas* 1991, **12:**93–94.
30. Hass V, Riedl A, Hofman T, Nischan A, Burghardt R, Boschmann M, Klapp B: **Bioimpedance and bioimpedance vector analysis in patients with anorexia nervosa.** *Europ Eat Disord Rev* 2012, **10:**1002. Epub ahead of print.
31. Marra M, Caldara A, Montagnese C, De Filippo E, Pasanisi F, Contaldo F, Scalfi L: **Bioelectrical impedance phase angle in constitutionally lean females, ballet dancers and patients with anorexia nervosa.** *Eur J Clin Nutr* 2009, **63**(7):905–908.

32. Marra M, De Filippo E, Signorini A, Pasanisi F, Contaldo F, Scalfi L: **Phase angle is a predictor of basal metabolic rate in female patients with anorexia nervosa.** *Physiol Meas* 2005, **26**:S145–S152.
33. Van Wymbeleke V, Brondel L, Marcel Brun J, Rigaud D: **Factors associated with the increase in resting energy enpenditure during refeeding in malnourished anorexia nervosa patients.** *Am J Clin Nutr* 2004, **80**:1469–1477.

Uncontrollable behavior or mental illness? Exploring constructions of bulimia using Q methodology

Kate Churruca*, Janette Perz and Jane M Ussher

Abstract

Background: In medical and psychological literature bulimia is commonly described as a mental illness. However, from a social constructionist perspective the meaning of bulimia will always be socially and historically situated and multiple. Thus, there is always the possibility for other understandings or *constructions* of bulimia to circulate in our culture, with each having distinct real-world implications for those engaging in bulimic behaviors; for instance, they might potentially influence likelihood of help-seeking and the success of treatment. This study used Q methodology to explore culturally-available constructions of bulimia nervosa.

Methods: Seventy-seven adults with varying experience of eating disorders took part in this Q methodological study. Online, they were asked to rank-order 42 statements about bulimia, and then answer a series of questions about the task and their knowledge of bulimia. A by-person factor analysis was then conducted, with factors extracted using the centroid technique and a varimax rotation.

Results: Six factors satisfied selection criteria and were subsequently interpreted. Factor A, "bulimia as uncontrolled behavior", positions bulimia as a behavioral rather than psychological issue. Factor B, entitled "bulimia is a distressing mental illness", reflects an understanding of bulimic behaviors as a dysfunctional coping mechanism, which is often found in psychological literature. Other perspectives position bulimia as about "self-medicating with food" (Factor C), "the pathological pursuit of thinness" (Factor D), "being the best at being thin" (Factor E), or as "extreme behavior vs. mentally ill" (Factor F). These constructions have distinct implications for the subjective experience and behavior of those engaged in bulimic behaviors, with some constructions possibly being more useful in terms of help-seeking (Factor B), while others position these individuals in ways that may be distressing, for instance as shallow (Factor D) or to blame (Factor E).

Conclusions: This study has identified a range of distinct constructions of bulimia. These constructions are considered to have implications for the behaviors and experiences of those engaging in bulimic behaviors. As such, further research into constructions of bulimia may illuminate factors that influence help-seeking and the self-perceptions of such individuals.

Keywords: Bulimia, Social constructionism, Q methodology, Help-seeking

Background

Clinically diagnosable bulimia nervosa can be identified in approximately one in every hundred young women in Western societies [1,2]. There is evidence that the behaviors that characterize this condition, such as binge eating and purging, are becoming increasingly common, with a more than twofold rise in prevalence for both men and women between 1995 and 2005 [1]. Despite this general increase, bulimic behaviors still occur more commonly in women than in men [1,3,4]; as such, bulimia is viewed as predominately a woman's problem [5]. However, most women exhibiting bulimic behaviors do not seek help or treatment [6-8]. This is a matter of serious concern, given the numerous associated health risks, such as cardiovascular and gastrointestinal problems [9,10], as well as psychological distress and reduced quality of life [11-13]. As such, there is a need for

* Correspondence: k.churruca@uws.edu.au
Centre for Health Research, University of Western Sydney, Locked Bag 1797, Penrith South 2751, Australia

research that examines factors that may influence help-seeking for bulimic behaviors.

A variety of factors have been implicated in the development and maintenance of bulimia, which can be broadly characterised as biological [14], psychological [15,16] and sociocultural [5,17]. However, bulimia is a complex problem, and is not easily explained through one particular factor, or type of factor [18]. Instead, integrating factors together within a multifactorial bio-psycho-social model is considered necessary to more fully understand eating disorders [18-21]. For such an approach to be truly integrative, however, it should not only focus on the way social, psychological and biological factors intersect to determine eating disordered behaviors. Rather, as is recommended in the study of all categories of health and illness [22,23], it should also examine the way social meanings of eating disorders affect subjective experience. Research into bulimia has generally focused on the multifactorial aetiology of the behavior [24], rather than the social meaning [25]. This is typical for investigations into psychiatric diagnostic categories [26], as causal pathways and behaviours are more readily observed and quantified than meaning [22], and statistical analysis of such pathways is highly valued in psychological and medical research [27]. However, social constructionism provides a theoretical basis from which to explore the variety of social meanings of bulimia, and the implications that these different understandings have for those involved.

Proponents of social constructionist theory argue that meaning and knowledge are constructed in ongoing processes of social interaction [28]. As such, one's perspective on a concept, such as bulimia, is always socially and historically situated, and open to being contested by competing understandings [28]. Bulimia might therefore be understood in terms of a number of alternate *constructions*: these are coherent accounts, representations, or ways of thinking about a topic, that circulate widely in our culture [29]. This includes biomedical, psychological and many social theories of eating disorders, that despite their differences, reflect a dominant construction that circulates in research, popular culture, and self-help resources, in which bulimia is positioned as an individual pathology and categorically distinct from normal eating behaviors [30-32].

These different constructions have different real-world implications for the subjectivity of those individuals engaging in bulimic behaviors; social constructionism suggests that they frame feelings, experiences, sense of self and perceptions of one's own behavior, making certain actions possible, while simultaneously closing down others [23,29,33]. For instance, the construction of bulimia as a mental illness, a common conceptualisation in the research literature [18,34], positions individuals with a bulimic diagnosis as not responsible for the abnormal and distressing condition they experience, and opens up the possibility for particular forms of treatment. On the other hand, as has been suggested for women diagnosed with depression [35,36], this construction might minimize the potential for personal agency and recovery without such treatment. This understanding may also conflict with other constructions of bulimia, as suggested in a study of community attitudes to mental illness in the UK, where over one-third of participants considered individuals with eating disorders responsible for their condition and that they should "pull themselves together" [37]. A further contrasting understanding of bulimia is found in some feminist theorising, where behaviors categorised as eating disorders are viewed as part of a continuum of eating behaviors, with psychiatric diagnosis of particular behaviors as 'disordered' deemed to reflect a broader cultural objectification and pathologization of women's bodies, linked to cultural constructions of normative femininities [32].

Research driven by social constructionist theory has previously been used to explore some aspects of bulimia. For instance, social constructionism has highlighted the negative relationship between cultural constructions of bulimia and anorexia, with the former having connotations of being out-of-control and disgusting, whereas the latter is partially glamorised and admired [38-40]. Evidence of this binary has been found in the talk of both health professionals and individuals engaged in bulimic behaviors, which may contribute to distress experienced by the latter and potentially intensify their dysfunctional eating behaviors [38]. Finally, the identity of "the bulimic" may efface other aspects of self; as such, this construction may limit willingness for treatment, with recovery becoming akin to "self-annihilation" [25].

If constructions of eating disorders impact upon the experiences of those engaged in bulimia, with the potential to impact upon behaviours such as help-seeking, it is important to identify and explicate dominant constructions which operate in a particular historical and cultural context [32]. In addition to comparing constructions of bulimia with anorexia, researchers have drawn attention to ways in which eating disordered behaviors are normative, rather than abnormal: binging and purging are not viewed as distinct from dieting and exercising for aesthetic or health reasons, with both made possible through the same social and historical conditions [41,42]. In a related area, social constructionist research has explored how constructions of anorexia work in conjunction with constructions of femininity, and in particular the idealised thin body that is so valued in women [43].

While research using social constructionist theory has been important in exploring some of the personal and social meanings of eating disorders, there are limitations.

For instance, the focus is often on anorexia or eating disorders more generally, rather than bulimia and bulimic behaviors, specifically [40,42]. Further, much analysis is theoretical, and relies on secondary data such as media texts [39,40,42,44], or data from interviews with a relatively small sample [38,41]. Consequently, there is a need for further empirical work investigating social constructions of bulimia. This is the aim of the present study, which will use Q methodology to identify and describe the constructions of bulimia that circulate in a contemporary Western society, Australia. This will involve sampling a range of perspectives on the issue, held by individuals who have engaged in bulimic and other eating disordered behaviors, those who have had other personal experience of eating disorders (e.g. knowing a friend or family member to go through it), and those who have no personal experience with eating disorders.

Q methodology

Q methodology combines both qualitative and quantitative techniques to study the "subjectivity involved in any situation" ([45], p. 561). As a method, it works to identify a range of subjective viewpoints that are shared by a number of individuals through an inverted form of factor analysis [46]. These participants' *construction* of the issue can then be contrasted with that of other individuals, who share a different way of thinking about the topic [47]. In Q methodology the aim is to describe and interpret the point-of-view associated with each factor; as such, it is not "the 'constructors'—the participants—who are the focus of the approach but the 'constructions' themselves" ([29], p. 180).

The strength of Q methodology is drawn from both qualitative and quantitative research traditions [48], and has been suggested as a more robust and suitable technique for exploring subjective viewpoints than alternative methods such as surveys [29,49-51]. It has been used to investigate the subjectivity involved in a variety of health issues, including understandings of irritable bowel syndrome [52], constructions of sex and intimacy in the context of cancer [53], parental judgement on infant immunisation [54], and the weight-control self-efficacy beliefs of obese women [48].

This paper presents the results from a Q methodological study, which explored constructions of bulimia. While the starting point for this research is that a number of alternative constructions of bulimia exist, the principle of "finite diversity" suggests that the potential range of such constructions is limited by socio-historical forces [29,51,55]. As such, it was expected that, through Q methodology, a number of coherent accounts of bulimia would emerge, and these would be shared among a group of participants.

Methods

The first step in a Q methodological study is to produce a set of items or statements about the topic that participants will sort. This Q set is derived through exhaustive sampling, so as to be as representative as possible of the opinion domain [51]. Participants (the P set) are then chosen strategically, because of their ability to model a viewpoint on the topic through Q sorting, and because their viewpoint matters [29,51]. This study received ethical approval from the Human Research Ethics Committee of the University of Western Sydney, with protocol number H9909.

The participants rank items of the Q set according to their relative agreement or disagreement, such that each statement gains its full meaning only through how it is configured in relation to every other statement [56]. It is therefore the similarities across the overall arrangement of statements in participants' Q sorts that are the basis for factors in the inverted factor analysis [51]. These processes are described below for the current study, with further description of the features and method of Q methodology provided elsewhere [51].

Item sampling - the Q set

In creating the Q set, statements should be representative of the different perspectives circulating in the public domain about that topic [57]. A Q set should "cover all the ground within the relevant conceptual space" ([51], p. 58), while remaining balanced and unbiased to any particular viewpoint [51]. To this end, the Q set used in the present study was derived through sampling constructions of bulimia in a wide range of naturalistic contexts [58,59], including academic sources, media, websites and online communities. This sampling process, and further refinement of statements for the Q set, was completed by the first author, in consultation with the second and third authors. Sampling statements involved reading the first 20 academic papers on Google Scholar returned with the search term "bulimia"; these sources were supplemented by a larger literature review of bulimia carried out in preparation for this research. News media was reviewed through a web-based search of archived news reports (using Google News) and the websites of Australian print magazines that focus on health and/or women's issues (e.g. Cleo). Additionally, any user comments sections associated with these articles were also reviewed. The top ten websites that were returned for a search of bulimia in Google were also reviewed to derive statements. These texts typically presented content on bulimia concerning health information and help-seeking. A web search was also used to identify visual depictions of bulimia and eating disorders, which lead to a pool of five American made-for-television films produced over the last 30 years on bulimia and a number of episodes of a popular Australian soap opera that aired in 2006. This content was all accessible online through the video sharing website YouTube, again allowing for a review of user comments and opinions on these videos. Finally, the social media website Tumblr, which allows users to aggregate content according to topics (tagging), was also reviewed for mentions of the word "bulimia". This search resulted in an item-pool of approximately 200 statements about bulimia.

A structured approach was employed to reduce the number of items [51], conducted by the first author, through a process of discussion with the second and third authors. This involved organising items together based on their similar subject matter, and resulted in six fairly coherent themes, each comprising 20–30 statements. These themes were: bulimia as a problem, bulimia as a solution, bulimia as a choice, bulimia as a person, bulimia as normative, and bulimia as marginalised. Statements were then refined within each of these themes; this involved eliminating items that were repetitious, breaking up double-barrelled items, and editing and rewording statements to improve their readability [51]. In service of this, all statements used the term 'bulimia' rather than 'bulimia nervosa', as the latter is wordier, and arguably a more clinical and less widely known term.

The statement refining process resulted in a Q set of 54 items, which was piloted with volunteers using the web-based software Q-Assessor [60]. In response to their feedback on the items and the Q sorting task, this item pool was further shortened and refined to a final Q set of 42 statements.

Recruitment and participants – the P set

In Q methodology, recruitment of participants is a strategic, rather than random, process [51]. Participants in this study were recruited through two channels to maximize the possibility that a variety of perspectives could be expressed [46]. The first group comprised 71 individuals (59 women, 9 men, M_{age} = 22, SD = 6, a further three did not provide demographic details), who identified as having at least a general knowledge of bulimia; they were recruited through undergraduate psychology courses. It is standard practice in Q methodology to include individuals in the P set whose viewpoints are of particular significance to the research focus [51]. The first group of this sample fulfills this brief as it is skewed towards younger women, the demographic in which eating disorders are most common [3,4]; further, as psychology students, these individuals are assumed to have some knowledge and interest in mental health. To further satisfy this recommendation, the second group of participants consisted of six women who reported engaging in bulimic behaviors (M_{age} = 20, SD = 3). They were recruited through advertising on social media and through print material in public sites on university campuses across western Sydney.

The final P set of 77 participants ranged in age from 17 to 50 (65 women, 9 men, M_{age} = 22, SD = 6). Three participants did not provide demographic details, something that may have been due to technical difficulties associated with online data collection, human error (e.g. missing a question or closing the window early), or to a resistance to providing any personal or potentially identifying information. While this sample size might be considered small for conventional factor analysis, the nature of the statistical technique in Q methodology, where the analysis is inverted, makes this sample perfectly adequate [46]. Indeed, the rule of thumb offered for use in Q methodology studies [29] indicates that a participant pool of between 40 and 60 is satisfactory for Q analysis. The majority of individuals in the P set indicated the cultural group with which they identified as Anglo-Australian (52%), followed by European (14%) and Middle-eastern (13%).

Procedure – Q sorting

Participants completed the Q sorting task online, using the website Q-Assessor [60]. On the introduction page they were asked to rank a set of 42 statements from those they most agreed (+4) with to those they most disagreed (−4) with, based on how well they represented their own understanding and thoughts about bulimia. The software directed participants through three stages of sorting. In the first, each participant organised the statements into three categories; those they agreed with, those they disagreed with, and those they were neutral about. At the second stage a fixed quasi-normal distribution (Figure 1) was introduced. This is a standard tool in Q sorting: the forced distribution simplifies later statistical procedures without impacting the factors that are produced [61], while the quasi-normal shape reflects that participants will feel comparatively strongly about a limited number of items [51]. Participants were first asked to sort the poles (+4 and −4); they were able to click through the statements, first in the "agree", and then "disagree", category, to select and "sort" the two they feel most strongly about. In the third stage, participants were free to rank the remainder of the statements into the distribution, moving them around and reviewing their placement up until they selected "submit". Following the sorting task, participants were asked a series of open-response questions. These allowed participants to elaborate on how they found the task and why they sorted the statements in the way they did (particularly the poles). There were also a number of questions asking participants about their own understanding of bulimia, their level of personal involvement with the topic and how they came by most of their knowledge about bulimia.

Q analysis and factor interpretation

Factor analysis is a common statistical method for classifying variables; in Q methodology these variables are

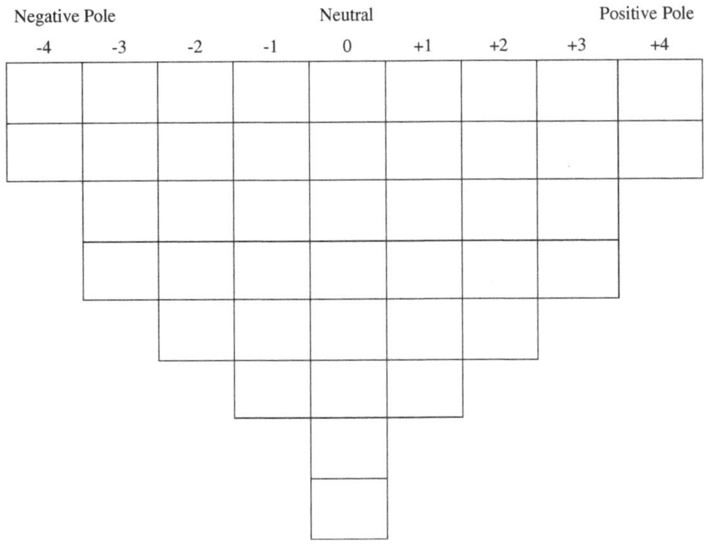

Figure 1 Participant response grid (Q grid).

participants' Q sorts [61]. Through correlating in this by-person way "any sizeable portions of common or *shared* meaning" ([51], p. 98) across Q sorts are identified; these portions of shared meaning become factors.

Factor analysis was, conducted by the first and second author in collaboration, in Q-Assessor, which after correlating all Q sorts together, uses the centroid method to extract factors. This technique is favored by Q methodologists [51,61] and aims to account for as much of the study variance as possible with each successive factor that is extracted. Extracted factors were then subjected to a varimax rotation. This method positions factors so that the overall solution accounts for as much of the explained variance as possible, while having each Q sort load significantly on only one study factor [51]. Varimax rotation is accepted as a sound method of factor rotation and was a suitable choice in this study as it reveals "a subject matter from viewpoints that almost *everybody* might recognize and consider to be of importance" ([51], p. 126). Following this rotation, a factor was selected if it possessed an eigenvalue greater than one, and had at least two Q sorts loading significantly upon it [51,61]. This joint criteria is an accepted standard in Q methodology, reflecting the focus on *shared* meaning, where a shared viewpoint is one that is common to more than one individual [51]. Significant factor loadings were assessed using the Fuerntratt criterion, which is more stringent than many others used in Q methodology (see [51,61]), as it takes into account both the factor loading of a Q sort *and* its communality (i.e. the Q sort variance explained by all factors): a loading is significant if the amount of a Q sort's variance explained by one factor exceeds 50% of the total variance explained (Fuerntratt, 1969, cited in [62]). Given that Q methodology is a novel approach exploring eating disorders, a more conservative criterion was considered appropriate. Six factors met these criteria, and were subjected to interpretation.

Interpretation of factors was facilitated by the creation of factor arrays; these are computed for each factor based on a composite of the Q sorts that load on it. By examining the meaning, ranking and overall configuration of statements in these arrays we begin to understand the construction of bulimia associated with that factor. The ranking of statements was compared across factors to determine similarities and points of divergence among the perspectives [51]. Finally, to supplement the interpretation, and more fully examine the context in which these constructions had come about, the socio-demographic data and the answers to the open-response questions about bulimia were examined for those participants who loaded significantly on a factor. This process of interpretation was initially conducted by the first author, with the second and third author making suggestions for elaboration and revisions, resulting in a final analysis which was agreed by all three authors.

Results

The centroid technique extracted seven factors that accounted for 60.5% of the total variance in this study. After varimax rotation all seven factors had eigenvalues in excess of one (≥4.12), however, only six had at least two significant Q sorts. Construct validity for each factor was indicated by the composite reliability coefficient (r_c), with all exceeding the acceptable value of 0.7. In Table 1 the characteristics for these factors are displayed. Table 2 shows the socio-demographic data for the participants

Table 1 Q factor characteristics

Characteristic	Factor					
	A	B	C	D	E	F
Number of defining sorts	4	7	4	7	2	2
Composite reliability	0.94	0.97	0.94	0.97	0.89	0.89
Eigenvalue	7.36	9.77	5.28	10.16	5.15	4.71
% of explained variance	9.56	12.69	6.86	13.20	6.68	6.11

whose Q sorts defined each factor. Factor scores of each statement across each factor are presented in the factor arrays in Table 3. In the following description of factors, bracketed notation is used to signify a statement's ranking within a factor array; for instance "(5: −4)" indicates that statement 5 was ranked at the −4 (most disagree) position.

Factor A: "bulimia as uncontrolled behavior"

Factor A explained 9.6% of the study variance. Four participants significantly loaded on this factor. Two were women aged 18 and 20, with one mentioning having a friend who had bulimia. Unfortunately, the two other factor exemplars did not supply any demographic data.

In Factor A, bulimia is positioned as a serious and distressing condition (1: +2; 36: −2; 3: +4) of being out of control of one's behavior. Cultural standards of an ideal body shape are deemed to play a large role in bulimia's development (38: +3; 33: +1), with people with bulimia seen as being obsessed with being thin (22: +1). Defining participants agreed that while bulimia affects both women and men (40: +4), and may be underestimated in men (31: +2), the desire for a thin body is ranked as being more typically an issue for women (28: +3). As one 18 years old defining participant's response to a question about the gender disparity associated with eating disorders suggests, "men also care about the way they present themselves, but they do not seem to go to the extremes that women do". For the perspective associated with Factor A, bulimia is about extremes: while issues with weight and shape are prevalent in our culture, the concerns and behaviors that characterise bulimia are considered to be far more extreme, and distinct from regular dieting and exercise (28: +3; 29: +1).

Participants defining Factor A endorsed the view that the path to bulimia might begin with individuals experimenting with binging and purging behaviors (12: +2), perhaps falsely believing that it will help them achieve their desired body shape, with the notion that this behavior works as a method to eat what you want and stay thin rejected (11: −2). Instead bulimia becomes increasingly severe (3: +4), and individuals lose their self-control (25: +2), becoming unable to stop their behavior (13: −4) and, ultimately, sacrifice their health (37: +1). In this vein, a defining participant (20 years of age) described a friend with bulimia as "they wanted to be thin and weren't happy with how they looked, ended up in hospital over it".

In the perspective associated Factor A, bulimia is characterised not only by a lack of control over one's behavior, but also a lack of insight into it, with participants endorsing the view that people with this condition don't understand why they binge and purge (4: +3). Bulimia is also positioned a distressing experience (1: +2), one from which recovery is desired (16: +3). However, as this requires a person to regain control over their behavior (25: +2), it is deemed to be difficult to achieve. This process, in which bulimia seems to begin with a choice but quickly becomes out-of-control, perhaps make the extent to which these individuals are victims difficult to judge (2: 0).

Participants defining Factor A prioritised sociocultural influences, while psychological issues were viewed as secondary (7: +1; 10: 0; 17: +1), or even rejected entirely, with food and eating not viewed as having any relationship to

Table 2 Socio-demographic for Q sorts (participants) defining each factor

Variable	Factor A (*n* =4)* (Count, %)	Factor B (*n* =7) (Count, %)	Factor C (*n* =4) (Count, %)	Factor D (*n* =7)* (Count, %)	Factor E (*n* =2) (Count, %)	Factor F (*n* =2) (Count, %)
Gender						
Woman	2 (100)	7 (100)	3 (75)	4 (66.7)	2 (100)	1 (50)
Man	0	0	1 (25)	2 (33.3)	0	0
Other	0	0	0	0	0	1 (50)
Age (*Mean, S.D.)*	19 (1)	22.3 (6.4)	20.3 (2.9)	19.8 (2.4)	18.5 (0.5)	20.5 (0.5)
Disordered eating experience						
Direct#	0	3 (42.8)	0	2 (33.3)	0	1 (50)
Friend/family member	1 (50%)	2 (28.6)	2 (50)	1 (16.7)	0	0
Impersonal	1 (50%)	2 (28.6)	2 (50)	3 (50)	2 (100)	1 (50)

*As some defining participants did not provide demographic data, calculations are based on the participants who did provide this information.
#Direct means that a participant stated they have engaged in bulimic behaviors.

Table 3 Q-set statements and factor array

Item		Factor A	Factor B	Factor C	Factor D	Factor E	Factor F
1	People with bulimia are distressed by their symptoms.	2	2	−1	1	0	0
2	Individuals with bulimia are victims of their disorder.	0	3	3	2	−1	1
3	Bulimia is a disease that gets worse over time.	4	0	−2	1	**3**	−1
4	People with bulimia don't know why they binge and purge.	3	−1	−1	−1	0	0
5	For those with bulimia, food is a means of escape.	−3	2	3	−1	−1	2
6	A person with bulimia attempts to improve their mood by eating.	−3	0	**4**	0	0	0
7	Bulimia might start as a way for a person to express feelings they are afraid to deal with.	1	1	1	1	0	1
8	People with bulimia are afraid of living without their condition.	0	0	−2	0	−1	2
9	Binging and then purging might give a person with bulimia a sense of control.	−1	**3**	1	0	1	3
10	Many people with bulimia have experienced some sort of past trauma.	0	1	−1	1	−2	0
11	Bulimia is getting to eat what you want and still stay thin.	−2	−1	−2	−3	**3**	1
12	Bulimia is something someone might try out after hearing about it e.g. on TV, social media, friends.	2	−2	0	0	1	3
13	A person with bulimia could stop their behaviors if they really wanted to.	**−4**	**−4**	2	0	−1	−3
14	People with bulimia have failed to get anorexia.	−2	−3	−3	−2	−2	−1
15	Bulimia is a lifestyle choice.	**−3**	**−4**	**−3**	0	−2	1
16	People with bulimia want to recover.	3	0	0	1	1	−2
17	In bulimia, binging and purging are ways of punishing yourself.	1	**4**	−1	−1	2	−1
18	People with bulimia are success-orientated, seeking physical and mental control.	−2	1	1	−2	**4**	1
19	Dieting only develops into bulimia when a person has other predisposing characteristics.	0	−2	0	0	−1	**4**
20	Individuals with bulimia use food like addicts use drugs.	−1	1	2	−1	−2	−2
21	Binging is a sign of weakness in people with bulimia.	−2	−1	−1	0	0	−2
22	People with bulimia are obsessed with being thin.	1	0	1	2	1	0
23	People with bulimia are impulsive.	−1	1	−2	−1	−3	−1
24	People with bulimia are self-centered.	−3	**−3**	−1	−2	0	**−3**
25	Recovering from bulimia requires having self-control.	2	0	2	1	1	1
26	Purging after eating a big or fattening meal is no big deal.	−1	−3	0	**−4**	**−4**	−1
27	Bulimia is an understandable response in a society with lots of high calorie foods.	0	0	0	−2	−2	−3
28	Bulimia is an extreme example of the weight and eating concerns that affect many women in our society.	3	2	3	3	3	0
29	Bulimia is very different from dieting and normal concerns about shape and weight.	1	2	0	3	0	−2
30	Nobody really knows what normal eating, or a healthy relationship with food, is.	2	−1	−2	−2	**−3**	**3**
31	Society probably underestimates the number of men who have bulimia.	2	3	1	2	1	**4**
32	Bulimia occurs because our whole society has an attitude that supports eating disorders.	−1	−1	2	−3	**3**	0
33	Bulimia is more common in women because our culture puts more pressure on them to be thin.	1	1	**4**	**4**	**4**	2
34	Bulimia is something to be ashamed of.	−1	−2	**−4**	**−3**	0	**−4**
35	Bulimia is more socially acceptable than anorexia nervosa.	−4	−2	0	−1	−3	3
36	Bulimia is not that serious.	−2	**−3**	−4	**−4**	−3	**−4**
37	People with bulimia trade health for looking good.	1	−1	0	2	2	−1
38	Media portrayals of an 'ideal' body shape contribute to the occurrence of bulimia.	**3**	2	2	**4**	2	2
39	Our society's increased focus on physical appearance will likely lead to a rise in bulimia in men.	0	3	1	2	−1	−2
40	Bulimia is not just a women's problem.	**4**	0	3	3	2	0
41	Bulimia is biological in nature.	0	−2	−3	−3	**−4**	−3
42	Bulimia is a mental illness.	0	**4**	−3	3	2	2

Bolded scores are for statements with normalized factor scores ≥ ±1.4, indicating the most powerful exemplars for each factor.

coping or mood improvement (5: –3; 6: –3). Thus bulimia is not about gaining control (9: –1), but about being unable to control one's behavior, to the point of being unable to stop (13: –4). As this perspective considers bulimia in terms of behavior, and the lack of control over ones behavior, the possibility that its underlying nature is biological or psychological is either uncertain or unimportant (41: 0; 42:0).

Factor B

Factor B accounted for 12.7% of the study variance. Seven participants had Q sorts that loaded significantly on this factor, with one being a negative relationship. These participants were all women, with an average age of 22.3 years and an age range of 18–37; three reported that they were engaged in bulimic behaviors currently, and another two had other personal experience (i.e. a close friend having bulimia). That one of the defining participants was negatively associated with this factor indicates that two coherent, but highly opposing perspectives on bulimia are subsumed under the one factor [51]. The first perspective to be considered is the one the majority of defining participants endorsed, the second is the converse position endorsed by only one of the participants who exemplified this factor.

"Bulimia is a distressing mental illness"

The first perspective that emerged from Factor B was a highly psychological account of bulimia. Defining participants endorsed the view that bulimia is a serious mental illness (36: –3; 42: +4), distinct from normal practices of weight control and concerns about one's body shape (29: +2; 30: –1). While sociocultural pressure for a thin body is deemed to have a hand in its development (38: +2; 28: +2), the desire for thinness is not positioned as the main issue in bulimia (22:0; 11: –1). Rather, participants defining this factor endorsed the idea that bulimic behaviors form as a means of dealing with upsetting issues in one's life, such as past trauma (10: +1). This view is expressed in the open-response of one of the defining participants (18 years of age) "...for me at least, bulimic behavior isn't solely due to concerns about my appearance – it's a method of coping with overwhelming, negative feelings and self-loathing". Further, as is suggested by this participant's statement, individuals are considered to have some insight into their condition, and the reasons behind their bulimia, as defining participants disagreed with the idea that people in this state don't know why they binge and purge (4: –1).

In this perspective, bulimia is positioned as a "coping mechanism"; defining participants endorsed the view that individuals may find solace in food (5: +2), and gain a sense of control from bulimic behaviors (9: +3). However, this situation is ultimately deemed to be maladaptive, as the experience of bulimia is positioned as distressing (1: +2), and bulimic behaviors are ranked as being self-punishing (17: +4). As bulimic behaviors both alleviate and contribute to distress, it is difficult to say whether or not people with bulimia want to recover (16: 0).

Participants defining the perspective of Factor B slightly endorsed the idea that the personality of the person dealing with bulimia has a role in their condition; they were, thus, likely to be high achievers (18: +1) or impulsive (23: +1). At the same time, and as with many biological illnesses, bulimia is positioned as something that anyone, man or woman, could develop (31: +3), as no predisposing characteristics are necessary (19: –2); an individual does not choose it (15: –4; 12: –2), has little control over their condition (2: +3), and is unable to just stop it (13: –4).

"Bulimia is a way to lose weight"

In the second perspective to emerge from Factor B, bulimic behaviors are positioned as a method an individual, most likely a woman (31: –3), uses to lose weight (11: +1). While there may be particular characteristics that make someone more likely to engage in bulimia (19: +2), these are unlikely to be psychological in nature (42: –4; 17: –4; 9: –3). It is very much something that an individual has control over (13: +4); their choice to engage in binging and purging (15: +4; 12: +2) is motivated by a desire to improve their appearance (37: +1). As the open-response by the woman (19 years of age), who defined this perspective, indicates, "they like to look skinny to impress men". This behavior is deemed to be quite shameful (34: +2), perhaps because it is viewed as selfish (24: +3), or because these individuals have failed at restricting their food intake, like an anorexic (14: +3), and binging is therefore a sign of weakness (21: +1). On the other hand, bulimia is not positioned as a serious problem (26: +3; 36: +3), and is more accepted socially than anorexia (35: +2).

Factor C: "self-medicating with food"

Factor C explained 6.9% of total variance with 4 participants significantly associated with this factor, three of whom were women. The average age of these participants was lower than the overall sample at 20.3 years, with a range of 17–25. Two defining participants indicated that they knew a friend who engaged in bulimic behaviors.

The participants defining Factor C rejected the notion that bulimia is a mental illness (42: –3). Instead, individuals with bulimia are deemed to be the victims (2: +3) of a culture that basically encourages eating disordered behaviors (32: +2). Defining participants rankings suggest that this may be because of the way thin bodies are idealised (38: +2); therefore, while men experience bulimia (40: +3), from the viewpoint of participants defining

Factor C, women are more commonly affected because they are usually under more pressure to be thin (33: +4; 28: +3). The ubiquity of a culture that provides the preconditions for an eating disorder means, for participants exemplifying this perspective, that all individuals are affected to varying extents; thus while they rejected the idea that there is no standard for a normal relationship with food (30: −2), they did not deem bulimia to be so far removed from commonplace practices of dieting and weight control (28: +3; 29: 0).

While similar sociocultural issues are emphasised in other factors, the perspective in Factor C is distinguished by the important role of food. Defining participants endorsed the view that people with bulimia use food to improve their mood (6: +4), to get a high (20: +2), and to withdraw from problems in their lives (5: +3). Thus food is positioned as having a medicinal quality; one defining participant (woman, 25 years of age), in her open-response to a question about how she acquired her knowledge of bulimia, described a friend who "every time she gets angry, she eats a huge amount of junk food, then she regrets it and vomits everything she ate".

According to one of the defining participants (woman, 25 years of age) in Factor C, bulimia involves a "struggle between the desire to lose weight and binge eating". This tension between longing for a particular body (22: +1) and *using* food makes compensatory behaviors necessary in this viewpoint. Thus purging behavior is considered secondary to the disordered eating and seemingly less problematic, as unlike the perspectives for every other factor, participants defining Factor C did not out rightly reject the idea that purging after a large meal was "no big deal" (26: 0). The cycle of binging and purging is something the person with bulimia is ultimately positioned as responsible for (13: +2) and so in order to recover they must regain control of their disordered eating (25: +2). On the other hand, while the idea that bulimia is a serious problem is endorsed in this perspective (36: −4), defining participants indicated that the behaviors are not necessarily distressing (1: −1) and suggested that the reasons behind them are not unknown to the person with bulimia (4: −1). As such, individuals with bulimia may or may not wish to recover (16: 0).

Factor D: "the pathological pursuit of thinness"

Factor D accounted for 13.2% of the variance and was defined by seven participants. Four of these were women and two were men, with a further participant failing to provide socio-demographic data. The average age of these participants was again slightly lower than the overall average, at 20.5 years (range 18–25). Two of these participants, recruited as first year psychology students, indicated having engaged in some level of disordered, or what they considered to be distressing, eating behavior in the past, though they did not provide specific details. Another participant stated that they had a friend who had experienced both anorexia and bulimia.

In the perspective associated with Factor D, the way a thin body is prized in our culture is deemed to be the biggest influence on the development of bulimia (33: +4). In particular, the role of the media in creating this ideal, and then pressuring individuals to attain it, is heavily endorsed in both defining participants ranking of statements (38: +4) and their open-responses: "I think people have it because of the pressure from the media to look a certain way" (woman, 18 years of age), "they (Women) want to look 'skinny' because according to most of society (mainly the (entertainment) media), only skinny girls are attractive and more feminine" (man, 19 years of age). Thus for participants loading on Factor D, what separates people with bulimia from their normal and healthy peers is that they are overly influenced by these messages, to the point of obsession (22: +2). People with bulimia are also positioned as willing to go to more extreme and serious lengths to attain this physique (26: −4; 36: −4), trading their health for looking good (37: +2). Therefore, bulimia is conceptualised outside the realm of normal eating (30: −2), dieting and weight management practices (29: +3), and cannot be explained by prevalent socio-historical conditions (27:-2; 32: −3). This unequivocal stance can be contrasted with Factor C, where bulimic behaviors are not positioned as deviant or abnormal.

While the cause of these behaviors might be societal, for the participants defining Factor D, binging and purging constitute a mental illness (42: +3); as one of these participants (woman, 19 years of age) suggested, it "affect(s) not just the body, but the mind of the individual as well". Thus bulimia is deemed to be a distressing experience (1: +1), with individuals becoming the victim of their own extreme desire for thinness (2: +2). This situation of being a victim of one's desire is perhaps why, for the participants defining Factor D, the extent to which a person with bulimia has chosen to be in that state (12: 0; 15: 0), or has the ability to get out of it (13: 0), is difficult to judge.

In Factor D, defining participants position bulimia as a problem that affects both women and men (40: +3; 39: +2), and may even be underestimated in the latter group (31: +2). However, the ranking of statements also suggests that, as a thin body is much more a standard of beauty for women, bulimia is likely still more of an issue for them too (33: +4; 28: +3). Indeed, defining participants' comments indicate that being a woman puts an individual at risk for bulimia, because women are more "self-conscious" and "sensitive to other people's thoughts about their weight/shape" (man, 19 years of age), "paranoid about (their) appearance" (woman, 19 years of age), and tend "compare themselves to other women" (woman, 20 years of age). Therefore the pathological pursuit of thinness, which bulimia is positioned as in Factor D, is something more likely to be engaged in by women.

Factor E: "being the best at being thin"

Factor E accounted for 6.68% of total variance and was defined by two participants; both were women, aged 18 and 19 years, and neither indicated having any firsthand experience with eating disorders.

This perspective is in some ways similar to Factor D, with bulimia again considered a mental illness involving the extreme pursuit of thinness (33: +4; 28: +3; 42: +2; 38: +2). However, there are subtle distinctions. For Factor D, those who develop bulimia are positioned as more *susceptible* to media and cultural messages; they are victims of these messages promoting a thin body, and the extreme behaviors they use to acquire it. On the other hand, the participants defining Factor E viewed people with bulimia not as victims (2: −1). Rather, these participants endorsed the idea that people with bulimia are seeking control (18: +4), particularly of their bodies because they are determined to be thin (9: +1; 22: +1). They are methodical in their attainment of this goal, with the idea that people with bulimia are impulsive rejected (23: −3). Bulimia is therefore positioned by the participants defining Factor E as a method that allows individuals to eat what they want while still achieving a thin body (11: +3). Though attempts to be thin become increasingly destructive (17: +2; 37: +2), the socially valued nature of this goal, and the measured way in which these individuals pursue it, perhaps makes it more difficult in this perspective than others to decide whether a person with bulimia is self-centred (24: 0).

For the participants defining Factor E, bulimia involves the rigid dedication to being thin, at any cost. While still conceptualised as a mental illness in this account, psychological issues are not viewed as important to either the development or maintenance of bulimia, with the notion that a person with bulimia experiences distress being treated neutrally or with mild disagreement (1: 0; 5: −1; 6: 0; 7:0; 8: −1; 10: −2), in contrast to Factor B. On the other hand, the rankings of defining participants suggest that as bulimia becomes worse as time goes on (3: +3), and results in the deterioration of health (37: +2), individuals with this condition generally want to recover (16: +1).

Factor F: "extreme behavior vs. mentally ill"

Factor F explained 6.11% of the variance with two participants defining this factor; one of these participants was a woman of 20 years of age, while the other was a woman of 21 years who was recruited as part of the group that had engaged in bulimic behaviors. However, she did not label them as bulimia.

The perspective of the participants defining Factor F is in some ways similar to that of Factor A, with both positioning bulimia as something one chooses to begin (15: +1), due to pressures within culture (33: +2; 38: +2). However, while in Factor A bulimia is positioned as a behavioral problem, for those participants defining Factor F, it is conclusively positioned as a mental illness (42: +2). Indeed the ranking of a number of statements by the participants loading on Factor F suggests that it not so much bulimic behaviors that are the issue, but the underlying mental illness. For instance, defining participants suggested purging to be less problematic in this account than in most other factors, though it was still ranked negatively (26: −1). Further, the notion that bulimic behaviors are different from dieting and normal concerns about shape and weight is rejected (20: −2), with the whole notion of 'normal' being questioned (30: +3). Bulimic behaviors are also positioned as more socially acceptable than anorexia (35: +3). Thus, while bulimia forms around weight-management behaviors, for the participants defining Factor F, it may not be these behaviors that distinguish a person with bulimia, but other "predisposing characteristics" (19: +4). This idea is supported by one of the defining participants for Factor F, who reported engaging in binging, restricting, purging, and extensive amounts of exercise, but actively denied that they were bulimia or an eating disorder.

The factors distinguishing extreme eating behaviors from the mental illness bulimia are deemed to be psychological; defining participants endorsed the view that bulimia provides an individual with a means of coping with difficulties in their life (9: +3; 8: +2; 5: +2; 7: +1). As such, while for Factor F bulimia is likely underestimated in men (31: +4), an increased concern about physical appearance for men will not necessarily increase the number of men with bulimia (39: −2).

While bulimia is positioned as a mental illness by the participants defining Factor F, the notion that it is also an ongoing lifestyle choice (15: +1) receives more agreement here than in any other factor. This may be because people with bulimia are deemed to not really want to recover (16: −2), as bulimia provides not only a method of dealing psychologically with any issues, but also a means of staying thin while being able to eat what you want (11: +1). At the same time, even if a person with bulimia wanted to get better, it wouldn't be so easy to just stop (13: −3), as the psychological issues involved in this condition make the thought of recovery frightening (8: +2).

Consensus statements

Some of the statements were ranked in a similar way across factors. A number of items were included to examine individuals' ideas about the gender disparity often found in statistics on the prevalence of eating disorders [63]. Two statements in particular (31 and 40) dealt with this issue. Though overall the ranking of each statement varied quite considerably across factors (31: +1 to +4; 40: 0 to +4), each factor ranked at least one of these statements at +2 or above, indicating an acknowledgement that men engage in bulimic behaviors. Across factors there was also a general agreement that bulimia is a serious issue (36: −2 to −4).

Discussion

This research study explored cultural constructions of bulimia using Q methodology. As is anticipated within social constructionist theory, this investigation found that understandings of bulimia were not confined to one singular account, but made possible through a number of alternate constructions. Further, and in line with the Q methodological principle of finite diversity [29], the number of these constructions was limited, with six distinct but overlapping accounts of bulimia identified.

These constructions differ in a variety of ways, including influencing factors, how bulimic behaviors are positioned, and the extent to which the individual engaging in such behavior is viewed as responsible. By examining the configuration of statements within and across factors, in conjunction with the comments and demographic details of defining participants, a richer and more contextualized account for each factor was produced.

In the perspective of Factor A, entitled "bulimia as uncontrolled behavior", individuals engaging in bulimia lack both control and insight into what they are doing. A potential implication of this construction is that they are unable to stop their behaviour alone, and, therefore, require the intervention of others to recover.

On the other hand, for Factor B, bulimia is not just about behaviour, but is the manifestation of an underlying mental illness. This conceptualization is common in both popular and specialized texts [64] and has been put forward by organizations that are authorities in the area of eating disorders [34]. It is also a position that is taken in Factors D, E, and F; however, Factor B is perhaps the most psychological account among these factors. This construction of bulimia as a dysfunctional coping mechanism is common in the research literature on eating disorders [65,66].

That almost half of the participants defining Factor B were women who reported engaging in bulimic behaviors suggests that these individuals may draw upon this construction to make sense of their own experiences. Perhaps, this is because this account offers a way of understanding bulimia that avoids blaming the individual, by positioning it as something separate from the self and outside normal behavior (a mental illness they carry within them), and gives high priority to emotional/psychological issues and the experience of distress. Thus, an appropriate response to individuals experiencing bulimia is compassion and help. Further, similar to the perspective of Factor A, the potential for a person with bulimia to exert agency, or recover alone from their condition, is foreclosed upon, as it is positioned as something outside of their control.

The other perspective associated with Factor B, defined by only one participant, has exactly the opposite implications. By positioning a person with bulimia as responsible for their condition, and able to recover if they wish, there is an explicit sense of blame not evident in other constructions, and also no implication that people with bulimia deserve sympathy.

For the understanding of bulimia in Factor C, entitled "self-medicating with food", the mood improving qualities of eating are prioritized; this echoes an area of research that explores pleasure and the negative affect regulating capacities of food in bulimia [67,68]. This construction of bulimia positions the person as an agent of their disorder, but does so in a way that effectively minimizes blame (e.g. highlighting the functional aspects of binge eating as necessary mood improver, positioning the person with bulimia as a victim of their culture). As such, this construction might be useful, even emancipatory, for those persons engaged in bulimia, but it would appear that it is not readily drawn upon, as research finds considerable self-blame amongst these individuals [69].

The perspectives of Factors C and D both strongly endorse the influence of culture on bulimia, and particularly the idealization of a thin body; however, they do so to remarkably different effect. For Factor C, bulimic behaviors, in particular purging, are not positioned as especially abnormal or problematic. This can be contrasted with the perspective of Factor D, "the pathological pursuit of thinness", where bulimic behaviors are viewed as unequivocally deviant. This clear-cut difference between normal and abnormal ties into how bulimia is commonly conceptualized in practice, where the categorical nature of diagnosis suggests that eating disorders are "discrete entities, demarcated by firm boundaries between one another and normality" ([31], p. S124). On the other hand this perspective conflicts with both feminist and social constructionist explanations of bulimia, and theoretical models in the research literature that view eating disordered behaviors as existing along a continuum with dieting and normal unrestrained eating (e.g. [70,71]).

The way in which bulimia is pathologized in Factor D may be less beneficial to people engaging in bulimic behaviors than other constructions identified here. Because it strongly connects bulimic behaviors with an extreme obsession with thinness, it positions the person as irrational, potentially even shallow, rather than, for instance, psychologically distressed, and thus worthy of sympathy or support (as in Factor B).

The construction of bulimia in Factor E, entitled "being the best at being thin", there is a more explicit sense of blame, as the person with bulimia is positioned as actively and methodically engaging in behaviors that allow them to stay thin. The endorsement that a certain type of person develops bulimia is also present in research into personality traits and eating disorders [72]. The consistent nature of personality means that the potential for an individual within this construction to change ones behavior is inhibited with this construction.

Finally in the perspective of Factor F, "extreme behavior vs. mentally ill", the issue of responsibility is determined by whether an individual is positioned as having the mental illness bulimia, or is simply engaging in behaviors that are culturally categorized as 'bulimic'. There is a potentially dangerous implication of drawing upon this construction: if bulimic behaviours are not positioned as especially problematic, despite their associated health risk, then the likelihood of seeking help may be minimized.

While there are some points of convergence across a number of these perspectives, they remain fairly distinct. Only two issues were perceived similarly across factors: first that bulimic behaviors are also an issue for men, and second that bulimia is serious. The unanimous positioning of men within a construction of bulimia is interesting, and works against the idea that eating disorders are predominately, or only, an issue for women [5,73]. Thus any of the constructions used here may be readily drawn upon by men engaging in bulimic behaviors to make sense of their experiences. Also, endorsement of the idea that bulimia is serious amongst the defining participants for all factors is encouraging, given the health risks and psychological distress associated with such behaviors.

This research study has demonstrated that there are a multitude of different ways of understanding bulimia and bulimic behaviors. Social constructionist theory suggests that these different constructions are not inert, but have the potential to impact on the practices of those engaged in bulimic behaviors, and on those around them. That is, by providing a lens through which people understand behavior and experience, different constructions may open up or limit the possibility for certain kinds of actions.

The strength of this research lies in its combining of qualitative sensitivity to meaning with robust quantitative statistical analysis, to explore constructions of bulimia. However, it is only a first step. In no way is the sample of participants used in this study representative of the wider population. This is not a major concern for Q methodology, which aims to study constructions in their available diversity, rather than attempting to generalize about the proportions to which these constructions are distributed in the population [74]. However, to more fully explore the *range* of culturally circulating constructions of bulimia, it would be beneficial for future research to use a more diverse sample, in terms of age, gender and cultural background, as well as knowledge and experience of eating disorders. It would also be useful for future researchers to directly examine the relationship between constructions of bulimia and help-seeking behavior, combining Q methodology with other qualitative and quantitative research methods.

Constructions of bulimia will frame not only the experiences of those engaged in bulimic behaviors but also the experiences and behaviors of those around them. As such, it is important for future research to incorporate other stakeholders, such as family members and health professionals who deal with eating disorders. While it is entirely possible that these groups make use of similar constructions to those identified in this study, this is unknown. Indeed individuals sharing a similar socio-historical location in relation to this issue may draw upon one particular construction, as was the case here for women reporting bulimic behaviors defining Factor B; other studies have found similarly, with particular stakeholder groups becoming associated with one factor perspective (e.g. [53]).

Conclusions

In conclusion, this study has shown that bulimia is not understood uniformly in our culture, but is a concept made sense of through a number of alternate constructions. The six constructions of bulimia that have been identified here share some things in common but have important differences too, such as in how much control/responsibility/blame the person is considered to have for their behavior or illness. These constructions potentially have distinct implications for how individuals engaged in bulimic behaviors think and behave, as well as how those around them may respond to them. As such, further study of constructions of bulimia may be able to provide insights into how and why, or why not, individuals seek help for their bulimic behaviors, and also the success of any treatment. While the assumptions of Q methodology hold that no one construction of bulimia is more valid than any other [33], some will certainly be more useful in reaching these goals.

Competing interests

The authors declare that they have no competing interests.

Authors' contributions

KC devised, planned and coordinated the study, with guidance by JP and JMU. KC carried out data collection, performed Q analysis and interpretation and drafted the manuscript, in ongoing consultation with JP and JMU. All authors read, revised and approved the final manuscript.

Acknowledgements

This research was made possible through an Australian Postgraduate Award.

References

1. Hay P, Mond J, Buttner P, Darby A: **Eating disorder behaviors are increasing: findings from two sequential community surveys in South Australia.** *PLoS ONE* 2008, **3**(2):e1541.
2. Hay P: **The epidemiology of eating disorder behaviors: an Australian community-based survey.** *Int J Eat Disorder* 1998, **23**(4):371–382.
3. Hoek HW, van Hoeken D: **Review of the prevalence and incidence of eating disorders.** *Int J Eat Disorder* 2003, **34**(4):383–396.
4. Fairburn CG, Harrison PJ: **Eating disorders.** *Lancet* 2003, **361**(9355):407–416.
5. Striegel-Moore RH, Silberstein LR, Rodin J: **Toward an understanding of risk factors for bulimia.** *Am Psychol* 1986, **41**(3):246–263.
6. Mond JM, Hay PJ, Darby A, Paxton SJ, Quirk F, Buttner P, Owen C, Rodgers B: **Women with bulimic eating disorders: when do they receive treatment for an eating problem?** *J Consult Clin Psych* 2009, **77**(5):835–844.
7. Mond JM, Hay PJ, Rodgers B, Owen C: **Health service utilization for eating disorders: findings from a community-based study.** *Int J Eat Disorder* 2007, **40**(5):399–408.
8. Hepworth N, Paxton SJ: **Pathways to help-seeking in bulimia nervosa and binge eating problems: a concept mapping approach.** *Int J Eat Disorder* 2007, **40**(6):493–504.
9. Pomeroy C, Mitchell JE: **Medical complications of anorexia nervosa and bulimia nervosa.** In *Eating disorders and obesity: a comprehensive handbook.* 2nd edition. Edited by Fairburn CG, Brownell KD. New York: The Guilford Press; 2002:278–285.
10. Kaplan AS, Woodside DB: **Biological aspects of anorexia nervosa and bulimia nervosa.** *J Consult Clin Psych* 1987, **55**(5):645–653.
11. Hay P: **Quality of life and bulimic eating disorder behaviors: findings from a community-based sample.** *Int J Eat Disorder* 2003, **33**(4):434–442.
12. Beumont PJV: **Clinical presentation of anorexia nervosa and bulimia nervosa.** In *Eating disorders and obesity: a comprehensive handbook.* 2nd edition. Edited by Fairburn CG, Brownell KD. New York: The Guilford Press; 2002:162–170.
13. Padierna A, Quintana J, Arostegui I, Gonzalez N, Horcajo M: **The health-related quality of life in eating disorders.** *Qual Life Res* 2000, **9**(6):667–674.
14. Kaye WH: **Neurobiology of anorexia and bulimia nervosa.** *Physiol Behav* 2008, **94**(1):121–135.
15. Cooper MJ, Wells A, Todd G: **A cognitive model of bulimia nervosa.** *Brit J Clin Psychol* 2004, **43**(1):1–16.
16. Vitousek K, Manke F: **Personality variables and disorders in anorexia nervosa and bulimia nervosa.** *J Abnorm Psychol* 1994, **103**(1):137–147.
17. Keel PK, Klump KL: **Are eating disorders culture-bound syndromes? implications for conceptualizing their etiology.** *Psychol Bull* 2003, **129**(5):747–769.
18. Polivy J, Herman CP: **Causes of eating disorders.** *Annu Rev Psychol* 2002, **53**(1):187–213.
19. Striegel-Moore RH, Bulik CM: **Risk factors for eating disorders.** *Am Psychol* 2007, **62**(3):181–198.
20. Davis C: **Eating disorders and hyperactivity: a psychobiological perspective.** *Can J Psychiat* 1997, **42**(2):168–175.
21. Striegel-Moore RH, Cachelin FM: **Etiology of eating disorders in women.** *Counsel Psychol* 2001, **29**(5):635–661.
22. Yardley L: **Reconciling discursive and materialist perspectives on health and illness.** *Theor Psychol* 1996, **6**(3):485–508.
23. Willig C: **A discourse-dynamic approach to the study of subjectivity in health psychology.** *Theor Psychol* 2000, **10**(4):547–570.
24. Theander SS: **Trends in the literature on eating disorders over 36 years (1965–2000): terminology, interpretation and treatment.** *Eur Eat Disord Rev* 2004, **12**(1):4–17.
25. Malson H, Finn DM, Treasure J, Clarke S, Anderson G: **Constructing 'The eating disordered Patient': a discourse analysis of accounts of treatment experiences.** *J Community Appl Soc* 2004, **14**(6):473–489.
26. Gone JP, Kirmayer LJ: **On the wisdom of considering culture and context in psychopathology.** In *Contemporary directions in psychopathology: scientific foundations of the DSM-V and ICD-11.* Edited by Millon T, Krueger RF, Simonsen E. New York: The Guilford Press; 2010:72–96.
27. Breen LJ, Darlaston-Jones D: **Moving beyond the enduring dominance of positivism in psychological research: implications for psychology in Australia.** *Aust Psychol* 2009, **45**(1):67–76.
28. Burr V: *Social constructionism.* 2nd edition. Sussex: Routledge; 2003.
29. Stainton Rogers R: **Q methodology.** In *Rethinking methods in psychology.* Edited by Smith JA, Harré R, Langenhove LV. London: SAGE Publications Ltd; 1995:178–192.
30. Malson H, Swann C: **Prepared for consumption: (Dis) orders of eating and embodiment.** *J Community Appl Soc* 1999, **9**(6):397–405.
31. Wilfley DE, Bishop ME, Wilson GT, Agras WS: **Classification of eating disorders: toward DSM-V.** *Int J Eat Disorder* 2007, **40**(Suppl 3):123–129.
32. Malson H, Burns M: **Re-theorising the slash of dis/order: an introduction to critical feminist approaches to eating dis/orders.** In *Critical feminist approaches to eating dis/orders.* Edited by Malson H, Burns M. East Sussex: Routledge; 2009:1–6.
33. Stainton Rogers R, Stainton Rogers W: **What the Brits got out of the Q: and why their work may not line up with the american way of getting into it.** *Electron J Commun* 1990, **1**(1):1–11.
34. Klump KL, Bulik CM, Kaye WH, Treasure J, Tyson E: **Academy for eating disorders position paper: eating disorders are serious mental illnesses.** *Int J Eat Disorder* 2009, **42**(2):97–103.
35. Lafrance MN: *Women and depression: recovery and resistance.* East Sussex: Routledge; 2009.
36. Lafrance MN: **A bitter pill: a discursive analysis of Women's medicalized accounts of depression.** *J Health Psychol* 2007, **12**(1):127–140.
37. Crisp AH, Gelder MG, Rix S, Meltzer HI, Rowlands OJ: **Stigmatisation of people with mental illnesses.** *Brit J Psychiat* 2000, **177**(1):4–7.
38. Burns M: **Eating like an ox: femininity and dualistic constructions of bulimia and anorexia.** *Fem Psychol* 2004, **14**(2):269–295.
39. Cooper T: **Anorexia and bulimia: the political and the personal.** In *Fed up and hungry: women, oppression and food.* Edited by Lawrence M. London: The Women's Press; 1987:175–192.
40. Squire S: **Anorexia and bulimia: purity and danger.** *Aust Feminist Stud* 2003, **18**(40):17–26.
41. Burns M, Gavey N: **'Healthy weight'at what cost? 'Bulimia'and a discourse of weight control.** *J Health Psychol* 2004, **9**(4):549–565.
42. Bordo S: *Unbearable weight: feminism, western culture, and the body.* Berkeley: University of California Press; 1993.
43. Malson H: *The thin woman: feminism, post-structuralism and the social psychology of anorexia nervosa.* London: Routledge; 1998.
44. Squire S: **The personal and the political: writing the theorist's body.** *Aust Feminist Stud* 2002, **17**(37):55–64.
45. Brown SR: **Q methodology and qualitative research.** *Qual Health Res* 1996, **6**(4):561–567.
46. Watts S, Stenner P: **Doing Q methodology: theory, method and interpretation.** *Qual Res Psychol* 2005, **2**(1):67–91.
47. Stephenson W: **The inverted factor technique.** *Brit J Psychol Gen Sect* 1936, **26**(4):344–361.
48. Dennis KE, Goldberg AP: **Weight control self-efficacy types and transitions affect weight-loss outcomes in obese women.** *Addict Behav* 1996, **21**(1):103–116.
49. Cross RM: **Exploring attitudes: the case for Q methodology.** *Health Educ Res* 2005, **20**(2):206–213.
50. Addams H, Proops JLR: *Social discourse and environmental policy: an application of Q methodology.* Northampton, MA: Edward Elgar Publishing; 2000.
51. Watts S, Stenner P: *Doing Q methodological research: theory, method & interpretation.* London: SAGE Publications Ltd; 2012.
52. Stenner P, Dancey CP, Watts S: **The understanding of their illness amongst people with irritable bowel syndrome: a Q methodological study.** *Soc Sci Med* 2000, **51**(3):439–452.
53. Perz J, Ussher J, Gilbert E: **Constructions of sex and intimacy after cancer: Q methodology study of people with cancer, their partners, and health professionals.** *BMC Cancer* 2013, **13**(1):270.
54. Harvey H, Good J, Mason J, Reissland N: **A Q-methodology study of parental understandings of infant immunisation: implications for health-care advice.** *J Health Psychol* 2013, **0**(0):1–12.
55. Stenner P, Watts S, Worrell M: **Q methodology.** In *The SAGE handbook of qualitative research in psychology.* Edited by Willig C, Stainton-Rogers W. London: SAGE Publications Ltd; 2008:215–239.
56. Stephenson W: **The foundations of psychometry: four factor systems.** *Psychometrika* 1936, **1**(3):195–209.
57. Curt BC: *Textuality and tectonics: troubling social and psychological science.* Buckingham: Open University Press; 1994.
58. McKeown B, Thomas D: *Q methodology: quantitative applications in the social sciences.* Newbury Park, CA: SAGE Publications Ltd.; 1988.

59. Shemmings D: **'Quantifying' qualitative data: an illustrative example of the use of Q methodology in psychosocial research.** *Qual Res Psychol* 2006, **3**(2):147–165.
60. **Q-assessor.** [http://q-assessor.com/]
61. Brown SR: *Political subjectivity: applications of Q methodology in political science.* New Haven, CT: Yale University Press; 1980.
62. Antretter E, Dunkel D, Haring C, Corcoran P, De Leo D, Fekete S, Hawton K, Kerkhof AJ, Lönnqvist J, Renberg ES: **The factorial structure of the suicide intent scale: a comparative study in clinical samples from 11 european regions.** *Int J Meth Psych Res* 2008, **17**(2):63–79.
63. Hsu LKG: **The gender gap in eating disorders: Why are the eating disorders more common among women?** *Clin Psychol Rev* 1989, **9**(3):393–407.
64. **National Eating Disorder Collaboration: Bulimia Nervosa Fact Sheet.** 2011, [http://www.nedc.com.au/files/logos/0638_NEDC_FS_BN_v4.pdf]
65. Troop NA: **Eating disorders as coping strategies: a critique.** *Eur Eat Disord Rev* 1998, **6**(4):229–237.
66. Rorty M, Yager J: **Histories of childhood trauma and complex post-traumatic sequelae in women with eating disorders.** *Psychiat Clin N Am* 1996, **19**(4):773–791.
67. Christensen L: **Effects of eating behavior on mood: a review of the literature.** *Int J Eat Disorder* 1993, **14**(2):171–183.
68. Johnson C, Larson R: **Bulimia: an analysis of moods and behavior.** *Psychosom Med* 1982, **44**(4):341–351.
69. Troop NA, Holbrey A, Treasure JL: **Stress, coping, and crisis support in eating disorders.** *Int J Eat Disorder* 1998, **24**(2):157–166.
70. Polivy J, Herman CP: **Diagnosis and treatment of normal eating.** *J Consult Clin Psych* 1987, **55**(5):635–644.
71. Mintz LB, O'Halloran MS, Mulholland AM, Schneider PA: **Questionnaire for eating disorder diagnoses: reliability and validity of operationalizing DSM—IV criteria into a self-report format.** *J Couns Psychol* 1997, **44**(1):63–79.
72. Cassin SE, von Ranson KM: **Personality and eating disorders: a decade in review.** *Clin Psychol Rev* 2005, **25**(7):895–916.
73. Drummond MJN: **Men, body image, and eating disorders.** *Int J Men's Health* 2002, **1**(1):89.
74. Stainton Rogers W: *Explaining health and illness: an exploration of diversity.* Harvester Wheatsheaf: Hemel Hempstead; 1991.

9

Emotion dysregulation, self-image and eating disorder symptoms in University Women

Elin Monell[1,2*], Louise Högdahl[1], Emma Forsén Mantilla[1] and Andreas Birgegård[1]

Abstract

Background: We studied associations between emotion dysregulation, self-image and eating disorder (ED) symptoms in university women, and contrasted two indirect effect models to examine possible intervening mechanisms to produce ED symptoms.

Methods: 252 female Swedish university students completed the Difficulties in Emotion Regulation Scale (DERS), the Structural Analysis of Social Behavior (SASB) self-image measure, and the Eating Disorder Examination Questionnaire (EDE-Q). Correlations between scales were followed by five simple mediation analysis pairs with two possible pathways using five ED symptom variables as outcome. The models posited either self-image or emotion dysregulation as mediator or independent variable, respectively. ED symptoms were EDE-Q Global score, objective binge eating episodes (OBE), subjective binge eating episodes (SBE), and two variants of EDE-Q excessive exercise.

Results: Emotion dysregulation and self-image were strongly correlated, and both correlated moderately with EDE-Q Global score. There were distinct indirect effects through self-image on the relationship between emotion dysregulation and ED symptoms, but not vice versa. These indirect effects were evident in relation to cognitive ED symptoms and both OBE and SBE, but not in relation to excessive exercise.

Conclusions: Results suggest that even if closely related, emotion dysregulation and self-image both contribute unique knowledge in relation to ED symptoms. Self-image as an intervening mechanism between emotion dysregulation and ED symptoms is relevant for models of the development, maintenance and treatment of ED, as well as treatment focus.

Keywords: Eating disorders, Emotion dysregulation, Self-image, Mediation, DERS

Background

Eating disorders (EDs) are relatively common among young women. A recent cohort-based study using Swedish population and healthcare registers found that adolescence is a high-risk period for the development of an ED, where the incidence of any ED by 2009 was 457.4 cases per 100,000 persons in the peak 16–17 year old age category in women [1]. A recent meta-analysis of community- and health-care based studies on prevalence of EDs found that the expected lifetime prevalence for any ED in women varies between 4.3 and 8.6 % depending on diagnosis and diagnostic criteria [2]. A comprehensive understanding of the etiology and maintenance of EDs is yet to be developed. Many researchers emphasize emotion regulation as important to move forward, although the longitudinal data needed for causal models is as yet largely lacking [3–5]. The present study related ED symptoms to emotion regulation and self-image, two factors previously shown to be related to ED when examined separately [6–8]. Briefly, emotion regulation is the ability to make sense of and manage one's emotions, and self-image is an organizing principle guiding habitual intrapersonal behavior and interpretation of and responses in social interaction. Both emotion regulation

* Correspondence: elin.monell@ki.se
[1]Department of Clinical Neuroscience, Karolinska Institute, Norra Stationsgatan 69 7th floor, 113 64 Stockholm, Sweden
[2]Centre for Research & Development, Uppsala University/Region Gävleborg, Uppsala, Sweden

and self-image are thought to be formed in interaction with significant others [9, 10], and both relate to social behavior and self-directed behavior, suggesting that the constructs might be interconnected or partly overlapping. Emotion regulation and self-image have been proposed to contribute to both development and maintenance of EDs [11–13]. However, the interrelationships between emotion regulation, self-image and EDs are currently unclear.

Emotion regulation

Emotion regulation refers to the acquired ability to recognize, understand, and accept one's emotions, as well as strategies to modulate the experience and expression of emotions in line with long-term goals and values [14]. This ability develops over time, and early childhood interactions with caregivers seem to be of great importance [10, 15]. Emotion dysregulation is suggested to be a central factor in the development and maintenance of various problematic behaviors like self-harm and violence towards others, where the most comprehensive theoretical work is Linehan's bio-psychosocial model of emotion dysregulation in borderline personality disorder (BPD) [16]. This model has also been used to describe similar processes in anorexia nervosa (AN) [3]. The model describes the development of emotion dysregulation as a transactional process between individual emotional vulnerabilities and invalidating responses from the social and family environment [15, 17]. Individual emotional vulnerability consists of relatively stable influences of temperamental affective tendencies (e.g. emotional sensitivity, reactivity, and time needed to recover from emotional events) as well as more transient factors related to sleeping habits, diet, physical health, etc. Invalidating response relates to interpersonal interactions where an individual's emotional and cognitive experiences are overlooked, misunderstood, or criticized by others. A vicious circle of vulnerability and invalidation where increased emotional arousal, and ensuing increased difficulty to accurately communicate emotional states, then risks maintaining and reinforcing emotion dysregulation and usage of dysfunctional regulatory strategies, for example self-harm in BPD patients [3, 15]. In sum, unfortunate transactional processes over time are thought to create pervasive trait-like patterns of emotion dysregulation. In everyday life, high intensity and/or long duration of emotional arousal tend to heighten the risk of emotion dysregulation in response to everyday emotional events [3].

Emotion dysregulation and EDs

The ability to identify and describe emotions is decreased among women with EDs [4, 18]. There is evidence for the BPD model of emotion dysregulation in AN, with respect to both individual vulnerabilities such as emotional sensitivity and reactivity, as well as experiences of invalidating response [3]. Women with EDs are also more likely to use dysfunctional regulation strategies such as rumination and suppression in response to negative affect [11, 19]. Fairburn, Zafran and Cooper suggest an inability to cope with intense emotional states as a transdiagnostic feature in some ED-patients and also state that ED behaviors may serve as maladaptive forms of emotion regulation, comparable to the use of self-harm in BPD [20]. The most widespread theory on the function of ED-behaviors suggests that binge eating, with or without subsequent purging, provides distraction from or amelioration of painful inner states, negatively reinforcing the behavior [20, 21]. In line with this theory, several experimental studies have found that negative mood precedes episodes of binge eating among women with bulimia nervosa (BN) [22, 23], binge eating disorder (BED) [24–26], and non-clinical women [27], even though the ameliorative functon of binge eating is yet to be consistently experimentally shown [28]. There is some support that restricting behaviors and excessive exercise may serve a similar function as suggested for binge eating [29, 30].

However, the relation between emotion dysregulation and EDs is still unclear, partly since conceptualizations and measurements of emotion dysregulation have differed in previous research. A growing number of ED researchers have used the Difficulties in Emotion Regulation Scale (DERS), measuring difficulties in awareness, acceptance and understanding of emotions, as well as lack of strategies to manage emotions, control impulses and problems engaging in goal-directed behavior while in distress. Recent studies using the DERS show that for women with either AN or BN, more ED symptoms was significantly correlated with more emotion dysregulation [6, 31]. Other studies show that individuals with AN or BN have significantly more difficulties with all DERS aspects compared to healthy comparison groups [7, 32, 33], and that higher DERS scores (i.e. more emotion dysregulation) after AN treatment predicted maintenance of AN psychopathology over time [34]. In addition, more ED symptoms were related to higher DERS scores in an ED group, a healthy comparison group, and two psychiatric groups [12], as well as in groups of healthy young women [35, 36].

Emotion regulation and self-image

Interpersonal factors that impact emotion regulation are increasingly in focus in ED research. For example, two recent meta-studies found that aspects of interpersonal difficulties affecting emotion regulation may serve as maintaining factors for EDs, these difficulties including for example the avoidance of expressing feelings to others, interpersonal distrust, more negative interactions with others, insecure attachment and perceived social inferiority [18, 37]. As indicated, the term "interpersonal" includes not only patterns of interaction with others, but also intrapsychic experiences related to self and others. A fruitful approach, not utilized in previous research, may then be to study emotion regulation within an interpersonal framework, drawing on theory concerning how the sense of self is formed and maintained in a social context. Such theoretical approaches can be found in the field of interpersonal theory, where self-image is a central concept [38].

Self-image is mainly described as self-directed behaviour, i.e. how an individual treats him-/herself. These behaviours will have cognitive, emotional and social implications since the self-image will guide how interactions with others are perceived and interpreted by the individual [39]. Further, people tend to behave in ways that evokes responses from others that are in line with the self-image, leading to its confirmation and preservation [9]. According to theory, the self-image is developed over time when patterns of social interaction are introjected, i.e. the way others (especially attachment figures) treat you will model your future self-treatment [9]. An individual's emotional vulnerabilities, as noted from theories on emotion regulation, will affect others' responses. This may in turn affect the sense of self as capable or deficient, as worthy of care, encouragement, criticism, or neglect. This self-view will likely impact emotional experiences and their expression, leading to a transactional and mutually reinforcing development of emotion regulation strategies and self-image, in an interpersonal context.

Self-image and EDs

Self-evaluation, especially measured as self-esteem, in ED patients has been studied before where ED patients frequently evaluate themselves more negatively than healthy comparison groups [18]. Other aspects of self-evaluation studied in relation to EDs are for example self-efficacy, self-directedness and self concept [40, 41]. The Structural Analysis of Social Behavior (SASB) is a model of self-image (and social behavior) based on interpersonal theory [42]. According to the SASB, the self-image has both trait and state aspects: there is considerable stability in self-image and evidence of associations with relationships to early significant others, but there is also variability in response to current stressors and situations [43–45], as exemplified by the fact that self-report is sometimes used with instructions to rate the self-image "at best" and "at worst" [46]. The SASB self-image thus differs from other self-related concepts in going beyond self-evaluation and self-directed feelings, to also include self-directed behavior and the implications of self-image for social behavior.

The SASB model (and its set of measurements) organize self-image in a circumplex with two dimensions: horizontal *Affiliation* axis ranging from self-love to self-attack and vertical *Autonomy* axis from enmeshment to differentiation. A positive self-image (predominantly self-love) is characterized by self-affirmation, self-love and self-protection whereas a negative self-image (predominantly self-attack) is characterized by self-blame, self-attack and self-neglect.

ED research using the SASB has found that patients with an ED have a more negative self-image compared to healthy and subclinically depressed comparison groups [8]. Initial SASB self-attack among ED patients further predicted treatment outcome after 3 years, being a stronger predictor than initial ED symptoms, general psychopathology, interpersonal relationships, and occupational status [47]. Specific self-image aspects also predicted outcome in different ED diagnoses [13] as well as treatment dropout [48]. Specific self-image aspects relate much more strongly to ED symptoms in young adolescent ED patients than in healthy young adolescents, a pattern also evident in older female adolescents and young women (the latter result was partly based on the same sample as the present study) [49, 50]. Also, relevant for outcomes relating to emotion dysregulation research, self-image has shown associations with suicidal behavior in ED patients [51].

Aim

In summary, interactions with significant others are an important way to acquire emotion regulation strategies, while at the same time, emotion regulation affects how such interactions occur. Interactions with others over time also model self-image, defined as internal self-directed behaviour, which from a here-and-now perspective has cognitive, emotional and social implications. Previous research has found significant connections between EDs and both emotion dysregulation and self-image when examined separately. As described, both emotion dysregulation and self-image develop over time starting in early childhood, with likely intertwined developmental paths. They may be risk factors for later ED development, and may impact ED symptoms in the present by emotion regulation affecting one's sense of self, which may impact ED symptoms, or the sense of self may affect emotion regulation, which in turn impacts ED symptoms.

No previous research has examined the association between self-image and emotion dysregulation. The aim of the present study was to do this and to associate both concepts to ED symptoms. We aimed to investigate which theoretical model best fits the data by contrasting two possible models to evaluate indirect effects (mediation): self-image as a mechanism for emotion regulation, or emotion regulation as a mechanism for self-image, to produce each of five different types of ED symptoms. Knowledge in this area may inform prevention and etiological models by suggesting hypotheses concerning mechanisms of vulnerability and how they are expressed during development, and what symptoms are likely to ensue. Also, findings may have implications for treatment efforts, by identifying more proximal and distal intervention targets to ameliorate symptoms.

Method

Participants

The sample consisted of 252 female Swedish university students with a mean age of 23.7 years (*SD* 3.58, range 19–35) and a mean BMI of 22.4 (*SD* 3.68, range 15.6–44.4). 374 students were given questionnaires whereof 288 (77 %) completed participation (i.e. returned the completed questionnaires). Thirty-six of these (12.5 %) were excluded prior to analysis: eight due to missing data (one without background information, seven with missing data for too many items on single instruments) and 28 due to age >35 years (this maximum age was decided *a priori* to match the sample to typical clinical ED populations). No final participant had more than two missing items for any one instrument. Since variables from the relevant measures could be computed with some missing items no imputation of data was conducted. Of the final sample, 181 (71.8 %) participants were recruited at lectures, 34 (13.5 %) at fixed occasions for drop in participation, and 37 (14.7 %) by advertisement around the campus area. There were no significant differences between subsamples depending on recruitment method on any variable (all ANOVA and post hoc p's > .05, data not shown).

Instruments

Eating Disorder Examination Questionnaire (EDE-Q, version 4.0) was used to assess ED symptoms [52]. The EDE-Q contains 36 items focused on the past 28 days and provides a Global score, four subscales (Eating concern, Shape concern, Weight concern, Restraint), and information regarding ED behavior. The Global score, where higher scores indicate more severe eating pathology, is used as an outcome for cognitive ED symptoms. The other outcomes were the following ED behavior items: presence/absence of objective binge eating episodes (OBEs), subjective binge eating episodes (SBEs), and excessive exercise. OBEs are defined as reporting rapidly eating objectively large amounts of food combined with loss of control over eating. SBEs are defined as loss of control but not eating large amounts. Excessive exercise is defined as intense exercise with the purpose to control weight or shape. We included both presence/absence of excessive exercise, as well as frequency of excessive exercise ≥ twice/week corresponding to the diagnostic cut-off in DSM-IV for BN. The latter was included in order to test exercise at diagnostic criterion level since any episodes of excessive exercise was reported by a substantial proportion of participants. We did not include vomiting as an outcome since only 11 participants (4.4 %) reported this behavior, and even fewer reported diuretic and laxative use (four participants for each). The EDE-Q has good psychometric properties [53], with satisfactory concurrent validity [52, 54], acceptable temporal stability and acceptable internal consistency [53, 55]. The Swedish version of the EDE-Q has shown satisfactory validity and acceptable reliability [56]. Mean Cronbach's α for the EDE-Q subscales in the present sample was .84 (range .81–.91).

Difficulties in Emotion Regulation Scale (DERS) consists of 36 items measuring aspects of emotion dysregulation, and provides a Total score and six subscales (Non-acceptance, Goals, Impulse, Awareness, Strategies, Clarity) [14]. The Total score, where higher scores indicate more difficulties with emotion regulation, is used in the statistical analysis. In its original form, the items in each subscale are summed to calculate the scores and the subscale scores are then summed to calculate the Total score. Since the subscales consist of different numbers of items and sums are therefore difficult to compare, we used mean scores that are comparable and interpretable in terms of the response scale metric, and the Total score was calculated as the average of the subscale scores. The DERS has shown good internal consistency and good test-retest reliability [14]. The DERS was translated from English to Swedish for the present study, using two independent translators (authors EM and AB) as well as back-translation from Swedish to English by a native English speaker. Preliminary factor analysis results for the current sample fairly reproduced the six-factor structure of the original (Birgegard: Factor structure of a Swedish version of the Difficulties in Emotion Regulation Scale, in preparation). Mean Cronbach's α for the DERS subscales in the present sample was .84 (range .75–.90).

Structural Analysis of Social Behavior introject, Swedish version 2.0 (SASB intrex version 3rd surface, self-image) was used to assess self-image [57]. The SASB introject consists of 36 items operationalizing self-directed behavior and attitudes. Responses form eight variables (clusters), six of which form the Affiliation score (by weighting the variables according to their proximity to the horizontal axis and dividing by the sum of the weights). SASB Affiliation is used in the statistical analysis and ranges from −100 to 100 where scores below zero indicate more self-directed attack and scores above zero indicate more self-directed love. The English language version of SASB intrex has shown good reliability and internal consistency [57]. The Swedish version of SASB intrex is highly consistent with the American version

(Armelius et al., unpublished manuscript, 1993) and has shown good internal consistency (Armelius, unpublished manuscript, 2001). Mean Cronbach's α for variables used to compute the SASB Affiliation score in the present sample was .78, range .65–.86.

Procedure

Questionnaires were administrated as a booklet in the following order: informed consent and contact details, questions about age, height, and weight, SASB, DERS and EDE-Q followed by four additional questionnaires not included in the present study. Time for participation was estimated to 30–40 min. Participants who were recruited at lectures got the booklet and a postage paid envelope, those who responded to advertisements emailed their address and were sent the materials, and recruitment information about the study was equated. Occasions for drop in on-site participation (at a university department) were announced by bulk email and on notice boards. All participants gave informed consent regarding storage and use of data, and were rewarded by gift certificate (approx. 15 USD) or course credit. The study was approved by the Stockholm Regional Ethics Review board (2013/243-31/3).

Statistical analysis

Statistical analyses were performed in SPSS Statistics version 21.0 for Mac. Scale correlations were Pearson r for continuous measures, point biserial coefficients (r_{pb}) when one variable was dichotomous, and the phi coefficient (r_{φ}) for two dichotomous variables, all interpreted the same. Simple mediation analysis with two possible pathways was conducted to evaluate indirect effects, using the PROCESS macro for SPSS by Hayes, Model 4 (mediation of independent variable X on outcome Y by mediator M) [58]. Following guidelines provided by Hayes, all mediation analyses were conducted using unstandardized variables. Therefore the pathway coefficients calculated by PROCESS are expressed in the metric of the variables. The first pathway posited DERS Total score as X and SASB Affiliation as M, and the second pathway did the opposite. Five model pairs with five different (ED-related) outcomes (Y) were tested: 1) EDE-Q Global score (EDE-Q), 2) presence/absence of OBEs, 3) presence/absence of SBEs, 4) excessive exercise ≥ twice/week (Regular EE), and 5) any excessive exercise (Any EE). The first outcome, EDE-Q Global score, was continuous and the other four were dichotomous. PROCESS is based on ordinary least squares regression for mediation models with continuous outcomes and logistic regression for dichotomous outcomes. Statistical inference for potential indirect effects was conducted through bias-corrected bootstrap confidence intervals based on 10.000 bootstrap samples [59]. The effect size for indirect effect (mediation path) for the continuous outcome model was Preacher and Kelley's Kappa-squared (κ^2) [60], ranging from 0 to 1, where small ≥ .01, moderate ≥ .09, and large effect size ≥ .25 conventions are applicable. Effect sizes for indirect effects with dichotomous outcomes are not available.

Results

Sample characteristics and scale correlations

Correlations between measures used in the indirect effect (mediation) models are shown in Table 1. Emotion dysregulation and self-image were strongly negatively correlated, and both correlated moderately with cognitive ED symptoms (EDE-Q Global score). All DERS subscales were also significantly correlated to EDE-Q Global Score ($r = .117$ to .369, not shown in Table 1). For the behavior-related ED variables, 47 (18.7 %) of all participants reported objective binge eating episodes, 61 (24.2 %) reported subjective binge eating episodes, 47 (18.7 %) reported regular excessive exercise, and 90 (35.7 %) reported any excessive exercise. All behavior-related ED variables correlated significantly with EDE-Q Global Score, but only the binge eating variables correlated significantly with emotion dysregulation and self-image. Since a significant correlation is not required for mediation analysis according to recent literature [61], all were tested for indirect effects.

Indirect effect (mediation) models

Results for the indirect effect (mediation) models are reported in unstandardized metric. The first pathway (where emotion dysregulation as X indirectly influenced the five different ED-variables as Y through its effect on self-image as M) had bias-corrected bootstrap confidence intervals for the indirect effect entirely above zero for three models (Table 2). Those models were the ones with outcome 1) EDE-Q Global score, 2) OBE, and 3) SBE. Coefficients are presented in Figs. 1, 2 and 3, where all unstandardized coefficients are expressed in the metric of the dependent variable, except for path a, which is expressed in the metric of the mediator. Standardized coefficients computed by regression analysis are presented in parentheses alongside their unstandardized counterparts in the figures.

For the model with outcome 1 (Fig. 1), the more emotion dysregulation, the less positive self-image, and the higher degree of ED symptoms. There was a moderate indirect effect of emotion dysregulation through self-image on ED symptoms (indirect effect, path ab: $\kappa^2 = .204$), but emotion dysregulation did not influence degree of ED symptoms independent of its effect on self-image (direct effect, path c'). For models with outcomes 2 (Fig. 2) and 3 (Fig. 3), emotion dysregulation indirectly influenced both OBE and SBE through its effect on self-image. Again,

Table 1 Descriptive statistics and Pearson correlations (r for 1–3, r_{ob} for 1–3 vs. 4–6, and r_{φ} for 4–6) and correlations (all including 4–7) among emotion dysregulation, self-image and eating disorder symptom variables

	M (SD); range	EDE-Q	DERS.	SASB	OBEs	SBEs	Reg. EE
EDE-Q	1.65 (1.21); 0–5.32	–					
DERS	2.32 (.58); 1.01–4.01	.391***	–				
SASB	41.93 (29.45); –47.3–96.8	–.462***	–.717***	–			
OBEs	–	.486***	.257***	–.317***	–		
SBEs	–	.532***	.212**	–.266***	.441***	–	
Reg. EE	–	.290***	.027	–.036	.029	.130*	–
Any EE	–	.323***	.096	–.087	.071	.178**	.642***

EDE-Q Eating Disorder Examination Questionnaire Global Score; *DERS* Difficulties in Emotion Regulation Scale Total score; *SASB* Structural Analysis of Social Behavior Affiliation Score; *OBE* Objective Binge eating Episodes; *SBE* Subjective Binge eating Episodes; *Reg. EE* Regular Excessive Exercise; *Any EE* Any Excessive Exercise

Note: * = $p < .05$, ** = $p < .01$, *** = $p < .001$

emotion dysregulation did not significantly influence OBE or SBE episodes independent of its effect on self-image.

The bias-corrected bootstrap confidence intervals for the indirect effect of the models with outcome 4) Regular EE, and 5) Any EE both included zero (–.391 to .626 and -.342 to .563, respectively) and thus were not supported. Similarly, all indirect effect confidence intervals for models positing self-image as independent (X) and emotion dysregulation as mediator (M) included zero (Table 3).

Discussion

The study examined the association between self-image, emotion dysregulation, and ED symptoms, and investigated which theoretical model best fits the data by contrasting two possible indirect effect (mediation) models. We found significant correlations between ED symptoms and emotion dysregulation and negative self-image, respectively. Emotion dysregulation was also highly correlated with self-image, suggesting that these constructs are closely related. The results however suggested that both contribute unique knowledge in relation to ED symptoms: there were distinct indirect effects through self-image on the relationship between emotion dysregulation and ED symptoms in university women. No direct effect of emotion dysregulation on ED symptoms was found, suggesting that emotion dysregulation has its effect via self-image as an intervening variable. As for the alternate model, no indirect effect through emotion dysregulation was found for the relationship between self-image and ED symptoms.

The indirect effects were evident for cognitive ED symptoms and for presence/absence of both objective and subjective binge eating, but not for excessive exercise. This may be because exercise reported in this sample might be related more to positive and healthy motivations, not being as symptomatic as the much less frequent binge eating. Although the exercise item asks about intense exercise with the purpose to control weight or shape, exercise responses may have a different quality in a non-clinical group than in clinical samples. Although significant, correlations between both exercise variables and EDE-Q Global score were weaker than those of the binge-eating variables. Binge eating as measured here therefore may be a more disordered behavior, and thus more representative of ED symptoms in this sample. As noted, we could not however test purging due to relative rarity of the behavior. It would be important therefore to examine possible indirect effects in relation to these behaviors in a clinical ED sample, where purging is more frequent and exercise may be more compulsive and symptomatic in nature.

The significant relationship between ED symptoms and emotion dysregulation measured by the DERS are in

Table 2 Mediation models summary: DERS as independent (X), SASB as mediator (M), and five different ED-related measures as dependent variables (outcomes; Y)

Outcome variable	Total effect (*c*)	SE	*p*	Direct effect (*c'*)	SE	*p*	Indirect effect (*ab*)	SE	95 % CIs
EDE-Q Global score (EDE-Q)	.810	.128	<.001	.253	.188	.180	.558	.127	.312 to .807
Objective binge eating episodes (OBE)	1.082	.278	<.001	.252	.400	.529	.840	.291	.315 to 1.448
Subjective binge eating episodes (SBE)	.822	.252	.001	.166	.362	.646	.659	.282	.141 to 1.259
Regular excessive exercise (Reg. EE)	.117	.275	.670	.007	.396	.985	.109	.260	–.391 to .626
Any excessive exercise (Any EE)	.343	.225	.128	.248	.323	.444	.095	.228	–.342 to .563

All coefficients are unstandardized and expressed in the metric of the outcome variable

CIs = bias-corrected bootstrapped confidence intervals based on 10000 bootstrap samples

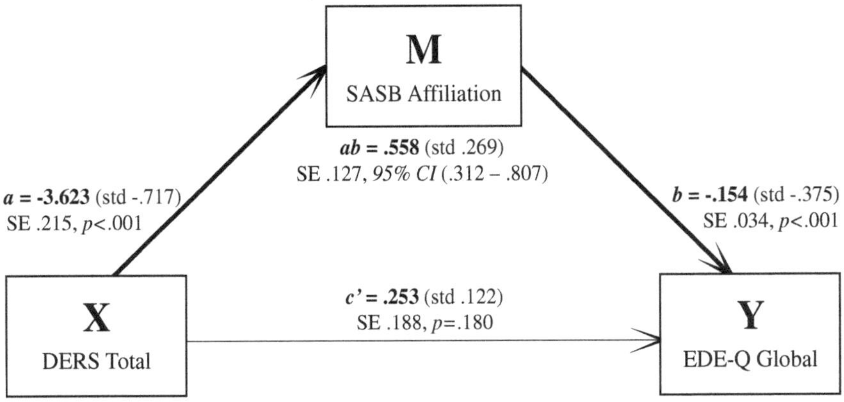

Fig. 1 Unstandardized and standardized coefficients mediation model 1; DERS Total score as independent (X), SASB Affiliation score as mediator (M), and EDE-Q Global score as dependent (Y). N = 252. SE = Standard Error. 95 % CI = 95 % Confidence Interval

line with previous research in both clinical and healthy samples [7, 33, 36]. Higher levels of emotion dysregulation as related to more ED symptoms seem to be a robust finding across several studies including this one. There is also a large body of research relating aspects of emotion dysregulation, such as reduced ability to identify and describe emotions and usage of dysfunctional strategies to regulate emotions, to the presence of ED symptoms [3–5, 11]. In relation to the theories on ED behavior, in particular binge eating, as maladaptive emotion regulation strategies [20, 21], our results did show significant, although rather weak, relationships between emotion dysregulation and binge eating. Lastly, there are hypotheses that emotion dysregulation may both precede and maintain ED [3, 11, 19]. Our results, being based on self-reported cross-sectional data, cannot clarify causality but are consistent with emotion dysregulation as important for ED symptoms, even in this non-clinical sample.

The significant relationship between ED symptoms and self-image measured by the SASB is also in line with previous research, where a more negative self-image was associated with more ED symptomatology in both clinical and healthy samples of different ages [8, 49, 50]. Our result of negative self-image being related to more ED symptoms is also in line with results from studies using related but less complex measures of different types of self-evaluation [18, 40]. In a broader perspective, our results on ED symptoms and self-image, being a concept of interpersonal origin, are also consistent with the notion that interpersonal factors are relevant for development and expression of ED [18, 37].

As for the conceptual and theoretical similarities between emotion dysregulation and self-image presented in the introduction [9, 18, 37, 39], the strong significant correlation between the DERS and the SASB indicates that they are indeed closely related. The findings regarding indirect effects may further suggest a hypothesis that emotion regulation is a more basic vulnerability factor that affects self-treatment. Although these factors are likely to evolve interactively, emotion regulation may be

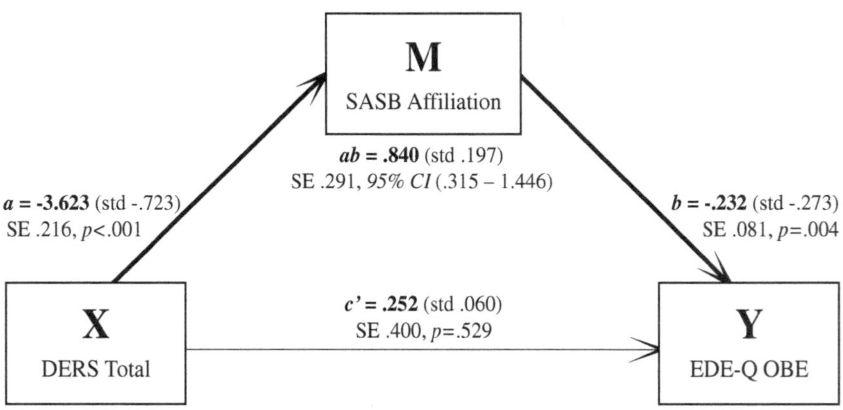

Fig. 2 Unstandardized and standardized coefficients mediation model 2; DERS Total score as independent (X), SASB Affiliation score as mediator (M), and EDE-Q Objective Binge eating Episodes as dependent (Y). N = 248. SE = Standard Error. 95 % CI = 95 % Confidence Interval

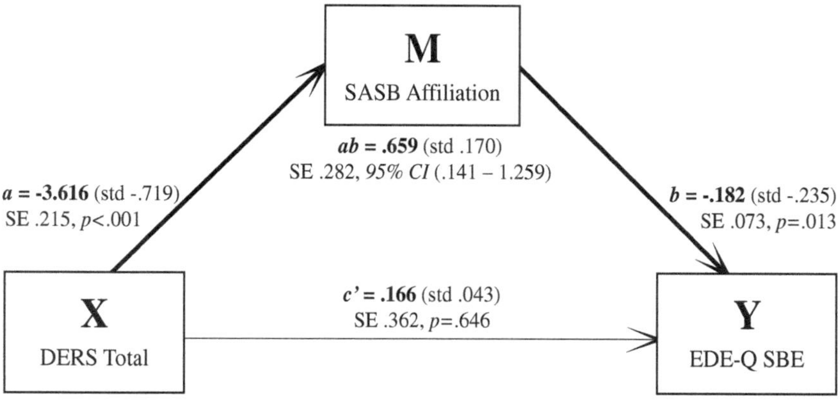

Fig. 3 Unstandardized and standardized coefficients mediation model 3; DERS Total score as independent (X), SASB Affiliation score as mediator (M), and EDE-Q Subjective Binge eating Episodes as dependent (Y). N = 248. SE = Standard Error. 95 % CI = 95 % Confidence Interval

a lower-level set of skills and self-image a higher-level set of conceptions of the worth and capabilities of oneself as a person, analogous perhaps to how throwing a ball relies on individual muscles in the arm and torso, but whose subjective relevance relates to length and accuracy of the throw.

Taken at face value, our findings indicate that a young woman with difficulties regulating emotions is vulnerable to ED symptoms if those difficulties negatively impact her self-image, but that emotion dysregulation per se will not lead to ED symptoms. For example, intense disappointment or feelings of rejection may lead to negative self-appraisal concerning weight and shape, and possibly binge eating as a problematic means of regulating the emotion, if it arises in the context of habitual self-blame, self-attack and lack of self-affirmation. If such factors are not present, our findings indicate that ED symptoms are less likely to occur. Importantly also, the SASB self-image measure operationalizes self-directed behavior, and not merely evaluations, attitudes or cognitions. Thus, ED symptoms may be construed, given our data, as negative self-treatment arising in the context of negative emotion that cannot be regulated adaptively. Besides affecting the individual, such a process will most likely have interpersonal consequences. Building on the transactional nature of emotion regulation proposed by Linehan [16], ED symptoms are unlikely to be met by others as an accurate expression of the emotion that triggered them. Instead, others may signal worry, frustration, or irritation (i.e. invalidating responses). This might give rise to feelings of guilt and alienation that, building on interpersonal theory [9, 39], could confirm a negative self-image. These kinds of processes could contribute to the increased social vulnerability experienced by individuals with EDs [18, 37], as well as exacerbating the risk of negative emotional arousal in new situations [3]. While broadly consistent with developmental models of psychopathology stressing interactions between temperamental traits (e.g. emotional vulnerability) and relational processes [3, 15, 17], this description is speculative and requires further refinement and research.

Implications

Our findings may indicate targets for treatment and prevention of ED. The indirect effects suggest for example that emotion regulation training, suggested as an important treatment intervention [31, 32, 34], needs to (also) target self-image, i.e. habitual self-directed behavior and the impact of difficult situations on patients' conceptions of themselves as individuals. Our findings

Table 3 Alternate mediation models summary: SASB as independent variable (X), DERS as mediator (M), and five different ED-related measures as dependent variables (outcomes; Y)

Outcome variable	Total effect (*c*)	SE	*p*	Direct effect (*c'*)	SE	*p*	Indirect effect (*ab*)	SE	95 % CIs
EDE-Q Global score (EDE-Q)	–.190	.023	<.001	–.154	.033	<.001	–.036	.027	–.091 to .013
Objective binge eating episodes (OBE)	–.269	.058	<.001	–.232	.081	.004	–.036	.056	–.148 to .072
Subjective binge eating episodes (SBE)	–.206	.051	<.001	–.182	.073	.013	–.024	.054	–.133 to .081
Regular excessive exercise (Reg. EE)	–.031	.054	.565	–.030	.078	.699	–.001	.052	–.101 to .105
Any excessive exercise (Any EE)	–.061	.045	.168	–.026	.064	.682	–.035	.046	–.127 to .055

All coefficients are unstandardized and expressed in the metric of the outcome variable
CIs = bias-corrected bootstrapped confidence intervals based on 10000 bootstrap samples

posit self-image as the more proximal construct in relation to presenting ED symptoms. Therefore, the relationship of self-image to body dissatisfaction, control of food intake, and compensatory behavior may be clearer to the patients themselves. On such a shared understanding and alliance basis, investigating the influence of negative emotion, and explicit emotion regulation skills training, may be more successful. Continuing the ball-throwing analogy, if a person consistently misses the target it may become relevant to train individual muscles, but such coaching must be based on, and continually return to, the higher-level synthetic ability to hit the mark. In addition, to prevent confirmation of the patient's problematic self-image by processes described by Benjamin [9], and thereby risk maintaining both ED symptoms and emotion dysregulation, the therapist may profitably consider interpersonal interactions both within and outside the therapeutic relationship from this perspective.

In addition to implications for treatment, our results points to the importance of attending to emotion regulation and self-image as a way of preventing ED. The ability to recognize, understand, and accept one's emotions, as well as having adaptive strategies to modulate the experience and expression of emotions, might be protective against negative self-treatment and possible subsequent ED symptoms. Also, prevention efforts may profit from explicitly addressing how problems handling emotions translate into self-treatment. For example, offering alternatives to subjective contingencies such as "I always react hysterically to things and ruminate on them, I'm a stupid and useless person" could prevent further translation into perfectionistic or impulsive attempts to deal with anxiety. A general awareness of the transactional associations between emotions, self-directed behavior and interpersonal interactions should be helpful [9, 16]. This might be of special importance among professionals encountering young individuals, for example in primary care, student health services, or family counseling. On a basic level, individuals can be informed on how to decrease the risk of too intense emotional arousal by properly managing sleep, diet, and physical health [3, 16]. For those who have been caught in vicious interactional patterns and dysfunctional ways of managing emotions, a greater understanding and clarification of the processes involved may be helpful. The presence of ED symptoms, i.e. negative self-treatment arising in the context of dysregulated negative emotion, puts the focus on improving social interactions and strengthening positive self-treatment as an important adjunct to development of skills to tolerate and manage a wide range of emotions.

Strengths and limitations

The results of the study are based on data from well-established and clinically relevant scales; the EDE-Q, the DERS and the SASB, all previously used in both ED research as well as research on various forms of psychopathology. Response rate was fair, and psychometric properties of the scales in our sample were generally acceptable to excellent. However, we had only cross-sectional data and cannot infer causality. Also, while response rate was fair, no attrition analyses could be performed, and it is possible that those who participated were systematically different from those who chose not to. Cronbach's α for one the six subscales forming SASB Affiliation was relatively low (.65), possibly attenuating associations with other variables (although the strong r vs. the DERS may speak against this). However, the remaining subscales all had acceptable internal consistency (Cronbach's α >.79), suggesting that the full Affiliation variable was reasonably internally consistent. The DERS was translated from English to Swedish for the present study, leaving the Swedish version of DERS so far relatively untested. However, preliminary psychometric investigation (including factor structure) suggests satisfactory properties (Birgegard: Factor structure of a Swedish version of the Difficulties in Emotion Regulation Scale, in preparation). We also ran a large number of analyses, leading to Type I error risk. This coupled with the fact that the present study is the first on the included interrelationships underlines the need for cautious interpretation and future replication. Of note however, p values were mostly substantially below .05 and the pattern of results was fairly consistent (e.g. exercise variables were not implicated overall but cognitive and binge-related ED symptoms were, and indirect effects was clearly found in one direction but not the other), suggesting some reliability in our findings. Nonetheless, given the complexity of the theoretical background, the aim of this study as well as the chosen methods, general caution is warranted for both interpretation and possible implications of the results.

Conclusion

The present study suggests that emotion dysregulation and self-image are closely related but both contribute unique knowledge in relation to ED symptoms: emotion dysregulation may contribute to ED symptoms via the self-image. This finding expands current knowledge on the relationship between emotion dysregulation and ED symptoms, with relevance for theories on the development and maintenance of ED, and may also contribute to more effective ED treatments. For the latter, further research on clinical samples is important, and to accurately infer causality between the constructs, experimental or longitudinal/sequential data are needed.

Abbreviations

ED: eating disorder; AN: anorexia nervosa; BN: bulimia nervosa; BED: binge eating disorder; DERS: Difficulties in Emotion Regulation Scale; SASB: Structural Analysis of Social Behavior; EDE-Q: Eating Disorder Examination Questionnaire; OBE: objective binge eating episodes; SBE: subjective binge eating episodes; EE: excessive exercise.

Competing interests
The authors declare that they have no competing interests.

Authors' contributions
EM and AB designed and carried out this study collaboratively. EM conducted the statistical analysis, supervised by AB. The manuscript was written collaboratively and all authors have approved the final manuscript.

Acknowledgements
The authors wish to thank David Clinton for help with back translation of the Difficulties in Emotion Regulation Scale.

References
1. Javaras KN, Runfola CD, Thornton LM, Agerbo E, Birgegard A, Norring C, et al. Sex- and Age-Specific Incidence of Healthcare-Register-Recorded Eating Disorders in Sweden: A Total Population Study. Int J Eat Disord. 2015; 48(8):1070–81. doi:10.1002/eat.22467.
2. Smink FR, van Hoeken D, Hoek HW. Epidemiology of eating disorders: incidence, prevalence and mortality rates. Curr Psychiatry Rep. 2012;14(4): 406–14. doi:10.1007/s11920-012-0282-y.
3. Haynos AF, Fruzzetti AE. Anorexia Nervosa as a Disorder of Emotion Dysregulation: Evidence and Treatment Implications. Clin Psychol: Science and Practice. 2011;18(3):183–202. doi:10.1111/j.1468-2850.2011.01250.x.
4. Nowakowski ME, McFarlane T, Cassin S. Alexithymia and eating disorders: a critical review of the literature. J Eat Disord. 2013;1:21. doi:10.1186/2050-2974-1-21.
5. Oldershaw A, Lavender T, Sallis H, Stahl D, Schmidt U. Emotion generation and regulation in anorexia nervosa: a systematic review and meta-analysis of self-report data. Clin Psychol Rev. 2015;39:83–95. doi:10.1016/j.cpr. 2015.04.005.
6. Racine SE, Wildes JE. Emotion dysregulation and symptoms of anorexia nervosa: the unique roles of lack of emotional awareness and impulse control difficulties when upset. Int J Eat Disord. 2013;46(7):713–20. doi:10. 1002/eat.22145.
7. Brockmeyer T, Skunde M, Wu M, Bresslein E, Rudofsky G, Herzog W, et al. Difficulties in emotion regulation across the spectrum of eating disorders. Compr Psychiatry. 2014;55(3):565–71. doi:10.1016/j.comppsych.2013.12.001.
8. Bjorck C, Clinton D, Sohlberg S, Hällström T, Norring C. Interpersonal profiles in eating disorders: Ratings of SASB self-image. Psychol Psychother. 2003; 76(Pt 4):337–49. doi:10.1348/147608303770584719.
9. Benjamin LS. A clinician-friendly version of the interpersonal circumplex-Structural Analysis of Social Behavior (SASB). J Pers Assess. 1996;66(2): 248–66. doi:10.1207/s15327752jpa6602_5.
10. Eisenberg N, Cumberland A, Spinrad TL. Parental socialization of emotion. Psychol Inq. 1998;9(4):241–73. doi:10.1207/s15327965pli0904_1.
11. Aldao A, Nolen-Hoeksema S, Schweizer S. Emotion-regulation strategies across psychopathology: A meta-analytic review. Clin Psychol Rev. 2010; 30(2):217–37. doi:10.1016/j.cpr.2009.11.004.
12. Svaldi J, Griepenstroh J, Tuschen-Caffier B, Ehring T. Emotion regulation deficits in eating disorders: a marker of eating pathology or general psychopathology? Psychiatry Res. 2012;197(1–2):103–11. doi:10.1016/j. psychres.2011.11.009.
13. Birgegard A, Bjorck C, Norring C, Sohlberg S, Clinton D. Anorexic self-control and bulimic self-hate: differential outcome prediction from initial self-image. Int J Eat Disord. 2009;42(6):522–30. doi:10.1002/eat.20642.
14. Gratz KL, Roemer L. Multidimensional assessment of emotion regulation and dysregulation: development, factor structure, and initial validation of the difficulties in emotion regulation scale. J Psychopathol Behav Assess. 2004; 26(1):41–54. doi:10.1023/B:JOBA.0000007455.08539.94.
15. Yap MB, Allen NB, Sheeber L. Using an emotion regulation framework to understand the role of temperament and family processes in risk for adolescent depressive disorders. Clin Child Fam Psychol Rev. 2007;10(2): 180–96. doi:10.1007/s10567-006-0014-0.
16. Linehan MM. Cognitive-Behavioral Treatment of Borderline Personality Disorder. New York: Guilford Press; 1993.
17. Fruzzetti AE, Shenk C, Hoffman PD. Family interaction and the development of borderline personality disorder- A transactional model. Dev Psychopathol. 2005;17(4):1007–30. doi:10.1017/S0954579405050479.
18. Caglar-Nazali HP, Corfield F, Cardi V, Ambwani S, Leppanen J, Olabintan O, et al. A systematic review and meta-analysis of 'Systems for Social Processes' in eating disorders. Neurosci Biobehav Rev. 2014;42:55–92. doi:10.1016/j. neubiorev.2013.12.002.
19. Oldershaw A, Lavender T, Sallis H, Stahl D, Schmidt U. Emotion generation and regulation in anorexia nervosa: A systematic review and meta-analysis of self-report data. Clin Psychol Rev. 2015. doi:10.1016/j.cpr.2015.04.005.
20. Fairburn CG, Cooper Z, Shafran R. Cognitive behaviour therapy for eating disorders: a "transdiagnostic" theory and treatment. Behav Res Ther. 2003; 41(5):509–28. doi:10.1016/s0005-7967(02)00088-8.
21. Heatherton TF, Baumeister RF. Binge eating as escape from self-awareness. Psychol Bull. 1991;110(1):86–108. doi:10.1037/0033-2909.110.1.86.
22. Smyth JM, Wonderlich SA, Heron KE, Sliwinski MJ, Crosby RD, Mitchell JE, et al. Daily and momentary mood and stress are associated with binge eating and vomiting in bulimia nervosa patients in the natural environment. J Consult Clin Psychol. 2007;75(4):629–38. doi:10.1037/0022-006X.75.4.629.
23. Smyth JM, Wonderlich SA, Sliwinski MJ, Crosby RD, Engel SG, Mitchell JE, et al. Ecological momentary assessment of affect, stress, and binge-purge behaviors: day of week and time of day effects in the natural environment. Int J Eat Disord. 2009;42(5):429–36. doi:10.1002/eat.20623.
24. Chua JL, Touyz S, Hill AJ. Negative mood-induced overeating in obese binge eaters: an experimental study. Int J Obes Relat Metab Disord. 2004; 28(4):606–10. doi:10.1038/sj.ijo.0802595.
25. Stein RI, Kenardy J, Wiseman CV, Dounchis JZ, Arnow BA, Wilfley DE. What's driving the binge in binge eating disorder?: A prospective examination of precursors and consequences. Int J Eat Disord. 2007;40(3):195–203. doi:10. 1002/eat.20352.
26. Wegner KE, Smyth JM, Crosby RD, Wittock D, Wonderlich SA, Mitchell JE. An evaluation of the relationship between mood and binge eating in the natural environment using ecological momentary assessment. Int J Eat Disord. 2002;32(3):352–61. doi:10.1002/eat.10086.
27. Deaver CM, Miltenberger RG, Smyth J, Meidinger AMY, Crosby R. An evaluation of affect and binge eating. Behav Modif. 2003;27(4):578–99. doi: 10.1177/0145445503255571.
28. Haedt-Matt AA, Keel PK. Revisiting the affect regulation model of binge eating: a meta-analysis of studies using ecological momentary assessment. Psychol Bull. 2011;137(4):660–81. doi:10.1037/a0023660.
29. Vansteelandt K, Rijmen F, Pieters G, Probst M, Vanderlinden J. Drive for thinness, affect regulation and physical activity in eating disorders: a daily life study. Behav Res Ther. 2007;45(8):1717–34. doi:10.1016/j.brat.2006.12.005.
30. Wildes JE, Ringham RM, Marcus MD. Emotion avoidance in patients with anorexia nervosa: initial test of a functional model. Int J Eat Disord. 2010; 43(5):398–404. doi:10.1002/eat.20730.
31. Fiore F, Ruggiero GM, Sassaroli S. Emotional dysregulation and anxiety control in the psychopathological mechanism underlying drive for thinness. Front Psychiatry. 2014;5:43. doi:10.3389/fpsyt.2014.00043.
32. Harrison A, Sullivan S, Tchanturia K, Treasure J. Emotion recognition and regulation in anorexia nervosa. Clin Psychol Psychother. 2009;16(4):348–56. doi:10.1002/cpp.628.
33. Harrison A, Sullivan S, Tchanturia K, Treasure J. Emotional functioning in eating disorders: attentional bias, emotion recognition and emotion regulation. Psychol Med. 2010;40(11):1887–97. doi:10.1017/ S0033291710000036.
34. Racine SE, Wildes JE. Dynamic longitudinal relations between emotion regulation difficulties and anorexia nervosa symptoms over the year following intensive treatment. J Consult Clin Psychol. 2015;83(4):785–95. doi: 10.1037/ccp0000011.
35. Burns EE, Fischer S, Jackson JL, Harding HG. Deficits in emotion regulation mediate the relationship between childhood abuse and later eating disorder symptoms. Child Abuse Negl. 2012;36(1):32–9. doi:10.1016/j.chiabu. 2011.08.005.
36. Cooper JL, O'Shea AE, Atkinson MJ, Wade TD. Examination of the difficulties in emotion regulation scale and its relation to disordered eating in a young female sample. Int J Eat Disord. 2014;47(6):630–9. doi:10.1002/eat.22278.
37. Arcelus J, Haslam M, Farrow C, Meyer C. The role of interpersonal functioning in the maintenance of eating psychopathology: a systematic review and testable model. Clin Psychol Rev. 2013;33(1):156–67. doi:10.1016/ j.cpr.2012.10.009.
38. Benjamin LS. SASB: A bridge between personality theory and clinical psychology. Psychol Inq. 1994;5(4):273–316. doi:10.1207/s15327965pli0504_1.
39. Sullivan S. The interpersonal theory of psychiatry. New York: Norton; 1953.

40. Bardone-Cone AM, Schaefer LM, Maldonado CR, Fitzsimmons EE, Harney MB, Lawson MA, et al. Aspects of self-concept and eating disorder recovery: what does the sense of self look like when an individual recovers from an eating disorder? J Soc Clin Psychol. 2010;29(7):821–46. doi:10.1521/jscp.2010.29.7.821.
41. Cella S, Iannaccone M, Cotrufo P. How perceived parental bonding affects self-concept and drive for thinness: a community-based study. Eat Behav. 2014;15(1):110–5. doi:10.1016/j.eatbeh.2013.10.024.
42. Benjamin LS. Structural analysis of social behavior. Psychological Rev. 1974; 81(5):392–425. doi:10.1037/h0037024.
43. Henry WP. Structural analysis of social behavior as a common metric for programmatic psychopathology and psychotherapy research. J Consult Clin Psychol. 1996;64(6):1263–75.
44. Critchfield KL, Benjamin LS. Internalized representations of early interpersonal experience and adult relationships: a test of copy process theory in clinical and non-clinical settings. Psychiatry. 2008;71(1):71–92. doi: 10.1521/psyc.2008.71.1.71.
45. Critchfield KL, Benjamin LS. Assessment of repeated relational patterns for individual cases using the SASB-based Intrex questionnaire. J Pers Assess. 2010;92(6):480–9. doi:10.1080/00223891.2010.513286.
46. Benjamin LS, Rothweiler JC, Critchfield KL. The use of structural analysis of social behavior (SASB) as an assessment tool. Annu Rev Clin Psychol. 2006;2: 83–109. doi:10.1146/annurev.clinpsy.2.022305.095337.
47. Bjorck C, Clinton D, Sohlberg S, Norring C. Negative self-image and outcome in eating disorders: results at 3-year follow-up. Eat Behav. 2007; 8(3):398–406. doi:10.1016/j.eatbeh.2006.12.002.
48. Bjorck C, Bjork T, Clinton D, Sohlberg S, Norring C. Self-image and treatment drop-out in eating disorders. Psychol Psychother. 2008;81(Pt 1):95–104. doi: 10.1348/147608307X224547.
49. Forsen Mantilla E, Bergsten K, Birgegard A. Self-image and eating disorder symptoms in normal and clinical adolescents. Eat Behav. 2014;15(1):125–31. doi:10.1016/j.eatbeh.2013.11.008.
50. Mantilla EF, Birgegard A. The enemy within: the association between self-image and eating disorder symptoms in healthy, non help-seeking and clinical young women. J Eat Disord. 2015;3:30. doi:10.1186/s40337-015-0067-x.
51. Runfola CD, Thornton LM, Pisetsky EM, Bulik CM, Birgegard A. Self-image and suicide in a Swedish national eating disorders clinical register. Compr Psychiatry. 2014;55(3):439–49. doi:10.1016/j.comppsych.2013.11.007.
52. Fairburn CG, Beglin SJ. Assessment of eating disorders: interview or self-report questionnaire? Int J Eat Disord. 1994;16(4):363–70.
53. Mond JM, Myers TC, Crosby RD, Hay PJ, Rodgers B, Morgan JF, et al. Screening for eating disorders in primary care: EDE-Q versus SCOFF. Behav Res Ther. 2008;46(5):612–22. doi:10.1016/j.brat.2008.02.003.
54. Wilfley DE, Schwartz MB, Spurrell EB, Fairburn CG. Assessing the specific psychopathology of binge eating disorder patients- interview or self-report? Behav Res Ther. 1997;35(12):1151–9. doi:10.1016/S0005-7967(97)80010-1.
55. Luce KH, Crowther JH. The reliability of the eating disorder examination - Self-report questionnaire version (EDE-Q). Int J Eat Disord. 1999;25(3):349–51. doi:10.1002/(SICI)1098-108X(199904)25:3<349::AID-EAT15>3.0.CO;2-M.
56. Welch E, Birgegard A, Parling T, Ghaderi A. Eating disorder examination questionnaire and clinical impairment assessment questionnaire: general population and clinical norms for young adult women in Sweden. Behav Res Ther. 2011;49(2):85–91. doi:10.1016/j.brat.2010.10.010.
57. Benjamin LS. SASB Intrex user's manual. Utah: University of Utah; 2000.
58. Hayes AF. Introduction to Mediation, Moderation, and Conditional Process Analysis. New York: Guilford Press; 2013.
59. Hayes AF, Scharkow M. The relative trustworthiness of inferential tests of the indirect effect in statistical mediation analysis: does method really matter? Psychol Sci. 2013;24(10):1918–27. doi:10.1177/0956797613480187.
60. Preacher KJ, Kelley K. Effect size measures for mediation models: quantitative strategies for communicating indirect effects. Psychol Methods. 2011;16(2):93–115. doi:10.1037/a0022658.
61. Hayes AF. Beyond Baron and Kenny: statistical mediation analysis in the new millennium. Commun Monogr. 2009;76(4):408–20. doi:10.1080/03637750903310360.

10

PreDictor Research in Obesity during Medical care - weight Loss in children and adolescents during an INpatient rehabilitation: rationale and design of the DROMLIN study

Helene Sauer[1], Anna Krumm[1], Katja Weimer[1], Björn Horing[1], Nazar Mazurak[1], Marco D Gulewitsch[2], Frank Hellmond[3], Dirk Dammann[3], Walter Binder[3], Peter Linse[3], Stephan Zipfel[1], Stefan Ehehalt[4], Gerhard Binder[5], Aydin Demircioglu[1], Eric R Muth[6], Paul Enck[1] and Isabelle Mack[1,7*]

Abstract

Background: Obesity in adults and children is increasing worldwide at alarming rates. Obese children and adolescents are likely to become obese adults with increased risk of a number of comorbidities. In addition to preventing the development of obesity at young age, it is necessary to individualize the therapy of already obese children and adolescents in order to increase the likelihood of weight loss and maintenance. Therefore, the aim of this study is to identify predictors which play a significant role in successful weight loss and weight loss maintenance in children and adolescents.

Methods/Design: Over a one year period, 60 obese children and adolescents between 9 to 17 years of age shall be recruited at an inpatient children rehabilitation facility in Germany. They will be investigated twice within a few days following admission and prior to discharge. The study will be an integrated component of an established inpatient weight-loss and in part psychosomatic therapy. The collected data can be grouped into four clusters: 1) demographic, sociometric and psychometric data, 2) objective and subjective parameters of body condition, 3) autonomic nervous system regulated functions and 4) objective and subjective parameters for eating behavior. Primary outcome is the change of the body mass index standard deviation score (BMI-SDS). In order to evaluate the data appropriately, all examinations will be also conducted in a normal-weight reference group, matched for age and gender.

Discussion: For some of the collected parameters the time span between measures may be too short. Therefore, a 6 months, 1 year and 2 year follow-up will be performed for evaluating the different predictors and their influence in regard to a successful intervention. Further middle- and long-term follow-up studies are planned.

Trial Registration: The study protocol was approved by the Ethics Committee of the University Hospital Tübingen, Germany. This study is registered at the German Clinical Trials Register (DRKS) with the clinical trial number DRKS00005122.

Keywords: Children, Obesity, Weight loss, Weight loss maintenance, Predictors, Inpatient, Rehabilitation

* Correspondence: isabelle.mack@uni-tuebingen.de
[1]Department of Psychosomatic Medicine and Psychotherapy, University Medical Hospital, Tübingen, Germany
[7]Department of Psychosomatic Medicine and Psychotherapy, University of Tübingen, Medical Hospital, Frondsbergstrasse 23, 72070 Tübingen, Germany
Full list of author information is available at the end of the article

Background

Rationale of the study

Obesity and its associated effects are increasingly becoming a health problem worldwide – both in children and in adults [1]. In Germany – as in most other European countries – up to 15% of the children between 3 and 17 years are overweight and 6% are obese [2,3]. Obesity is characterized by an excessive increase in adipose tissue [4]. According to the World Health Organization (WHO) an individual is defined as overweight with a body mass index (BMI) ≥ 25 kg/m^2 and as obese with a BMI ≥ 30 kg/m^2 [5]. However, these ranges are not transferable to children and adolescent values because of the different phases of life as a function of growth and puberty. Therefore, in pediatric medicine gender and age specific standard value tables are used for classification. By definition children and adolescents are overweight if their value is within the top ten percent and as obese if within the top three percent of their age group [5].

There are different inpatient and outpatient therapies to treat obesity in children and adolescents. These target changes in the fields of behavior, nutrition and physical activity [6]. In some cases, inpatient treatment is indicated, e.g. in children with severe obesity coupled with disturbed eating behaviors and psychosocial problems. For many children, these therapies are initially successful. In addition to weight reduction parameters like physical fitness, blood pressure, lipid and insulin levels as well as the psychological status improve [6]. After the intervention, it seems to be difficult for many children to maintain the skills they have acquired and to continue with weight reduction or stabilization at home, especially if no follow-up therapy is provided [6].

This raises the question which factors are crucial for the development of obesity, as well as which factors play significant roles in successful weight loss and weight loss maintenance in children and adolescents.

Predictors of obesity, weight loss and weight loss maintenance

Different attempts have been made to identify potential predictors of weight loss and weight loss maintenance in the past [7-10]. Besides epigenetic and genetic approaches, these strategies can be subdivided into four clusters of investigations depending on the main focus of the researchers and research groups. These clusters include 1) demographic, psychometric and sociometric data, 2) objective and subjective parameters of physical condition, 3) autonomic nervous system regulated functions and 4) objective and subjective parameters of eating behavior. In most cases, interest has been limited to variables within one cluster rather than across clusters.

In addition, clinical variables such as actual weight, diagnosis, comorbidities [11], medication [12], metabolic status (e.g. fasting glucose levels and glucose tolerance) [13], and endocrine variables [14,15] have frequently been used to try to predict success of dietary management, but yielding little predictive ability. Often, a number of predictors are associated with obesity. Most often these include psychological, but rarely physiological [14], psycho-physiological [16] or neurocognitive functions [17]. Furthermore, few of these predictors have been studied for their predictive value of weight reduction and weight loss maintenance as part of inpatient or outpatient treatment.

Demographic, sociometric and psychometric predictors

It is known that in general the social environment of the child plays a crucial role in weight control [18,19]. This applies to aspects such as ethnic origin [20], income [21], health of parents [22] as well as their eating habits [23]. The EvAKuJ study showed - in a sample of 1916 overweight and obese children and adolescents - that in inpatient treatments only the BMI at admission was predictive of the short and long-term treatment success, whereas gender, all collected psychosocial variables and the parental BMI played no significant role [24].

Subjective and objective parameters for body condition

The total energy requirement of an organism is made up of the resting energy requirement, the activity dependent energy consumption, and food-induced thermogenesis [25]. This balance is substantially altered in adult obesity [26] and potentially in children as well [27].

An increase in physical fitness has a positive effect on body composition and weight, which has also been shown for children during an inpatient treatment for weight loss [28].

In childhood, sleep duration appears to have a significant impact on body composition. Gonnissen and colleagues (2013) showed an inverse correlation between changes in BMI and changes in sleep duration in puberty which resulted in neuroendocrine variations during adulthood. These variations were reflected in a positive energy balance with a coexistence of sleep disturbance [29]. Furthermore, it could be shown that increased sleep duration and an increase in physical activity were associated with positive changes in sleep behavior in inpatients during weight reduction [30].

It was recently shown in young people that parents, peers, media, and religious influences have an impact on the nature and extent of body satisfaction and influence the type and amount of consumed food and the frequency of physical activity [31-33]. Disturbances of body image are frequent in eating disorders [34] and also affect other parts of body awareness [35]. Sarisoy and colleagues (2012) compared obese individuals to healthy controls and found negative correlations between self-esteem, body image, and harm avoidance scores, and a positive correlation between body image and self-directedness in the obese population [36]. As yet, only few studies investigated the development of body image disturbances in children and report controversial results [37].

Disordered interoception (perception of intrinsic bodily sensations, e.g. hunger and satiety) has been reported as a secondary marker of diseases such as cancer cachexia and depression in the elderly. An interoception test (Schandry [38]) should allow investigating whether increased body weight and therapy changes are associated with bodily perception and whether these parameters influence the course of weight loss or regain.

Autonomic nervous system regulation

The autonomic nervous system (ANS) controls the maintenance of the balance of vital functions such as breathing, heart rate, and digestion and plays a crucial role in the regulation of acute and chronic stress responses [39]. BMI has a direct influence on heart rate variability (HRV) at rest and during exercise [40,41] and during fasting in healthy subjects [42]. Patients with obesity often show a changed balance between the (decrease) activity of the parasympathetic and the (increased) sympathetic nervous system [43] that normalizes after weight loss [44]. Another potentially relevant measure of ANS activity is the electrogastrogram (EGG) recording gastric myoelectrical activity [45,46] closely associated with cardiac HRV [47].

Psychosocial stressors such as parental divorce [48,49], poor mental health of parents [50,51] or of children themselves [52,53], are often associated with negative health outcomes [54-56], but appear to act as moderators rather than mediators of weight-loss. To our knowledge, the ANS response to acute (experimental) stress [57] has not been evaluated as a potential predictor of weight-loss and weight-loss maintenance in children and adolescents.

Subjective and objective measures of eating behavior

Smell and taste are often altered in patients with eating disorders and obesity, even in children [58,59], but data are controversial. It is not clear whether children who participate in weight loss programs have pathological sensory thresholds and whether these changes are normalized after treatment.

In obese children, hyperactivity of the limbic and paralimbic brain areas was observed during presentation of food stimuli in the hungry state. These areas remain activated after a meal and after the presentation of food stimuli [60]. It is not clear whether and how processing of food stimuli plays a role in weight loss treatment.

When subjects were asked to fill the same amount of water in a low, wide glass and in a tall, narrow one tend to fill more water in the low, wide glasses due to an optical illusion [61,62]. This implies that the estimation of food portion sizes may be affected by their visual appearance [61,62]. It is not known whether the number of correct/incorrect estimates of quantities of food and liquids is different in our study population and whether this has an impact on prediction of weight loss and weight maintenance.

An indirect measurement of eating behavior is the eating rate (run of a spoon or a fork to the mouth per time unit) [63]. Moreover, an increased eating rate may be associated with excess weight [64]. It was shown [65] that the movement of eating is different to other accidental or deliberate motor activities of the dominant hand or arm. On this basis, a device was developed called "bite-counter" [66] which can measure the eating rate. The bite-counter had not been evaluated in children and adolescents.

While the list of potential measurements within and across these clusters is virtually unlimited, their selection can be determined based on two criteria: a) feasibility in a pediatric inpatient setting at the beginning and the ending of a therapy within a limited time frame, and b) having been shown previously to bear relevance in (childhood and adolescent) obesity.

Methods/Design

Aims of the study

The aim of the study is to identify potential pre-treatment predictors of successful weight loss in obese children and adolescents during a standardized therapeutic treatment in an inpatient rehabilitation setting. In addition, repeated measures of the same variables at the end of treatment may demonstrate whether psychophysiological measures that respond to weight loss are associated with therapy success and whether they may serve to predict long-term weight-loss maintenance at follow-up. In addition, clinical parameters will be taken from the hospital charts and examined as potential predictor variables. We are aware that for some of the collected parameters the time span between measures may be too short. Therefore, follow-up studies are planned for evaluating the success of intervention.

Study population

Patients and the inpatient setting

The obesity therapy concept at the Children Rehabilitation Hospital for Respiratory Diseases, Allergies and Psychosomatics, Wangen i.A., Germany is aimed at recovery from comorbid diseases associated with obesity, rediscovering joy of life, developing a forward-looking perspective, independent living, and growing up unencumbered. The children and young people are treated in accordance with the latest developments in medicine, especially pediatrics and in close cooperation with regional educational institutions such as the obesity academy (Adipositas-Akademie Baden-Württemberg e.V.), an atopic dermatitis academy (Neurodermitisakademie München/Wangen/

Gaißach) and an asthma academy (Asthmaakademie Baden-Württemberg e.V.). Infants, children and adolescents are housed and cared for in small therapeutic groups with peers of the same age and in residential units situated on a park-like hospital ground. The clinic has its own kindergarten and a school with regular classes for all types of curricula.

Pediatricians, allergists, psychologists, social workers and nursing staff, teachers, trainers, dietetic professionals, occupational and speech therapists and staff for physical therapy work together as one team. The special obesity training is an integral part of therapy. The individual modules of the training are rooted in the concept of the clinic, including exercise and sports, change to a healthy diet, and weight-loss.

The nutrition concept is based on a balanced diet or "optimized mixed diet". In nutrition training, patients meet weekly in small groups of 6–8 age-matched participants. In a training kitchen, all children and adolescents learn how to prepare food and cook with the aim of proper food handling and preparation when they return home. Additionally, they complete "shopping training" in a supermarket.

The hospital treats approximately 200 obese children and adolescents per year. The average duration of stay is 42 days.

Inclusion criteria

Children and adolescents with an indication for hospitalization for the purpose of weight loss - as set by their responsible primary or secondary care physicians - and with a BMI scoring higher than the 97th percentile specific for age and gender will be included [67]. The age range is set between 9 to 17 years. An indication for inpatient rehabilitation is given if the child suffers from diseases that are relevant or have negative impact on education, training or earning capacity (emotional, social development, personal development), especially for disorders/diseases that could have negative effects on the functioning of the particular age-appropriate levels of activity and social participation in all spheres of life. Medical rehabilitation is part of a long-term management of chronically ill children and adolescents and their families. The goal is an improvement, but at least to prevent deterioration (stabilization) of the health status-quo with regard to the current or future needs in education, training and profession. Requirement for inpatient rehabilitation is that the available outpatient options have been exploited and that a beneficial effect of the disease process can be expected.

Exclusion criteria

Children with severe psychiatric comorbidities, linguistic or intellectual limitations (by judgment of the treating physician or therapist), type-1 diabetes, tumors, systemic disorders, or severe cardiovascular diseases will be excluded.

Control group

A healthy normal weight reference group of 30 children with the same exclusion criteria will be recruited for potential predictor parameters for which age and gender-specific norm data are missing in the literature. These children will come from the catchment area of the University Hospital Tübingen, Germany.

Outcomes

Primary outcome

The primary outcome measure is the change of the body mass index standard deviation score (BMI-SDS) [68]. SDS values indicate how many standard deviations an individual's BMI lays above or below an age and gender matched median of BMI, a deviation of the value about two standard deviations above (+2) corresponds to the 97.7 percentile of the reference group [69]. Reference data for German children are used [67]. In order to calculate the BMI, the body weight and body height will be measured upon admission and upon discharge of their inpatient stay using calibrated instruments.

Secondary outcomes

Secondary outcomes measures include the changes in body composition and motor performance. Body composition is measured by a lipometer© (Möller Messtechnik, Graz, Austria) [70-72]. The motor performance is assessed by the Dordel-Koch-Test [73].

Appointments

After informed consent, the hospital planning office will receive a screening form with psychophysiological assessments and will include the child into the study, depending on the particular time-slots available for the child. Afterwards, it will integrate four half-day assessments into the individual therapy plan. This procedure avoids time conflicts with other therapies and insures that the investigations are completed within the first week after admission and during the last week prior to discharge.

The children will pass two test sessions upon admission, one in the morning and one in the afternoon, and the same test sessions will be repeated prior to discharge. On both occasions, a series of investigations will be performed which can be grouped into four clusters: 1) demographic, sociometric and psychometric data 2) objective and subjective parameters of body condition, 3) autonomic nervous system regulated functions and 4) objective and subjective parameters for eating behavior (see below).

Psychophysiological investigations

Within and across the discussed clusters, the number of measures chosen is based on theoretical (previous data available) as well as pragmatic reasons (feasibility, availability). For logistic reasons, the investigations are split into two groups, one of which is conducted during a morning session (9.00 h to 12.00 h), while the other one is conducted on a separate day in the afternoon (14.00 h to 16.00 h) (see Table 1). In addition, clinical data from the medical charts will be collected for the analysis. A list of all used questionnaires (of all clusters) is provided in Tables 2 (children) and 3 (parents).

Cluster 1: Sociometrics and psychometrics

Besides conventional sociodemographic data (family history and status, social status, education etc.) all children will complete the following psychometric questionnaires, usually in validated German translations: a health-related quality-of-life scale (ILK, children and adults) [77], a depression scale (DIKJ) [83], a somatization scale in dependence on the International Children's Somatization Inventory (CSI/SI-KJ) [79,80], the trait anxiety scale (STAI-C) [81,82], screenings for emotional and behavioral problems (SDQ) [90,91], and the self-esteem scale according to Rosenberg [92].

Cluster 2: Physical condition measures

The children will complete the Sleep Self Report (SSR) [74,75] which records sleep problems, and the Pediatric Daytime Sleepiness Scale (PDSS) [76]. Parents will fill in the Pediatrics Sleep Habits Questionnaire (PSQ) [85], a screening tool for sleep behavior, the ESS-E [86,87] determining daytime sleepiness, and the Children's Sleep Habits Questionnaire (CSHQ) [88,89] once at the beginning of the therapy.

The Dordel – Koch test [73] will be used to capture the basic functions and motor performances of children and adolescents. The test battery consists of lateral jumping back and forth (coordination under time pressure, speed), sit and reach (flexibility of the hips and lower spine), standing long jump (explosive strength of the lower extremity), sit-ups (strength of the abdominal muscles and hip flexors), standing on one leg (coordination with precision tasks), push-ups (strength of the shoulder, chest and arm muscles) and the 6-minute walk distance (aerobic endurance). Additionally, physical fitness will be recorded by a regular bicycle ergometry program supervised by specially trained staff during the regular course of therapy. Body composition will be recorded by a lipometer© (Möller Messtechnik, Graz, Austria) that enables a non-invasive, fast, accurate, and reliable measurement of the thickness of subcutaneous fat [70-72] including hip and waist circumference. Moreover, the method is evaluated by a data set of 1351 juveniles of which 101 were obese [93]. In addition, anthropometric measures of various body parts will be collected by tape, calipers, and a scale. Thoracic breadth and depth will be assessed in order to detect the type of physiques according to the "Metric-Index" [94].

Table 1 Measurement protocol

Time a.m.	First session	Approximate duration	Time p.m.	Second session	Approximate duration
8:50	Welcome/general questions	5-10 min	14:30	Welcome	5-10 min
	Anthropometry	5-10 min		Media consumption questionnaire	5-10 min
	Sleep Self Report (SSR)/Pediatric Daytime Sleepiness Scale (PDSS)	7-10 min		Interoception test	5 min
	Taste test	5-10 min		ECG/EGG/SCL Baseline	20 min
	Inventory for recording the Quality of life in Children and Adolescents (ILK)	3-5 min			
	Smell test	15-20 min		Stress test	5 min
	Inventory of Eating and Weight problems Inventory for Children (EWI-C/IEG-K)	15-20 min		Post stress test	20 min
	Dordel- Koch test	15-20 min			
	Somatization Inventory for Children and Adolescents (SI-KJ)/State-Trait Anxiety Inventory (STAI-C)	5-10 min		Water load test Post water load	2-5 min 20 min
	Cognitive ability to discriminate volumes of food and liquids	15-20 min		Eating behavior test with snacks	20 min
	Depression Inventory for Children and Adolescents (DI-KJ)	10-15 min			
	Body image	10-15 min		Stress and Stress Coping Questionnaire for Children and Adolescents (SSKJ-J)	15-20 min
	Self-esteem scale by Rosenberg	2-5 min			
11:30	Farewell		17:00	Farewell	

Table 2 Questionnaires for children

Questionnaires	Short description
Sleep Self Report (SSR) [74,75]	28 items; three thematic areas; three answer options ranging from "common" to "uncommon"
Pediatric Daytime Sleepiness Scale (PDSS) [76]	32 items; six thematic areas; five Answer options ranging from "always" to "never"
Inventory for recording the Quality of life in Children and Adolescents (ILK) version for children [77]	10 items; seven thematic areas; five answer options ranging from "very good" to "very bad"
Inventory of Eating and Weight problems Inventory for Children (EWI-C/IEG-K) [78]	60 items; ten subscales; four answer options ranging from "not true at all" to "totally agree"
Somatization Inventory for Children and Adolescents (SI-KJ) [79,80]	35 items; list of symptoms; five answer options ranging from "not at all" to "much"
State-Trait Anxiety Inventory (STAI-C) [81,82]	20 items; two scales; three answer options ranging from "almost never" to "often"
Depression Inventory for Children and Adolescents (DI-KJ) [83]	26 items; queries gradations of symptoms; decision between three predefined answer alternative
Stress and Stress Coping Questionnaire for Children and Adolescents (SSJK) [84]	84 items; three subscales; five answer options ranging from "never" to "always"
Revised self-esteem scale by Rosenberg	10 items; total score from 10–40, the higher the score the higher the level of self-esteem; Four answer options ranging from "strongly disagree" to "strongly agree"

The interoception test according to Schandry [38] will test the ability of the children to correctly perceive body-internal cardiac signals (heart beat) [47,95]. During four intervals of 25, 35, 45, and 55 seconds duration, separated by 30 second resting periods, an electrocardiogram (ECG) will be recorded and children shall count their own heartbeats. A start and stop cue signals beginning and end of the counting phases. Participants are not allowed to take their pulse or to attempt any other manipulation that can facilitate the detection of heartbeats. Following the stop signals, children will be asked to report the number of counted heartbeats that will be evaluated against the recorded heart rate. Furthermore, a test for perception of their own body image will be performed by means of estimation of size of their body (total, parts) in relation to various external objects and sensory cues. Standardized tests for chemosensitivity (smell, taste) using validated tools (Burghart Messtechnik GmbH, Wedel, Germany) [96,97] to measure their respective thresholds, identification and discrimination ability will be conducted.

Cluster 3: Autonomic regulation

An electrocardiogram (ECG) will be recorded for off-line analysis of heart-rate variability (HRV) during rest (20 min) and following a mental stress test (counting backwards in steps of 7 from 1000, 300, or 100, depending on the age and intellectual level of the children; 20 min). Afterwards, the children will be asked to rate the perceived stress level on a scale between one (absolutely not stressed) to six (absolutely stressed). The ECG is recorded for inter-beat intervals (IBI) allowing Fast Fourier Transformation of data to estimate heart rate variability (HRV) parameters (high and low frequency (HF, LF)).

At the same time, three surface electrodes placed over the upper abdomen will record myoelectrical activity from the stomach (EGG) [98] for off-line analysis. At the end of the session, a water loading test [99,100] will be performed to determine the response of the stomach to an intragastric strain associated with gastric filling: subjects will be asked to drink as much water as possible within 5 minutes until the feeling of fullness is reached. The water load test

Table 3 Questionnaires for parents

Questionnaires	Short description
Pediatrics Sleep Habits Questionnaire (PSQ) [85]	22 items; three subscales; Answer options: Item 1 to 16: "yes", "no", "don't know"; item 17 to 22: four options ranging from "does not apply" to "meets most of time"
Epworth Sleepiness Scale (ESS-E) [86,87]	8 items; total score from 0–24; four answer options ranging from "would never doze" to "dozing high probability"
Children's Sleep Habits Questionnaire (CSHQ) [88,89]	33 items; eight subscales; three answer options ranging from "common" to "uncommon"
Subjective Strength and Weaknesses (SDQ) [90,91]	25 items; five subscales; three answer options ranging from "does not apply" to "clearly applicable"
Inventory for recording the Quality of life in Children and Adolescents (ILK) version for parents [77]	11 items; nine thematic areas; five answer options ranging from "very good" to "very bad"

will be followed by a 20 minutes measurement of the EGG. EGG signals will be analyzed with a Fast Fourier Transformation (FFT) procedure. A frequency of 3 cycles per minute (cpm) is regarded as normal gastric activity and between 4 to 10 cpm as tachygastria. This allows calculating the percentage spectral power from the total range of myoelectric gastric activity and computing the ratio between the percentage of the normogastria and the tachygastria band. This ratio has repeatedly been described as an indicator for disturbed myoelectric gastric activity, for example in patients with gastroparesis [99], but also in obesity [46].

Skin conductance will be measured parallel to ECG and EGG by using two separate finger electrodes on the dominant hand. For ECG, EGG and skin conductance measurement, a portable system (3991/3-GPP BioLog, UFI Company, Morrow Bay, CA, USA) will be used. Furthermore, a questionnaire survey of experience of stress and coping in childhood (SSKJ 3–8) [84] is added to cluster three.

Cluster 4: Eating behavior

For psychological assessment of eating behavior the inventory of eating and weight problems for children (EWI-C) [78] will be used, in addition, also a specific questionnaire asking for their food preferences and regular eating behaviors at home.

To validate eating behavior as indicated in the questionnaire, children will be allowed a 20-minute post-stress recovery (see above) while watching a movie on TV and taking snacks of different caloric density ad libitum, with the experimenter not present during that time. However, unbeknown to the children the snack plate will be filmed during this period. In addition, food will be weighted before and after the session and consumed calories will be calculated. In addition, some of the children will carry a novel "bite-counter" (Bite Technologies, Pendleton, South Carolina, USA) [66,101] that registers the numbers of arm and hand movements typical for eating behavior. Video-recordings will be used to validate the bite counting technology, as well.

Furthermore, the cognitive ability to discriminate volumes of food and liquids will be tested. Therefore, pairs of glasses (e.g. low, wide glass versus a slim, tall glass), of plates and bowls with pre-defined amounts of water or uncooked lentils (representing food) will be presented. The children and adolescents will be asked to estimate the quantities of the provided amounts. They will also be asked to estimate the amount of food needed to satisfy normal hunger.

Ethics and registration of the study

The study protocol was approved by the Ethics Committee of the medical faculty for the University Tübingen, Germany. This study is registered at the German Clinical Trials Register (DRKS) with the clinical trial number DRKS00005122. The DRKS is an approved primary register in the WHO network. Children and parents were informed about the study purpose during the admission interview by a physician or therapist and were asked to provide written consent prior to inclusion.

Statistics

We expect measures to be highly correlated within each cluster, and some variables within each cluster to be more sensitive or predictive to weight-loss during treatment than others. These key variables have been used as predictors for sample size calculation.

Cluster 1: Key variable: self-esteem scale according to Rosenberg
Cluster 2: Key variable: agility/motor activity (Dordel-Koch test)
Cluster 3: Key variable: ECG/IBI response to stress
Cluster 4: Key variable: caloric intake per time unit

To calculate optimal sample size, G*Power 3.1.7 [102] was used. To analyze the main research question (prediction of weight loss maintenance by key variables), sample size was derived for r^2 deviation from zero (F distribution, Linear multiple regressions: Fixed model, R^2 deviation from zero). Correlations of $r = .3$ (medium effect size [103]) were assumed for predictor-outcome associations as well as the predictor's intercorrelation matrix, resulting in a squared multiple correlation of $r^2 = .189$ and an $f^2 = .234$. With a level of significance at alpha = .05 and a statistical power (1-beta) of .8, a sample size of 57 would be optimal to decide on the predictive quality of the model.

Statistical analysis will be conducted in two steps: variables within each cluster will be tested for their intercorrelation, their responsiveness to weight change, and for their ability to predict weight loss in a one-by-one fashion (step 1). In cases of high within-cluster intercorrelation (as predicted), a hierarchical model will be constructed with the most sensitive variable per cluster to be entered into a multivariate regression model (step 2).

Follow-up

The obese children will be included in a voluntary web-based aftercare program. This pilot program provides a possibility of periodic input of the actual weight and a graphical feedback of weight development, a chat option with the administrator for special questions regarding weight development and nutrition, and information and links to self-aid and support.

Six months after discharge the children will be contacted by phone and questioned about weight development and about implementation of the learned tools during therapy (portion sizes, activity in everyday life, coping of stress). Twelve months after discharge, children will receive a questionnaire and a prepaid return envelope by mail with an additional form for weight verification that has to be filled-in by a local pharmacist or a physician. The effort is rewarded with a gift certificate. A two year follow-up, and further middle- and long-term follow-up studies are also planned.

Discussion

In conclusion, this study will discover potential psychophysiological predictors which play a significant role in successful weight loss in obese children and adolescents during a standardized therapeutic treatment in an inpatient rehabilitation setting. Carefully planned short-, middle- and long-term follow-up studies will be conducted in order to find predictors of successful weight-loss maintenance in obese children and adolescents. Some of the analyzed parameters may be useful as screening instruments to adjust future therapeutic intervention to the needs of the child.

Authors' information

Study was designed by a multiprofessional team. The first and last author are part of the research department Psychosomatic Medicine and Psychotherapy, University Medical Hospital, Tübingen, Germany and are interested in obesity in children and adolescents. For this reason, they approached the Fachkliniken Wangen i.A. and the present study design was established.

Acknowledgements

This study is funded by grants from the Else Kröner-Fresenius-Stiftung, Bad Homburg, Germany. We would like to thank all staff of the Fachkliniken Wangen i. A., especially Dr. Robert Jäschke and Rainer Beer, in advance for their support in carrying out the study, and all colleagues at the University Hospital Tübingen who helped us with planning and implementation. We acknowledge support by the Deutsche Forschungsgemeinschaft and the Open Access Publishing Fund of the Tuebingen University.

Author details

[1]Department of Psychosomatic Medicine and Psychotherapy, University Medical Hospital, Tübingen, Germany. [2]Department of Psychology, Clinical Psychology and Psychotherapy, University of Tübingen, Tübingen, Germany. [3]Fachkliniken Wangen i.A., Children Rehabilitation Hospital for Respiratory Diseases, Allergies and Psychosomatics, Wangen i.A., Germany. [4]Public Health Department of Stuttgart, Department of Pediatrics, Dental Health Care, Health Promotion and Social Services, Stuttgart, Germany. [5]Department of Pediatric Endocrinology and Diabetology, University Children's Hospital, Tübingen, Germany. [6]Department of Psychology, Clemson University, Clemson, South Carolina, USA. [7]Department of Psychosomatic Medicine and Psychotherapy, University of Tübingen, Medical Hospital, Frondsbergstrasse 23, 72070 Tübingen, Germany.

Abbreviations

ANS: Autonomic nervous system; BMI: Body mass index; BMI-SDS: Body mass index standard deviation score; ECG: Electrocardiogram;
EGG: Electrogastrogram; FFT: Fast Fourier Transformation; HRV: Heart rate variability; HF: High frequency; IBI: Inter-beat intervals; LF: Low frequency; SDS: Standard deviation score; WHO: World Health Organization.

Competing interests

The authors declare that they have no competing interests.

Authors' contributions

HS: responsible for conception and design of the study and will perform it, will acquire and analyze the data, drafted the paper. AK: will perform of the study, will acquire and analyze the data. KW: responsible for acquisition and preparation of the electrogastrogram part, will analyze the respective data. BH: responsible for preparation of statistics and will support the analysis of data. NM: responsible for acquisition and preparation of the heart rate variability, skin conductance data and will analyze it. MDG: responsible for preparation of the psychometry, stress behavior in children data, will support the analysis and interpretation of these data. FH: responsible for preparation and acquisition of clinical eating behavior data at the FW. DD: pediatrician responsible for the clinical logistics, supervision and preparation of the study at the FW. WB: responsible for clinical logistics, supervision, conception, preparation and participant recruitment of the study at the FW. PL: responsible for acquisition and preparation of clinical physical activity data at the FW. SZ: responsible for design and funding of the study. SE: pediatrician responsible for preparation of the study and will support analysis and interpretation of the data. GB: pediatrician responsible for preparation of the study and will support analysis and interpretation of the data. AD: responsible for construction and implementation of the follow-up website. ERM: provides technology and will analyze parts of the Bite-Counter data, as native speaker responsible for English writing. PE: responsible for conception, design and funding of the study and will support analysis of the data and paper writing. IM: responsible for conception, funding, design and preparation of the study, will acquire and analyze data, drafted the paper. All authors: read and approved the final manuscript.

References

1. Hotamisligil GS: **Inflammation and metabolic disorders.** *Nature* 2006, **444**(7121):860–867.
2. Kurth BM, Rosario SA: **The prevalence of overweight and obese children and adolescents living in Germany. Results of the German Health Interview and Examination Survey for Children and Adolescents (KiGGS).** *Bundesgesundheitsblatt Gesundheitsforschung Gesundheitsschutz* 2007, **50**(5–6):736–743.
3. World Health Organisation (WHO): *Prevalence of Overweight and Obesity and Adolescents.* Geneva: World Health Organization; 2009:Fact Sheet 23.
4. Trayhurn P: **Hypoxia and adipose tissue function and dysfunction in obesity.** *Physiol Rev* 2013, **93**(1):1–21.
5. World Health Organization: *Obesity: Preventing and Managing the Global Epidemic. report of a WHO Consultation WHO Technical Report Series 894.* Geneva: World Health Organization; 2000.
6. Oude Luttikhuis H, Baur L, Jansen H, Shrewsbury VA, O'Malley C, Stolk RP, Summerbell CD: **Interventions for treating obesity in children.** *Cochrane Database Syst Rev* 2009, **3**:1–57.
7. Lindvall K, Jenkins P, Emmelin M, Scribani M, Norberg M, Larsson C, Weinehall L: **Primary weight maintenance: an observational study exploring candidate variables for intervention.** *Nutr J* 2013, **12**(1):97.
8. Munro IA, Bore MR, Munro D, Garg ML: **Using personality as a predictor of diet induced weight loss and weight management.** *Int J Behav Nutr Phys Act* 2011, **8**:s129.
9. Myers VH, McVay MA, Champagne CM, Hollis JF, Coughlin JW, Funk KL, Gullion CM, Jerome GJ, Loria CM, Samuel-Hodge CD, Stevens VJ, Svetkey LP, Brantley PJ: **Weight loss history as a predictor of weight loss: results from Phase I of the weight loss maintenance trial.** *J Behav Med* 2012. in press.
10. Wang P, Holst C, Wodzig WK, Andersen MR, Astrup A, van Baak MA, Larsen TM, Jebb SA, Kafatos A, Pfeiffer AF, Martinez JA, Handjieva-Darlenska T, Kunesova M, Viguerie N, Langin D, Saris WH, Mariman EC: **Circulating ACE is a predictor of weight loss maintenance not only in overweight and obese women, but also in men.** *Int J Obes (Lond)* 2012, **36**(12):1545–1551.
11. Bramlage P, Wittchen HU, Pittrow D, Kirch W, Krause P, Lehnert H, Unger T, Hofler M, Kupper B, Dahm S, Bohler S, Sharma AM: **Recognition and management of overweight and obesity in primary care in Germany.** *Int J Obes Relat Metab Disord* 2004, **28**(10):1299–1308.

12. Vitiello B, Riddle MA, Yenokyan G, Axelson DA, Wagner KD, Joshi P, Walkup JT, Luby J, Birmaher B, Ryan ND, Emslie G, Robb A, Tillman R: **Treatment moderators and predictors of outcome in the Treatment of Early Age Mania (TEAM) study.** *J Am Acad Child Adolesc Psychiatry* 2012, **51**(9):867–878.
13. Talaei M, Sadeghi M, Marshall T, Thomas GN, Iranipour R, Nazarat N, Sarrafzadegan N: **Anthropometric indices predicting incident type 2 diabetes in an Iranian population: the Isfahan Cohort study.** *Diabetes Metab* 2013. in press.
14. Strohacker K, McCaffery JM, Maclean PS, Wing RR: **Adaptations of leptin, ghrelin or insulin during weight loss as predictors of weight regain: a review of current literature.** *Int J Obes (Lond)* 2013. in press.
15. Robinson JG, Ballantyne CM, Hsueh WA, Rosen JB, Lin J, Shah AK, Tomassini JE, Lowe RS, Tershakovec AM: **Age, abdominal obesity, and baseline high-sensitivity C-reactive protein are associated with low-density lipoprotein cholesterol, non-high-density lipoprotein cholesterol, and apolipoprotein B responses to ezetimibe/simvastatin and atorvastatin in patients with metabolic syndrome.** *J Clin Lipidol* 2013, **7**(4):292–303.
16. Bellisle F, Tremblay A: **Satiety and body weight control. Promise and compromise. Comment on 'Satiety. No way to slim'.** *Appetite* 2011, **57**(3):769–771. discussion 784–790.
17. de la Monte SM, Tong M, Nguyen V, Setshedi M, Longato L, Wands JR: **Ceramide-mediated insulin resistance and impairment of cognitive-motor functions.** *J Alzheimers Dis* 2010, **21**(3):967–984.
18. Gundersen C, Mahatmya D, Garasky S, Lohman B: **Linking psychosocial stressors and childhood obesity.** *Obes Rev* 2011, **12**(5):e54–e63.
19. Ahrens W, Bammann K, Siani A, Buchecker K, De Henauw S, Iacoviello L, Hebestreit A, Krogh V, Lissner L, Marild S, Molnár D, Moreno LA, Pitsiladis YP, Reisch L, Tornaritis M, Veidebaum T, Pigeot I; IDEFICS Consortium: **The IDEFICS cohort: design, characteristics and participation in the baseline survey.** *Int J Obes (Lond)* 2011, **35**(Suppl 1):S3–S15.
20. Caprio S, Daniels SR, Drewnowski A, Kaufman FR, Palinkas LA, Rosenbloom AL, Schwimmer JB: **Influence of Race, Ethnicity, and Culture on Childhood Obesity: Implications for Prevention and Treatment: a consensus statement of Shaping America's Health and the Obesity Society.** *Diabetes Care* 2008, **31**(11):2211–2221.
21. Gransky S, Stewart SD, Gundersen C, Lohman BJ, Eisenmann JC: **Family stressors and child obesity.** *Social Scince Research* 2009, **38**:755–766.
22. Gibson LY, Byrne SM, Davis EA, Blair E, Jacoby P, Zubrick SR: **The role of family and maternal factors in childhood obesity.** *Med J Aust* 2007, **186**(11):591–595.
23. Rhee K: **Childhood overweight and the relationship between parent behaviors, parenting style, and family functioning.** *The ANNALS of the American Academy of Political and Social Science* 2008, **615**(1):11–37.
24. Hoffmeister U, Molz E, Bullinger M, van Egmond-Frohlich A, Goldapp C, Mann R, Ravens-Sieberer U, Reinehr T, Westenhofer J, Wille N, Holl RW: **Evaluation of obesity treatment in children and adolescents (EvAKuJ Study). Role of therapeutic concept, certification, and quality indicators.** *Bundesgesundheitsblatt Gesundheitsforschung Gesundheitsschutz* 2011, **54**(5):603–610.
25. Landsberg L, Young JB, Leonard WR, Linsenmeier RA, Turek FW: **Do the obese have lower body temperatures? A new look at a forgotten variable in energy balance.** *Trans Am Clin Climatol Assoc* 2009, **120**:287–295.
26. Winkler S, Pico C, Ahrens W: **Physiological mechanisms in the development of adiposity.** *Bundesgesundheitsblatt Gesundheitsforschung Gesundheitsschutz* 2010, **53**(7):681–689.
27. Hansen JC, Gilman AP, Odland JO: **Is thermogenesis a significant causal factor in preventing the "globesity" epidemic?** *Med Hypotheses* 2010, **75**(2):250–256.
28. Rigamonti AE, Agosti F, De Col A, Marazzi N, Lafortuna CL, Cella SG, Muller EE, Sartorio A: **Changes in plasma levels of ghrelin, leptin, and other hormonal and metabolic parameters following standardized breakfast, lunch, and physical exercise before and after a multidisciplinary weight-reduction intervention in obese adolescents.** *J Endocrinol Invest* 2010, **33**(9):633–639.
29. Gonnissen HK, Adam TC, Hursel R, Rutters F, Verhoef SP, Westerterp-Plantenga MS: **Sleep duration, sleep quality and body weight: Parallel developments.** *Physiol Behav* 2013, **121**:112–116.
30. Lehnique Y, Locard E, Vivant JF, Mounier A, Serban A, Remontet L, Porquet D, Joly MO, Mamelle N: **Evolution of GH secretion in urine during an in-patient slimming course in obese children.** *Int J Obes Relat Metab Disord* 2000, **24**(3):363–368.
31. McCabe MP, Mavoa H, Ricciardelli LA, Schultz JT, Waqa G, Fotu KF: **Socio-cultural agents and their impact on body image and body change strategies among adolescents in Fiji, Tonga, Tongans in New Zealand and Australia.** *Obes Rev* 2011, **12**(Suppl 2):61–67.
32. Vocks S, Legenbauer T, Heil A: **Food intake affects state body image: impact of restrained eating patterns and concerns about eating, weight and shape.** *Appetite* 2007, **49**(2):467–475.
33. Cash TF: **Treatment of body image disturbances.** In *Handbook of Eating Disorders and Obesity.* Edited by Thompson JK. New Jersey: Wiley; 2004:515–541.
34. Hrabosky JI, Cash TF, Veale D, Neziroglu F, Soll EA, Garner DM, Strachan-Kinser M, Bakke B, Clauss LJ, Phillips KA: **Multidimensional body image comparisons among patients with eating disorders, body dysmorphic disorder, and clinical controls: a multisite study.** *Body Image* 2009, **6**(3):155–163.
35. Vancampfort D, Vanderlinden J, De Hert M, Soundy A, Adamkova M, Skjaerven LH, Catalan-Matamoros D, Lundvik Gyllensten A, Gomez-Conesa A, Probst M: **A systematic review of physical therapy interventions for patients with anorexia and bulemia nervosa.** *Disabil Rehabil* 2013. in press.
36. Sarisoy G, Atmaca A, Ecemis G, Gumus K, Pazvantoglu O: **Personality characteristics and body image in obese individuals.** *Asia Pac Psychiatry* 2012, :. in press.
37. Legenbauer T, Thiemann P, Vocks S: **Body image disturbance in children and adolescents with eating disorders.** *Z Kinder Jugendpsychiatr Psychother* 2014, **42**(1):51–59.
38. Schandry R: **Heart beat perception and emotional experience.** *Psychophysiology* 1981, **18**(4):483–488.
39. Baumann N, Turpin JC: **Neurochemistry of stress, an overview.** *Neurochem Res* 2010, **35**(12):1875–1879.
40. Vallejo M, Marquez MF, Borja-Aburto VH, Cardenas M, Hermosillo AG: **Age, body mass index, and menstrual cycle influence young women's heart rate variability -a multivariable analysis.** *Clin Auton Res* 2005, **15**(4):292–298.
41. Sztajzel J, Jung M, Sievert K, Bayes De Luna A: **Cardiac autonomic profile in different sports disciplines during all-day activity.** *J Sports Med Phys Fitness* 2008, **48**(4):495–501.
42. Mazurak N, Gunther A, Grau FS, Muth ER, Pustovoyt M, Bischoff SC, Zipfel S, Enck P: **Effects of a 48-h fast on heart rate variability and cortisol levels in healthy female subjects.** *Eur J Clin Nutr* 2013, **67**(4):401–406.
43. Muralikrishnan K, Balasubramanian K, Ali SM, Rao BV: **Poincare plot of heart rate variability: an approach towards explaining the cardiovascular autonomic function in obesity.** *Indian J Physiol Pharmacol* 2013, **57**(1):31–37.
44. de Jonge L, Moreira EA, Martin CK, Ravussin E: **Impact of 6-month caloric restriction on autonomic nervous system activity in healthy, overweight, individuals.** *Obesity (Silver Spring)* 2010, **18**(2):414–416.
45. Muth ER, Thayer JF, Stern RM, Friedman BH, Drake C: **The effect of autonomic nervous system activity on gastric myoelectrical activity: does the spectral reserve hypothesis hold for the stomach?** *Biol Psychol* 1998, **47**(3):265–278.
46. Riezzo G, Pezzolla F, Giorgio I: **Effects of age and obesity on fasting gastric electrical activity in man: a cutaneous electrogastrographic study.** *Digestion* 1991, **50**(3–4):176–181.
47. Herbert BM, Herbert C, Pollatos O, Weimer K, Enck P, Sauer H, Zipfel S: **Effects of short-term food deprivation on interoceptive awareness, feelings and autonomic cardiac activity.** *Biol Psychol* 2012, **89**(1):71–79.
48. Hamer M, Stamatakis E: **Inflammation as an intermediate pathway in the association between psychosocial stress and obesity.** *Physiol Behav* 2008, **94**(4):536–539.
49. Lorenz FOSR, Conger RD, Elder GH, Johnson C, Chao W: **Married and recently divorced mothers' stressful events and distress: tracing change across time.** *J Marriage Fam* 1997, **59**:219–232.
50. Gutman LMMV, Tokoyawa T: **Financial strain, neighborhood stress, parenting behaviors, and adolescent adjustment in urban African-American families.** *J Res Adolesc* 2005, **15**:425–440.
51. Hazel NA, Hammen C, Brennan PA, Najman J: **Early childhood adversity and adolescent depression: the mediating role of continued stress.** *Psychol Med* 2008, **38**(4):581–589.
52. Franko DL, Striegel-Moore RH, Thompson D, Schreiber GB, Daniels SR: **Does adolescent depression predict obesity in black and white young adult women?** *Psychol Med* 2005, **35**(10):1505–1513.
53. Goodman E, Whitaker RC: **A prospective study of the role of depression in the development and persistence of adolescent obesity.** *Pediatrics* 2002, **110**(3):497–504.

54. Dearing E, McCartney K, Taylor BA: **Within-child associations between family income and externalizing and internalizing problems.** *Dev Psychol* 2006, **42**(2):237–252.
55. Downey L, Van Willigen M: **Environmental stressors: the mental health impacts of living near industrial activity.** *J Health Soc Behav* 2005, **46**(3):289–305.
56. Eamon MK: **The effects of poverty on childrens socioemotional development: an ecological systems analysis.** *Soc Work* 2001, **46**(3):256–266.
57. Weimer K, Gulewitsch MD, Schlarb AA, Enck P: **Stressreaktivität von Kindern mit funktionellen Bauchschmerzen im Vergleich zu gesunden Kontrollen.** *Z Gastroenterol* 2012, **50:**K241.
58. Donaldson LF, Bennett L, Baic S, Melichar JK: **Taste and weight: is there a link?** *Am J Clin Nutr* 2009, **90**(3):800S–803S.
59. Rapps N, Giel KE, Sohngen E, Salini A, Enck P, Bischoff SC, Zipfel S: **Olfactory deficits in patients with anorexia nervosa.** *Eur Eat Disord Rev* 2010, **18**(5):385–389.
60. Bruce AS, Holsen LM, Chambers RJ, Martin LE, Brooks WM, Zarcone JR, Butler MG, Savage CR: **Obese children show hyperactivation to food pictures in brain networks linked to motivation, reward and cognitive control.** *Int J Obes (Lond)* 2010, **34**(10):1494–1500.
61. Ittersum K.v. W, B: **'Bottoms Up!' The Influence of Elongation on Pouring and Consumption Volume.** *J Consum Res* 2003, **30**(3):455–463.
62. Wansink B, van Ittersum K: **Shape of glass and amount of alcohol poured: comparative study of effect of practice and concentration.** *BMJ* 2005, **331**(7531):1512–1514.
63. Dong Y, Hoover A, Muth E: **A device for detecting and counting bites of food taken by a person during eating.** In *IEEE International Conference on Bioinformatics and Biomedicine*; 2009:265–268.
64. Mesas AE, Munoz-Pareja M, Lopez-Garcia E, Rodriguez-Artalejo F: **Selected eating behaviours and excess body weight: a systematic review.** *Obes Rev* 2012, **13**(2):106–135.
65. Dong YME: **Monitoring eating consumption via wrist motion tracking.** In *IEEE Transaction on information technology in biomedicine*; 2011. in press.
66. Dong Y, Hoover A, Scisco J, Muth E: **A new method for measuring meal intake in humans via automated wrist motion tracking.** *Appl Psychophysiol Biofeedback* 2012, **37**(3):205–215.
67. Kromeyer-Hauschild KWM, Geller F, Ziegler A, HC G z, Hesse V: **Percentiles of body mass index in children and adolescents evaluated from different regional German studies.** *Monatsschr Kinderheilkd* 2001, **149:**807–818.
68. Cole TJ: **The LMS method for constructing normalized growth standards.** *Eur J Clin Nutr* 1990, **44**(1):45–60.
69. Kunze D, Wabitsch M: *Konsensbasierte Leitlinie zur Prävention und Therapie von Übergewicht und Adipositas im Kindes- und Jugendalter*, 2012. [http://www.aga.adipositas-gesellschaft.de/fileadmin/PDF/Leitlinien/AGA_S2_Leitlinie.pdf], Version 04.10.
70. Tafeit E, Greilberger J, Cvirn G, Lipp RW, Schnedl WJ, Jurimae T, Jurimae J, Wallner-Liebmann SJ: **Estimating DXA total body fat percentage by lipometer subcutaneous adipose tissue thicknesses.** *Coll Antropol* 2009, **33**(2):391–396.
71. Jurimae T, Sudi K, Payerl D, Leppik A, Jurimae J, Muller R, Tafeit E: **Relationships between bioelectric impedance and subcutaneous adipose tissue thickness measured by LIPOMETER and skinfold calipers in children.** *Eur J Appl Physiol* 2003, **90**(1–2):178–184.
72. Tafeit E, Moller R, Sudi K, Reibnegger G: **Artificial neural networks as a method to improve the precision of subcutaneous adipose tissue thickness measurements by means of the optical device LIPOMETER.** *Comput Biol Med* 2000, **30**(6):355–365.
73. Jouck SKB, Graf C, Predel HG, Dordel S: **Dordel-Koch-Test (DKT) - zur Erfassung der motorischen Basisfunktionen im Kindes- und Jugendalter; ertse Ergebnisse der Normierung.** *Aktuuel Ernaerungsmed* 2006, **31:**27.
74. Owens JA, Spirito A, McGuinn M, Nobile C: **Sleep habits and sleep disturbance in elementary school-aged children.** *J Dev Behav Pediatr* 2000, **21**(1):27–36.
75. Schwerdtle BRK, Kübler A, Schlarb AA: **Screening Validation and psychometric properties of the German version of the Sleep Self Report (SSR-DE). A self-report questionnaire for the assessment of sleep disorders in children from 7–12 years old.** *Somnologie* 2010, **14:**267–274.
76. Perez-Chada D, Perez-Lloret S, Videla AJ, Cardinali D, Bergna MA, Fernandez-Acquier M, Larrateguy L, Zabert GE, Drake C: **Sleep disordered breathing and daytime sleepiness are associated with poor academic performance in teenagers. A study using the Pediatric Daytime Sleepiness Scale (PDSS).** *Sleep* 2007, **30**(12):1698–1703.
77. Mattejat F, Remschmidt H: *ILK Inventar zur Erfassung der Lebensqualität bei Kindern und Jugendlichen. Ratingbogen für Kinder, Jugendliche und Eltern.* Bern: Verlag Hans Huber; 2006.
78. Diehl JM: **Attitude to eating and body weight by 11- to 16-year-old adolescents.** *Schweiz Med Wochenschr* 1999, **129**(5):162–175.
79. Walker LS, Garber J, Greene JW: **Somatization symptoms in pediatric abdominal pain patients: relation to chronicity of abdominal pain and parent somatization.** *J Abnorm Child Psychol* 1991, **19**(4):379–394.
80. Garber IWL, Zeman J: **Somatization symptoms in a community sample of children and adolescents: Further vadildation of the Children's Somatization Inventory.** *Psychol Assess* 1991, **3:**588–595.
81. Spielberger CD, Drew EC, Lushene RE, Montuori J, Platzek D: *STAIC Manual.* Palo Alto: Consulting Psychologists Press; 1973.
82. Unnewehr S, Joormann S, Schneider S, Margraf J: **Deutsche Übersetzung des state-trait anxiety inventory for children.** In *Manuscript Drafting Process*; 1992.
83. Stiensmeier-Pelster JSM, Duda K: *DIKJ Depressions-Inventar für Kinder und Jugendliche.* Göttinge: Hogrefe Verlag; 2000.
84. Lohaus AEH, Kohlmann C-W, Klein-Heßling J: *SSKJ 3–8. Fragebogen zur Erhebung von Stress und Stressbewältigung im Kindes- und Jugendalter.* Göttingen: Hogrefe; 2006.
85. Chervin RD, Hedger K, Dillon JE, Pituch KJ: **Pediatric sleep questionnaire (PSQ): validity and reliability of scales for sleep-disordered breathing, snoring, sleepiness, and behavioral problems.** *Sleep Med* 2000, **1**(1):21–32.
86. Johns MW: **A new method for measuring daytime sleepiness: the Epworth sleepiness scale.** *Sleep* 1991, **14**(6):540–545.
87. Handwerker G: **Epworth-Sleepiness-Scale für Kinder (ESS-K).** In *Kompendium Schlafmedizin.* Edited by Schulz H. Landsberg/Lech: Ecomed-Verlag; 2002.
88. Owens JA, Spirito A, McGuinn M: **The Children's Sleep Habits Questionnaire (CSHQ): psychometric properties of a survey instrument for school-aged children.** *Sleep* 2000, **23**(8):1043–1051.
89. Schlarb AA SB, Hautzinger M: **Validation and psychometric properties of the German version of the Children's Sleep Habits Questionnaire (CSHQ-DE).** *Somnologie - Schlafforschung und Schlafmedizin* 2012, **14**(4):260–266.
90. Goodman R: **The Strengths and Difficulties Questionnaire: a research note.** *J Child Psychol Psychiatry* 1997, **38**(5):581–586.
91. Klasen H, Woerner W, Rothenberger A: **Goodman R: [German version of the Strength and Difficulties Questionnaire (SDQ-German)–overview and evaluation of initial validation and normative results].** *Prax Kinderpsychol Kinderpsychiatr* 2003, **52**(7):491–502.
92. Collani H: **Zur internen Struktur des globalen Selbstwertgefühls nach Rosenberg.** *Zeitschrift für Differentielle und Diagnostische Psychologie* 2003, **24:**3–7.
93. Moeller R, Horejsi R, Pilz S, Lang N, Sargsyan K, Dimitrova R, Tafeit E, Giuliani A, Almer G, Mangge H: **Evaluation of risk profiles by subcutaneous adipose tissue topography in obese juveniles.** *Obesity (Silver Spring)* 2007, **15**(5):1319–1324.
94. Greil H, Trippo U: **Physique and body composition: comparisons of methods and results.** *Coll Antropol* 1998, **22**(2):345–363.
95. Herbert BM, Pollatos O: **The body in the mind: on the relationship between interoception and embodiment.** *Top Cogn Sci* 2012, **4**(4):692–704.
96. Landis BN, Welge-Luessen A, Bramerson A, Bende M, Mueller CA, Nordin S, Hummel T: **"Taste Strips" - a rapid, lateralized, gustatory bedside identification test based on impregnated filter papers.** *J Neurol* 2009, **256**(2):242–248.
97. Hummel T, Sekinger B, Wolf SR, Pauli E, Kobal G: **'Sniffin' sticks': olfactory performance assessed by the combined testing of odor identification, odor discrimination and olfactory threshold.** *Chem Senses* 1997, **22**(1):39–52.
98. Miller KEME: **Efficacy of acupressure and acustimulation bands for the prevention of motion sickness.** *Aviat Space Environ Med* 2004, **75:**227–234.
99. Koch KL, Stern RM: *Handbook of Electrogastrography.* Oxford: Oxford University Press; 2004.
100. Friesen CALZ, Schurman JV, Andre L, Mc Callum RW: **Autonomic nervous system response to a solid meal and water loading in healthy children:**

its relation to gastric myoelectrical activity. *Neurogastroenterol Motil* 2007, **19**:376–382.
101. Scisco JL, Muth ER, Dong Y, Hoover AW: **Slowing bite-rate reduces energy intake: an application of the bite counter device.** *J Am Diet Assoc* 2011, **111**(8):1231–1235.
102. Faul FEE, Buchner A, Lang A-G: **Statistical power analyses using G*Power 3.1: Tests for correlation and regression analyses.** *Behav Res Methods* 2009, **41**:1149–1160.
103. Cohen J: *Statistical Power Analysis for the Behavioral Sciences.* secondth edition. Hillsdale, NJ: Lawrence Erlbaum Associates; 1988.

Reducing self-objectification: are dissonance-based methods a possible approach?

Carolyn Black Becker[1*], Kaitlin Hill[1], Rebecca Greif[2], Hongmei Han[3] and Tiffany Stewart[3]

Abstract

Background: Previous research has documented that self-objectification is associated with numerous negative outcomes including body shame, eating disorder (ED) pathology, and negative affect. This exploratory open study investigated whether or not an evidence-based body image improvement program that targets thin-ideal internalization in university women also reduces self-objectification. A second aim of the study was to determine if previous findings showing that body shame mediated the relationship between self-objectification and eating disorder pathology at a single time point (consistent with self-objectification theory) but did not mediate longitudinally (inconsistent with self-objectification theory) would be replicated in a new sample under novel conditions.

Methods: Ninety-six university women completed a peer-led dissonance-based intervention, along with assessment measures at pre-, post-intervention, 8-week and 8-month follow-up. To address the open trial nature of this study, a planned manipulation check was included to make sure that peer-led dissonance decreased thin-ideal internalization, body dissatisfaction, eating disorder pathology, and negative affect with effect sizes being similar to past randomized controlled trials. We hypothesized that all three subscales of the Objectified Body Consciousness Scale (i.e., self-surveillance, body shame, and appearance control beliefs) would be reduced. In addition, we hypothesized that body shame would mediate the relationship between self-objectification (i.e., self-surveillance) and eating disorder pathology at a both at a single time point and longitudinally.

Results: The planned manipulation check supported the interpretation that peer-led dissonance in this study largely yielded comparable changes to past controlled trials. In terms of changes in dependent variables, results supported all hypotheses with the exception of body shame, which remained unchanged. With regards to the mediation analyses, our first (cross-sectional) hypothesis but not our second (longitudinal) was supported.

Conclusions: Findings provide preliminary support for the use of dissonance interventions in reducing self-surveillance and body control beliefs. Results for body shame and the mediation analyses suggest that greater scrutiny of the body shame construct is warranted.

Keywords: Self-Objectification, Body shame, Cognitive dissonance-based interventions, Eating disorders, Mediation, Sororities

* Correspondence: cbecker@trinity.edu
[1]Department of Psychology, Trinity University, One Trinity Place, San Antonio, TX 78212-7200, USA
Full list of author information is available at the end of the article

Background

Objectification theory is a conceptual framework, rooted in feminist theory, regarding women's experience of their bodies [1-4]. Objectification theory posits that women's bodies are regularly objectified (i.e., depicted as sexual "objects to be viewed") in several cultures, including modern western culture. According to objectification theory, frequent experiences of objectification by others socialize women to engage in self-objectification, whereby a woman internalizes the outside perspective, and subsequently assesses the value of her body based on how others perceive it. Self-objectification can be viewed as adaptive to some degree in that it allows women to anticipate the social ramifications of their appearance [3]. Yet, when discrepancies exist between a female's body and the external standard she uses to judge her body, negative self-evaluation often ensues [1,4]. Thus, in societies, such as modern western culture, in which the ideal female body type is not only significantly thinner than the average woman but also largely unattainable by virtue of consisting of physically incompatible body attributes (e.g., low body fat and large breasts [4]), self-objectification often results in negative views of oneself.

Research supports the link between self-objectification and a number of negative outcomes for women [2,4,5]. For instance, consistent with objectification theory, habitual self-monitoring of one's appearance, which characterizes self-objectification, has been associated with increased body shame and appearance anxiety [1]. Furthermore, increased focus on one's appearance is hypothesized to decrease the mental resources utilized for other activities, subsequently decreasing performance on cognitive tasks, such as math [3]. Perpetual external focus also has been linked to decreased awareness of one's internal states and ability to obtain peak motivational states [6,7]. Finally, self-objectification appears to be associated with psychological disorders, including unipolar depression, sexual dysfunction, and eating disorders [1,8]. For instance, there is a large body of research supporting a relationship between self-objectification and eating disorders for women ranging in age from adolescence through later adulthood [9-12]. Further, consistent with proposed relationships in objectification theory, body shame appears to at least partially mediate the relationship between self-objectification and measures of eating disorders, albeit at a single time-point [13-15].

Objectification theory has been studied in a number of contexts, including sororities, because some evidence suggests that they may attract women with elevated levels of self-objectification and/or perpetuate or exacerbate this mentality [16,17]. A largely North American tradition, sororities are social institutions for university aged women that aim to meet university women's need to belong. In a recent study, Rolnik, Engeln-Maddox, and Miller [17] compared levels of self-objectification, body shame, and eating attitudes and behaviors between undergraduate women who participated in sorority recruitment (i.e., "rush") and those who did not participate at four time points (5 days before recruitment; 4 days into recruitment; bid day; and 1-month after bid day). Recruitment is a sort of courtship process whereby female students determine to which sorority they wish to apply, and sororities decide whom they wish to invite as new members. Rolnik et al. also examined the relationship between BMI and the sorority recruitment process. The authors hypothesized that women who participated in recruitment would show increased levels of self-objectification, body shame, and eating disorder behavior at all time points, as compared to those who did not participate. Further, they predicted that participation in recruitment and joining a sorority would increase self-objectification because recruitment represents a real world example of an objectifying process in that appearance (e.g., conforming to the thin-ideal) is often believed to be highly important during recruitment (see http://sororityrush.webs.com/preparationi.htm). They also predicted that women with higher BMIs would be more likely to drop out of and be less satisfied with recruitment. Results were mixed; findings indicated that women who participated in recruitment had increased levels of self-objectification and eating disorder behaviors and attitudes at all four time points. Evidence did not, however, indicate that recruitment worsened self-objectification. Rolnik et al. also found no difference in body shame between those who did and did not participate in recruitment, although sorority members showed an increase in body shame one month after joining a sorority. BMI negatively correlated with satisfaction with the recruitment process and predicted whether a participant dropped out of recruitment.

Rolnik et al. [17] also investigated proposed relationships in objectification theory (i.e., that self-objectification leads to increased body shame which increases one's risk for an eating disorder [5]). As noted above, previous cross-sectional research supports objectification theory's proposed relationships between self-objectification, body shame, and eating disorder pathology with body shame at least partially mediating the relationship between self-objectification and eating disorder pathology when relationships are tested at a single time point [13-15]. Con sistent with past research, Rolnik et al. found that body shame mediated the relationship between self-objectification and eating disorder pathology when the model was tested at baseline. Yet, when Rolnik et al. conducted a longitudinal mediation analysis with the same dataset and measures, they found that changes in self-objectification (which was operationalized using the self-surveillance subscale of the Objectified Body

Consciousness Scale [2]) did not predict changes in body shame, and that changes in shame did not predict eating disorder attitudes/behavior. In short, a relationship that has been consistently found at a single time point did not hold up when investigated longitudinally. This is an important finding because objectification theory proposes a longitudinal not cross-sectional relationship.

Studying objectification theory under conditions that are likely to increase self-objectification is one approach to investigating this theory. Another approach is to investigate objectification theory and self-objectification under conditions that may reduce self-objectification. For instance, it may be that programs that reduce variables strongly associated with self-objectification (e.g., body dissatisfaction, eating disorder pathology, negative affect [1,2,8-12]) may also reduce self-objectification and offer a novel way to investigate relationships proposed in this theory. Moreover, given the increased recognition about the problematic effects of self-objectification, it is important to begin to study methodologies for reducing self-objectification.

Research supports the use of a peer-led cognitive dissonance-based intervention (PL-DBI) in reducing body dissatisfaction and other eating disorder risk factors in university-based undergraduate communities, like sororities. PL-DBI is supported by both the general research on cognitive dissonance-based approaches [18-24] as well as by specific randomized trials conducted within the sorority context [25-28]. Cognitive dissonance, a well-studied psychological phenomenon, is an uncomfortable psychological state that occurs when actions and beliefs are misaligned [29]. It typically is resolved by altering beliefs to be consistent with one's actions. Dissonance-based interventions (DBIs) generally aim to induce cognitive dissonance with respect to the thin-ideal standard of female beauty by having participants speak and act against the thin-ideal during a series of small group activities and homework assignments. PL-DBI was started in partnership with an entire community of local sororities at one university, and then expanded in partnership with a national sorority in the United States. This approach also has been implemented in non-sorority settings on select campuses in the United States (e.g., dorms, with intramural trainers; see Becker, Stice, Shaw & Woda [30] for additional detail), as well as in the United Kingdom (www.succeedfoundation.org).

To date, PL-DBI has been implemented with at least one group on over 80 undergraduate campuses in the United States and two campuses in the United Kingdom. Prior randomized controlled research has demonstrated that PL-DBI reduces participants' levels of thin-ideal internalization, body dissatisfaction, dietary restraint, negative affect and bulimic pathology [27-29], and that sorority peer-leaders who have greater exposure to the program show even greater improvement in these domains [27]. Importantly, PL-DBI has been found to be superior to alternative, credible interventions at post-intervention [28] and at follow-up [26,31]. Further, PL-DBI has generated 14-month within group effect sizes [28] that are comparable to those found for the original version of dissonance prevention in Stice et al.'s [23] randomized controlled trial at 1-year. Follow-up analyses for this study by Stice et al. [21] also found that DBIs can reduce onset of eating disorders at three years.

As previously noted, self-objectification has been linked to body dissatisfaction and disordered eating. Further, self-objectification has been implicated as at least partially mediating the relationship between thin-ideal internalization and body dissatisfaction [32], and research indicates that self-objectification and thin-ideal internalization may have a bidirectional relationship on one another [33]. Thus, it seems plausible that DBIs, which explicitly seek to reduce thin-ideal internalization and have documented success in reducing body dissatisfaction in controlled trials, might decrease levels of self-objectification. DBIs may be particularly salient given that participants are encouraged to collectively battle the thin-ideal as a form of political body activism, an approach that should fit well with attempts to combat objectification. Despite this, DBI's impact on self-objectification largely has not been explored. To date, one study has examined whether or not a modified version of a DBI reduced self-objectification [33]. In this study, the DBI was specifically altered to include an increased focus on self-objectification and was found to reduce self-objectification. Yet, given that the original DBI (sans the extra focus on self-objectification) has been shown to influence so many factors associated with self-objectification (e.g., eating disorders pathology, body dissatisfaction, thin-ideal internalization, negative affect), it remains possible that the original form of the DBI will impact self-objectification rendering modifications unnecessary.

The first aim of this exploratory open trial was to investigate whether unmodified PL-DBI improves self-objectification. To study self-objectification, we utilized the Objectified Body Consciousness Scale [2], which is composed of three subscales that assess self-objectification and associated constructs: self-surveillance, body shame, and appearance control beliefs. We used this measure to facilitate comparison with Rolnik et al. [17] and to assist with our secondary aim (see below). Self-surveillance is the subscale that typically is used to operationalize self-objectification; thus in the present study, self-surveillance represents self-objectification. Body shame is often viewed as one domain of body dissatisfaction and was important for our secondary aim. Although the appearance control beliefs construct has been identified as less reliable than self-surveillance and body shame [34], given the exploratory nature of this study we chose to include it.

We investigated three hypotheses in the present study and included a manipulation check to address the open nature of this trial. For the manipulation check, we checked to make sure that, as in controlled studies, PL-DBI participants evidenced reductions in thin-ideal internalization, body dissatisfaction, negative affect, and eating disorder pathology. We also benchmarked effects sizes in the present study against effect sizes in previous controlled trials. Previous trials have demonstrated that DBI reduces these risk factors relative to control conditions including alternate interventions (i.e., thus accounting for demand, regression to the mean, placebo). Thus, if effects in the present study are comparable, we have some, albeit not perfect, evidence that reductions in the present trial are not merely a result of demand, regression to the mean etc. We next hypothesized that participants would show improvements in self-surveillance, body shame and appearance control beliefs (Hypothesis 1). If the manipulation check held and hypothesis 1 was supported, we would suggest that self-objectification, body shame, and appearance control beliefs be investigated in future controlled trials.

A secondary aim of this study was to see if the unexpected longitudinal mediation findings from the above-mentioned Rolnik et al. [17] study would be replicated. To our knowledge, Rolnik et al. conducted the first and only published longitudinal mediation analysis regarding self-objectification, body shame, and disordered eating. Thus, we sought to investigate if results would be similar when we investigated the same relationships longitudinally with a different sample that participated in a positive body image program. Like Rolnik et al., we first sought to determine if our sample yielded results consistent with previous cross-sectional research before examining objectification theory longitudinally. If this study does not replicate previous cross-sectional findings, this suggests that any longitudinal findings may be sample specific. However, if the study did replicate standard cross-sectional findings, but did not support a longitudinal relationship, this would represent a bigger challenge to the theory. For our mediation analyses, we first hypothesized that body shame would mediate the relationship between self-objectification and eating disorder pathology at baseline (Hypothesis 3). We next hypothesized that Rolnik et al.'s findings were a random finding, and that we would also find a mediation relationship longitudinally (Hypothesis 4).

Method

Participants

Participants were 96 female students at a small southwestern university in the United States who received PL-DBI [35] as part of new sorority member orientation and agreed to participate in a voluntary, associated study. The campus sororities annually and collectively require all new members (i.e., those who have accepted "bids" to join a specific sorority) to complete PL-DBI unless the new members have an excused absence (e.g., class conflict).

Participants' ages ranged from 18 to 21 years ($M = 18.76$, $SD = 0.77$). The body mass index (BMI) of participants, calculated using self-reported weight and height measurements, ranged from 17.33 to 36.32 ($M = 22.34$, $SD = 3.38$). We used the NIMH two-question approach to assess ethnicity and race. Twelve percent of respondents endorsed Hispanic/Latino ethnicity, 72% endorsed not Hispanic/ Latino and 16% did not respond. In response to the second question, 82% endorsed white, 3% Asian, 2% more than one race, 1% Black, and 12% did not respond. Because the focus of PL-DBI is on prevention and not treatment, as in past studies [25,26,28] we removed four participants from analysis for meeting probable eating disorder status based on the Eating Disorder Examination - Questionnaire (final analyzed sample N =92).

Procedure

Overview

Because the campus sororities require all new members to participate in the annual "Body Image Program," the "program" (i.e., the PL-DBI program) and "study" (i.e., the assessments only) were separated such that new members could attend the required program and opt out of the voluntary study. As appropriate, the program and overarching study were reviewed and approved by the Institutional Review Board (IRB), Sorority Presidents, Greek Council, and Student Affairs at Trinity University (e.g., Greek Council approved both study and program whereas IRB approved only the study).

Using lists of the new members for each sorority, new members were randomly allocated by undergraduate RAs into groups of 8 to 10, stratified by sorority. Thus, each group had roughly equal representation of members from each sorority. Each group was run by two to four peer-leaders, typically three, drawn from different sororities. At the beginning of the program, held in February, during new member orientation, new sorority members from each of the seven campus sororities attended a brief orientation session. Consenting participants for the voluntary study completed baseline questionnaires using a self-generated ID number to ensure confidentiality and then placed these in a large envelope. All participants were informed that if they chose to participate in the study, they could quit the study at any time without consequence. There was no compensation awarded for participation. To reduce coercion, we also informed all program participants that they could pretend to fill out the questionnaires and return blank questionnaires in the envelope. After completing questionnaires, participants met with their assigned groups to begin the first session. The second session took place exactly one week after the first session. Sessions were designed to last approximately 105 min plus time to complete questionnaires. Consenting participants filled out post-intervention questionnaires after the completion of the second session. Additional questionnaires were completed at 8-week and 8-month follow-up during sororities' weekly meetings.

Participant flow

Of the 92 participants at baseline, 70 (76%) completed questionnaires at post-intervention, 74 (80%) completed questionnaires at 8-week follow-up, and 64 (70%) completed questionnaires at 8-month follow-up.

Peer leader recruitment and training

PL-DBI was led by older sorority members. Active sorority members who had previously completed PL-DBI were recruited to be peer-leaders. Interested members were asked to self-screen for body image and eating disorder issues prior to volunteering and were asked not to volunteer if they felt these issues were severe or problematic. We also emphasized that if someone with an eating disorder or significant body image concerns did volunteer, she risked jeopardizing the entire program by making it appear hypocritical. The sororities take great pride in their annual body image program; thus we explicitly asked members to put the greater good of the program above their individual desire to lead a group. This is the same strategy that we have used in our past controlled trials [25-28].

Training for peer-leaders lasted a total of 9 hrs consisting of two 4½ hr sessions held one week apart. Peer-leaders were trained in small groups of 9–12, which were sub-divided into three training teams. Peer-leaders were trained by a doctoral level psychologist (CB) with the assistance of research assistants (RAs). The first session began with an introduction to the program and an overview of the history and impact of the program. Following this introduction, each training team was allotted an equal portion of time to run an abbreviated version of the first session in which they were instructed to follow the script provided in the PL-DBI manual [35]. Each team took turns being the peer-leaders while the other groups acted as mock-participants in the session; this allowed the peer-leaders to experience the session multiple times as well as lead it once.

Immediately after each group completed leading their session, they received supervision that focused on reinforcing group leadership skills and adherence to the manual, corrected any misconceptions or problematic parts of the session, and highlighted teamwork and individual group leader strengths and any observed weaknesses. The second training session was conducted in the exact same manner with each group performing an abbreviated second session while the other groups acted as mock participants.

The program

The PL-DBI began with an initial meeting orienting the new members to the program and the study, informing them about the history and structure of the program. Next, we explained the difference between the semi-mandatory program and the voluntary study. Following this, new members who chose to participate then completed consent forms and baseline questionnaires. The program was delivered to each cohort of new members in two 2-hour sessions that were held one week apart.

All groups were run simultaneously. After the initial orientation meeting, the peer-leaders for each group led their new members to the room designated for their sessions. Each room was provided a tape recorder for them to use to record the session; tapes were later used to check adherence. After introductions and icebreakers, the participants discussed the definition and origin of the thin-ideal. They also discussed how various messages from the media, peers, dating partners, families, and culture perpetuate the thin-ideal. Next, participants were given approximately 20 minutes to come up with a list of the costs of pursuing the thin-ideal in their workbooks, after which the group worked together to identify and thoroughly discuss the costs specific to six different areas such as self-esteem and academic costs, which were written on a board by a peer-leader.

Participants then identified examples of times where they encountered pressures to be thin and created verbal challenges for the situations. Each participant shared one of her examples with the whole group. Next, participants received a "mirror homework" assignment, which involved standing in front of a mirror wearing as little clothing as tolerable and writing down all of their positive qualities.

Participants began the second session by reviewing the mirror exercise they completed for homework following the last session, which included stating out loud one physical and emotional quality they liked about themselves. The participants then completed three role-plays with the peer-leaders. In this exercise, each peer-leader adopted a different persona obsessed with pursuing the thin-ideal. Once each character was introduced, participants broke into smaller groups and were given approximately 5 minutes to role-play intervening with each character, as though she was a close friend, with the goal of convincing her not to pursue the thin-ideal. Participants next discussed the role that fat talk plays in perpetuating the thin-ideal and how to challenge it. New members then created a top-10 list of ways to avoid or learn to battle the thin-ideal promoted by the society; this was titled "body activism." Next, they discussed and listed the ways in which their individual sorority or all of the sororities together could collectively battle thin-ideal; this was referred to as "sorority body activism." A core aspect of this exercise was to motivate participants to act on the collective sense of political outrage that naturally develops during PL-DBI.

At the end of the final session, members were encouraged to choose one self-affirmation exercise to participate in, either listed in their workbooks or one of their own, to promote more positive talk about, and behavior towards, their bodies. Finally, participants who volunteered for the study completed the post-intervention questionnaires and were dismissed.

Measures

Self-objectification, Body shame and Control beliefs

Self-objectification in the main analyses was operationalized using the14-item version [36] of the Objectified Body Consciousness Scale [2]. The OBCS is composed of three subscales with a total of 14 statements: self-surveillance (four items), body shame (five items), and appearance control beliefs (five items). The self-surveillance subscale is commonly conceptualized as a key indicator of self-objectification [34] and includes statements such as "I often compare how I look with how other people look." The body shame subscale identifies the degree to which the individual feels shamed by their evaluation relative to the cultural thin ideal, including such statements as "I feel like I must be a bad person when I don't look as good as I could." Statements under the appearance control beliefs subscale focus on the extent that the individual feels that they are in control of their appearance using statements such as "I think I could look as good as I wanted to if I worked at it." For each statement, the participant uses a 7-point Likert scale ranging from *strongly agree* to *strongly disagree* to rate the degree to which each statement corresponds with their own attitude towards their bodies. Responses on the OBCS are averaged for analysis. In college samples, internal consistency for the subscales in the short version of the OBCS ($\alpha = .66$-$.89$) has been found to be good and comparable to that of the classic version of the OBCS [34]. Likewise, two-week test-retest reliability has been found to be adequate ($r = .62$-$.81$) and subscale scores for the short version have been found to be highly correlated with the classic version ($r = .77$-$.82$) [36]. In this study, because of the way we handled reversed scored items for control beliefs, higher scores indicated more favorable appearance control attitudes whereas lower scores represent more positive attitudes with regards to self-surveillance and body shame. In the present sample internal consistency was good for self-surveillance ($\alpha = .86$-92 for all time points) and body shame ($\alpha = .80$-91). Consistent with past research, control beliefs had acceptable though weaker internal consistency ($\alpha = .53$-79). For the mediation analysis, we followed Rolnik et al.'s [17] approach of using the self-surveillance subscale as a sole indicator of self-objectification and the body shame subscale for the construct of body shame.

Thin-ideal internalization

Thin-ideal internalization was assessed with the Ideal Body Stereotype Scale-Revised (IBSS-R [37]). This scale consists of 10 items, in which participants endorse how much they agree (1 = *strongly disagree*, 5 = *strongly agree*; scale range: 1–5) with statements such as "thin women are more attractive." Scores from the items were averaged. In past studies, this scale has demonstrated adequate internal consistency ($\alpha = .89$) and test-retest reliability ($r = .63$) [38,39]. Internal consistency in the present sample was consistent with past research ($\alpha = .77$-$.92$).

Body dissatisfaction

We assessed body dissatisfaction with 9 items from the Satisfaction and Dissatisfaction with Body Parts Scale [40] as done in past dissonance trials by Stice et al [21,23]. Research supports the internal consistency ($\alpha = .94$), 3-week test-retest reliability ($r = .90$), and predictive validity for onset of bulimic symptoms [41]. In this sample, internal consistency was good ($\alpha = .89$-$.94$).

Eating disorder pathology

Eating disorder pathology was measured by taking a composite score of the diagnostic items from the Eating Disorder Examination-Questionnaire (EDE-Q [42]) as previously done in related studies [26,28]. The EDE-Q is a self-report version of the Eating Disorder Examination, which is currently considered the "gold standard" for assessing eating disorder pathology (EDE [43]). The EDE-Q, which has been extensively researched and tested for its psychometric properties [44-46] has been widely used. The 10 diagnostic items assess to what degree participants engaged in eating disordered behaviors over the past 28 days (e.g., "over the past 28 days, how many times have you taken laxatives as a means of controlling your shape or weight?"). Internal consistency for the eating disorder composite was adequate ($\alpha = .77$-$.81$) in the present sample.

Negative affect

We assessed negative affect using the fear, guilt, and sadness subscales from the Positive and Negative Affect Schedule-Revised (PANAS-X [47]). Participants indicated to what degree they had been feeling various emotional states (e.g., nervous, scared, and lonely) over the past few weeks by providing a rating from 1 = *very slightly or not at all* to 5 = *extremely* (scale range: 1–5). Scores from the 17 items were averaged. Prior research with this scale has demonstrated good internal consistency ($\alpha = .95$), convergent validity with affective measures, and predictive validity for bulimic symptom onset [38,47]. In the present study, internal consistency was good ($\alpha = .90$-94).

Results

Impact of PL-DBI (Manipulation check and hypothesis 1)

All analyses were conducted on an intent-to-treat basis. Missing data points were handled with PROC mixed procedure with maximum likelihood imputation procedures in SAS. Analyses of variance (ANOVAs) were conducted with time (pre-, post-, 8-week, and 8-month) as the repeated factor to test our main hypothesis that our intervention would improve all dependent measures at post-intervention and follow-up time points. Because the eating disorder pathology composite was skewed, we normalized using a square root transformation. Skewed PANAS data was normalized using a logarithmic transformation. We calculated Cohen's *d* effect sizes for post-intervention and all follow-ups to facilitate comparisons with previous trials (see Table 1 for means, standard deviations and Cohen's *d* effect sizes).

We first investigated whether our four traditional variables (i.e., thin-ideal internalization, body dissatisfaction, eating disorder pathology, and negative affect) showed the typical and expected reductions over time as a manipulation check. We found a statistically significant effect for all four traditional variables (thin-ideal internalization, $F\ (3,\ 214) = 19.95$, $p < .0001$; body dissatisfaction, $F\ (3,\ 212) = 5.29$, $p = .0015$; eating disorder pathology, $F\ (3,\ 213) = 10.35$, $p < .0001$; and negative affect, $F\ (3,\ 214) = 7.79$, $p < .0001$). Results of post-hoc comparisons for baseline to each follow-up are presented in Table 1. We then examined baseline to 8-month follow-up within group effect sizes from three previous trials to determine if effect sizes in the present study were comparable. Overall, effects were slightly lower in the present uncontrolled study at 8-months ($d = .20$ - $.33$) as compared to previous controlled studies (Becker et al. [26]: $d = .19$ - $.61$; Becker et al. [27]: $d = .28$-$.40$; 2010: $d = .30$ - $.59$), even though post hoc analyses at 8-months indicated that most effects were significantly different from baseline. Perhaps ironically, the effect size of the one outcome variable that was not significant at 8-months in the present study (see Table 1), thin-ideal internalization ($d = .31$) was virtually identical to that found in Becker et al. [28] ($d = .30$), where it was significant. Taken as a whole, results from this open trial were reasonably comparable to past research if slightly smaller, and support the interpretation that PL-DBI yielded a similar effect in this trial to past controlled studies.

We next examined our three new variables, each associated with objectification theory. For self-surveillance, we found a statistically significant improvement, $F\ (3,\ 211) = 8.04$, $p < .0001$, which was maintained at 8-month follow-up (see Table 1). The magnitude of effect was very similar to our traditional variables. We found a similar pattern when we examined control beliefs, $F\ (3,\ 211) = 10.17$, $p < .0001$. Thus, our hypotheses were supported with these two novel variables. Our hypothesis for body shame, however, was not supported. Body shame did not evidence any meaningful change ($d = .03$ at 8 months) during the course of PL-DBI, $F\ (3,\ 211) = 1.78$, $p = .1513$.

Mediation analyses (Hypotheses 2 & 3)

Mediation analysis tests whether the potential mediator variable (a third variable) influences the relationship between the two primary variables of interest. Mediation analyses were conducted to determine if body shame mediated the relationship between self-objectification (operationalized with the self-surveillance subscale) and eating disorder pathology at baseline (Hypothesis 2). We hypothesized that body shame would reduce the effect of self-objectification on eating disorder pathology, or in

Table 1 Means and standard deviations for dependent measures

Measures	Baseline *M (SD)*	Post intervention *M (SD)*	8-week follow-up *M (SD)*	8-month follow-up *M (SD)*	Post intervention *d*	8 weeks *d*	8 months *d*
Negative Affect	1.73(.60)	1.50(.49)	1.47(.55)	1.60(.62)	.40*	.38*	.20*
Thin-Ideal Internalization	3.56(.42)	3.05(.72)	3.26(.65)	3.43(.53)	1.2*	.69*	.31
Body Dissatisfaction	3.06(.80)	2.80(.75)	2.98(.76)	2.82(.70)	.35*	.08	.33*
EDE-Q	1.09(.74)	0.87(.63)	0.71(.62)	0.84(.67)	.36*	.47*	.32*
Body Shame	2.82(1.17)	2.78(1.25)	3.03(1.17)	2.84(1.11)	.05	.18	.03
Self-Surveillance	5.01(1.30)	4.55(1.27)	4.44(1.19)	4.70(1.10)	.38*	.43*	.31*
Control Beliefs	3.04(.85)	3.51(.98)	3.54(.75)	3.35(1.03)	.56*	.59*	.38*

Note: Improvement for all measures is indicated by decreasing scores with the exception of Body Control, for which higher scores indicate improvement.
* indicates $p < .05$ for post-hoc t-test comparison with baseline. Cohen's *d* effect size estimates: .2 = small; .5 = medium; .8 = large [48].

other words, we hypothesized that the amount of mediation (which is called the indirect effect) would be significant from zero. In order to evaluate if body shame mediated the relationship between self-objectification and eating disorder pathology at baseline, we tested four pathways: (a) self-objectification predicting body shame, (b) self-objectification predicting eating disorder pathology, (c) body shame predicting eating disorder pathology, and (d) body shame mediating the relationship between the other two variables. To facilitate comparison with Rolnik et al. [17], we used similar analyses and performed a series of regression models to test the above pathways as outlined by Baron and Kenny [40]. Next, a bias-corrected accelerated bootstrapping method was used to test if the indirect effect was zero [49].

At baseline, we tested the above pathways with 91 participants. First, it was confirmed that objectification significantly predicted body shame ($b = .41$, $t = 4.86$, $p < .0001$) and self-objectification significantly predicted eating disorder pathology ($b = .13$, $t = 3.92$, $p = .0002$). Next, there was a significant effect of body shame on eating disorder pathology ($b = .20$, $t = 6.12$, $p < .0001$). When controlling for body shame, the effect of self-objectification on eating disorder pathology became non-significant ($b = .056$, $t = 1.72$, $p = .089$). Finally, the indirect effect of self-objectification on eating disorder behavior through body shame was estimated to be .07, with 95% confidence interval from .03 to .12, using a bias-corrected accelerated bootstrap with 5,000 replications [50]. These findings suggest that body shame mediated the relationship between self-objectification and eating disorder pathology at baseline.

A cross-lagged panel model was constructed using PROC CALIS in SAS to examine whether the above-mentioned relationship existed longitudinally (Hypothesis 3). We used pre-, post-intervention, and 8-week data and chose not to use eight-month data so that data included in the model were more evenly spaced. In this model, each variable was allowed to predict its own occurrence at subsequent time points; other predictors were examined in addition to those previous effects that had been controlled for, as depicted in Figure 1.

The comparative fit index (CFI) and the standardized root mean square residual (SRMR) were reported. A CFI of .95 or higher and a SRMR of .08 or lower is considered ideal [51]. For the present model, the CFI had a value of .98 and the SRMR had a value of .07, which indicated that the model fit the data well. As shown in the Figure 1, self-objectification at Time 1 predicted self-objectification at Time 2, and the Time 2 value predicted self-objectification at Time 3 (all $ps < .001$). The same findings held for body shame and eating disorder pathology variables (all $ps < .001$). However, self-objectification failed to predict body shame when controlling previous occurrence ($ps > .05$). The results for body shame predicting eating disorder pathology was not consistent over time. Body shame at Time 1 positively predicted eating disorder pathology at Time 2 ($p < .001$) while body shame at Time 2 negatively predicted eating disorder pathology at Time 3 when previous eating disorder pathology was controlled ($p < .01$). Since there is no relationship between self-objectification and body shame when controlling for previous occurrence, basic conditions to establish the mediation were not met and the cross-sectional mediation relationship described earlier was not replicated for longitudinal data.

Discussion

The purpose of the present study was two-fold. First, we sought to determine whether or not self-objectification as measured by the OBCS was reduced in sorority members who participated in a PL-DBI program. Second, we wanted to determine if the mediation findings of Rolnik et al. [17] would replicate under very different circumstances (i.e., during implementation of a positive body image program versus sorority recruitment which could be viewed as increasing body scrutiny).

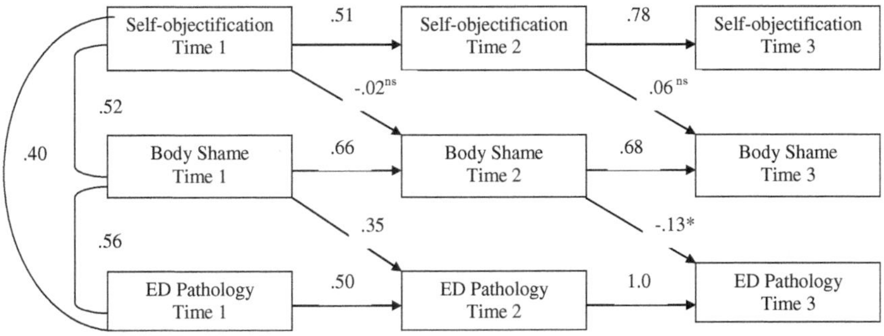

Figure 1 Cross-lagged panel model examining mediation longitudinally. Note: ns, not significant at .05 level; *, significant at .01 level; otherwise significant at .001 level.

Regarding the first objective, results indicated that self-surveillance, which is commonly viewed as the OBCS subscale most closely linked with the concept of self-objectification, and control beliefs were both reduced during the course of PL-DBI with effects maintained at 8-month follow-up in new sorority members. Although these findings will need to be replicated in controlled trials, this study provides preliminary evidence that DBIs which reduce thin-ideal internalization and body dissatisfaction may also impact self-objectification, with virtually identical effect sizes in this study. It should be noted that that effect size was relatively small, so additional research will be needed to determine the clinical significance of this finding. Importantly, however, the self-objectification effect size was virtually the same in this study ($d = .31$) at 8-months as in Kroon Van Diest & Perez [33] ($d = .29$) at 5-months. This strongly suggests that the modifications they made to increase the focus on self-objectification were unnecessary.

The current trial was not controlled; thus it could be argued that significant effects were not a result of the program but some other factor such as maturation or testing. Yet, in this trial, effect sizes for body dissatisfaction, thin-ideal internalization, negative affect, and eating disorder pathology were similar to past controlled trials in which dissonance outperformed alternative interventions under the same conditions (peer-led with new sorority members: Becker et al. [25-28]). Moreover, in the Rolnik et al. [17] sorority study, they found no statistically significant changes in self surveillance over time in either the sorority recruitment or control group, suggesting that self surveillance does not reduce merely as an effect of repeated testing over time.

Although participation in PL-DBI was associated with a reduction in self-surveillance and control beliefs, it was not associated with a reduction in body shame. This is a particularly interesting finding in that several constructs hypothesized in the literature to be closely related to body shame (e.g., body dissatisfaction, self-surveillance, eating disorder pathology, thin-ideal internalization) all showed significant and sustained reductions during the course of this study, whereas body shame showed absolutely no change. One possible explanation is that this is simply a random chance finding. This seems unlikely, however, in that Greif, Farris, You, Becker and Wilson [52] found a similar result in a small study of PL-DBI conducted with sororities at a university in the northeast section of the United States. In that study, both the self-surveillance and body control subscales improved, whereas body shame showed no improvement.

Alternatively, it could be that body shame would have naturally increased in this population without the PL-DBI program. Body shame was the one construct that significantly increased in sorority members over the course of Rolnik et al.'s study [17]. Thus, it could be that PL-DBI prevented that increase. This interpretation highlights the need for a follow-up trial that uses a no-intervention control group so that the natural course of body shame is observed.

Yet another explanation is that participants were already fairly low on body shame at baseline with a mean rating of 2.82 which falls between *disagree* and *somewhat disagree* on this scale (sample item: "I would be ashamed for people to know what I really weigh"). This is in contrast to the mean rating of 5.01 on the self-surveillance scale at baseline (sample item: "I often compare how I look with how other people look"), which is equivalent to *somewhat agree*. In other words, this finding could merely indicate a floor effect on this subscale. Interestingly, although baseline scores for self-surveillance are quite similar for the three sorority studies to include this measure (*M* range 5.01-5.29), mean body shame scores for Rolnik et al. [17] and the present study (M range 2.82-2.97) were quite a bit lower than in Basow et al. [16] which reported a mean of 4.03 in sorority members. This provides some support for a possible floor effect.

Another possible interpretation is that the body shame subscale of the OBCS is operationalizing a construct that does not fully map onto the construct originally conceptualized by Fredrickson and Roberts [3] and/or that the relationship between self-objectification, body shame, and eating disorder pathology is not as straightforward as previously thought. These latter interpretations are supported by the mediation findings of this present study and those of Rolnik et al. [17]. To review, Rolnik et al. found that body shame partially mediated the relationship between self-objectification (as measured by self-surveillance) and eating disorder pathology when the relationship was tested at a single time point. This finding was consistent with previous studies (see Tiggemann [53] for review) and consistent with self-objectification theory. Yet, when Rolnik et al. conducted, to our knowledge, the first longitudinal evaluation of the mediating role of body shame, the model was not supported. The present study found almost identical findings. Body shame mediated the relationship between self-objectification and eating disorder pathology at baseline. Yet, when we examined the relationship over time, the mediation model was not supported.

The relative consistency of findings between the present study and Rolnik et al. [17] are striking given that the longitudinal data were collected under quite different conditions. Rolnik et al. collected the data during sorority recruitment, which they argue is a real world situation that could be expected to increase self-objectification. In contrast, we collected our data during the implementation and follow-up of a well-established evidence-based body image improvement program that decreased self-surveillance. The fact that the mediating role of body shame was not supported longitudinally in either study suggests (a) that Rolnik et al.'s findings likely were not spurious, (b) further longitudinal research with other samples is needed, and (c) that researchers may need to rethink the conclusion that body shame as measured by the OBCS can be definitively said to at least partially mediate the relationship between self-objectification and eating disorder pathology in support of self-objectification theory. One interpretation of our study and Rolnik et al.'s is that objectification theory is simply wrong when it comes to the proposed pathway linking self-objectification to eating disorders. This seems a plausible hypothesis but clearly more research is needed before drawing this conclusion, particularly given the potential for floor effects mentioned earlier. It is clear, however, that we cannot assume that cross-sectional support is sufficient for a longitudinal model, and that researchers must begin to study this model longitudinally. Continued cross-sectional research serves little purpose at this point.

Lastly, it may be that body shame is more complex than previously realized. Another way to state this is that factors other than self-objectification may have a significant influence on body shame independent of self-objectification. For instance, Slater and Tiggemann [54] recently found that although time since menarche did not have an influence on self-objectification in adolescent girls, it did have an influence on body shame. More specifically, those girls who began menstruating more recently reported greater body shame. Thus, factors not measured in the present study may have had a significant influence on body shame while not affecting other dependent variables. Even if this is true, however, it suggests that revisions to objectification theory's proposed eating disorder pathway are likely in need to address this complexity.

This study has a number of limitations. First, as noted above this was an exploratory open trial with respect to the question of the impact of dissonance-based interventions on self-objectification. As such, findings need to be replicated in a controlled trial, ideally with a bigger sample, to address concerns about demand and other treats to internal validity. Although we conducted a manipulation check to make sure effect sizes were comparable to past trials for the traditional variables, controlled research is needed for the new variables. Second, there was some attrition. Although we accounted for that statistically and conducted intent-to-treat analyses, the use of incentives to retain a greater percentage of future samples at follow-up would be beneficial. Third, we were only able to use self-report measures in this study.

Conclusion

The present investigation provides preliminary evidence that DBIs may impact self-objectification, although further study is needed. This study also adds to a very limited literature suggesting that body shame may not mediate the relationship between self-objectification and eating disorder pathology longitudinally, despite significant evidence that the proposed mediating model is supported at a single time point. This, combined with the finding that body shame did not reduce over the course of the PL-DBI program while highly related constructs did improve, suggests that the body shame construct and the subscale of the OBCS deserve further critical scrutiny as does objectification theory and the proposed pathway from self-objectification to eating disorders.

Competing interests

Dr.'s Carolyn Black Becker and Rebecca Greif have received compensation in the past for time spent training people in the use of dissonance-based interventions. Dr. Becker is also co-director of the Body Project Collaborative, LLC which was formed to facilitate dissemination of dissonance-based interventions.

Authors' contributions

CB, RG, KH, and TS conceptualized this paper. CB and KH collected the original data for the paper. CB, RG, KH, and TS all contributed to the writing, editing, formatting of the paper. KH managed and organized the database. HH conducted the statistical analyses and reviewed write up of analyses. HH, CB, and TS reviewed and interpreted the results. All authors read and viewed the final version of this manuscript.

Acknowledgments

The authors thank the sororities of Trinity University for their support of this research.

Author details

[1]Department of Psychology, Trinity University, One Trinity Place, San Antonio, TX 78212-7200, USA. [2]Rutgers University, GSAPP, New Brunswick, NJ, USA. [3]Pennington Biomedical Research Center, Baton Rouge, LA, USA.

References

1. Fredrickson BL, Roberts T, Noll SM, Quinn DM, Twence JM: **That swimsuit becomes you: sex differences in self-objectification, restrained eating, and math performance.** *J Pers Soc Psychol* 1997, **75**(1):269–284.
2. McKinley NM, Hyde JS: **The objectified body consciousness scale: development and validation.** *Psychol Women Q* 1996, **20:**181–215.
3. Fredrickson BL, Roberts TA: **Objectification theory: toward understanding women's lived experience and mental health risks.** *Psychol Women Q* 1997, **21:**73–206.
4. Calogero RM, Tantleff-Dunn S, Thompson JK: **Objectification Theory: An Introduction.** In *Self-objectification in women: Causes, consequences, and counteractions*. 1st edition. Edited by Calogero RM, Tantleff-Dunn S, Thompson JK. Washington, D. C: American Psychological Association; 2011:3–22.
5. Noll SM, Fredrickson BL: **A meditational model linking self-objectification, body shame, and disordered eating.** *Psychol Women Q* 2004, **36:**195–203.
6. Csikszentmihalyi M: *Flow: The Psychology of Optimal Experience*. New York: Harper Perennial; 1990.
7. Quinn DM, Chaudoir SR, Kallen RW: **Performance and flow: A review and integration of self-objectification research.** In *Self-Objectification in Women: Causes, Consequences, and Counteractions*. 1st edition. Edited by Calogero RM, Tantleff-Dunn S, Thompson JK. Washington, D. C: American Psychological Association; 2011:19–38.
8. Prichard I, Tiggemann M: **Objectification in fitness centers: self-objectification, body dissatisfaction, and disordered eating in aerobic instructors and aerobic participants.** *Sex Roles* 2005, **53:**19–28.

9. Augustus-Horvath C, Tylka TL: **A test and extension of objectification theory as it predicts disordered eating: does women's age matter?** *J Couns Psychol* 2009, **56**:253–265.
10. Calogero R, Davis WN, Thompson JK: **The role of self objectification in the experience of woman with eating disorders.** *Sex Roles* 2005, **52**:45–49.
11. Harrison K, Fredrickson BL: **Women's sports media, self-objectification, and mental health in black and white adolescent females.** *J Commun* 2003, **53**(2):216–232.
12. Tiggemann M, Lynch JE: **Body image across the life span in adult women: the role of self-objectification.** *Dev Psychol* 2001, **37**(2):243–253.
13. Kozee HB, Tylka TL, Augustus-Horvath C, Denchik A: **Development and psychometric evaluation of the interpersonal sexual objectification scale.** *Psychol Women Q* 2007, **31**:176–189.
14. Slater A, Tiggemann M: **A test of objectification theory in adolescent girls.** *Sex Roles* 2002, **46**:343–349.
15. Tylka TL, Hill MS: **Objectification theory as it relates to disordered eating among college women.** *Sex Roles* 2004, **51**:719–730.
16. Basow SA, Foran KA, Bookwala J: **Body objectification, social pressure, and disordered eating behavior in college women: The role of sorority membership.** *Psychol Women Q* 2007, **31**(4):394–400.
17. Rolnik AM, Engeln-Maddox R, Miller SA: **Here's looking at you: Self-objectification, body image disturbance, and sorority rush.** *Sex Roles* 2010, **63**:6–17.
18. Matusek JA, Wendt SJ, Wiseman CV: **Dissonance thin-ideal and didactic healthy behavior eating disorder prevention programs: Results from a controlled trial.** *Int J Eat Disord* 2004, **36**:376–388.
19. Mitchell KS, Mazzeo SE, Rausch SM, Cooke KL: **Innovative interventions for disordered eating: evaluating dissonance-based and yoga interventions.** *Int J Eat Disord* 2007, **40**:120–128.
20. Stice E, Chase A, Stormer S, Appel A: **A randomized trial of a dissonance-based eating disorder prevention program.** *Int J Eat Disord* 2001, **29**:247–262.
21. Stice E, Marti CN, Spoor S, Presnell K, Shaw H: **Dissonance and healthy weight eating disorder prevention programs: long-term effects from a randomized efficacy trial.** *J Consult Clin Psychol* 2008, **76**:329–340.
22. Stice E, Mazotti L, Weibel D, Agras WS: **Dissonance prevention program decreases thin-ideal internalization, body dissatisfaction, dieting, negative affect, and bulimic symptoms. A preliminary experiment.** *Int J Eat Disord* 2000, **27**:206–217.
23. Stice E, Shaw H, Burton E, Wade E: **Dissonance and healthy weight eating disorder prevention programs: a randomized efficacy trial.** *J Consult Clin Psychol* 2006, **74**:263–275.
24. Stice E, Trost A, Chase A: **Healthy weight control and dissonance-based eating disorder prevention programs: Results from a controlled trial.** *Int J Eat Disord* 2003, **33**:10–21.
25. Becker CB, Smith LM, Ciao AC: **Reducing eating disorder risk factors in sorority members: a randomized trial.** *Behav Ther* 2005, **36**:245–253.
26. Becker CB, Smith LM, Ciao AC: **Peer-facilitated eating disorder prevention: a randomized effectiveness trial of cognitive dissonance and media advocacy.** *J Couns Psychol* 2006, **53**:550–555.
27. Becker CB, Bull S, Smith LM, Ciao AC: **Effects of being a peer-leader in an eating disorder prevention program: can we further reduce eating disorder risk factors?** *Eat Disord* 2008, **16**:444–459.
28. Becker CB, Wilson C, Williams A, Kelly M, McDaniel L, Elmquist J: **Peer-facilitated cognitive dissonance versus healthy weight eating disorders prevention: a randomized comparison.** *Body Image* 2010, **7**:280–288.
29. Festinger L, Fredrickson BL, Roberts T, Noll SM, Quinn DM, Twence JM: **That swimsuit becomes you: Sex differences in self-objectification, restrained eating, and math performance.** *J Pers Soc Psychol* 1998, **75**(1):269–284. *A theory of cognitive dissonance.* Oxford, England: Row, Peterson; 1957.
30. Becker CB, Stice E, Shaw H, Woda S: **Use of empirically-supported interventions for psychopathology: can the participatory approach move us beyond the research-to-practice gap?** *Behav Res Ther* 2009, **47**:265–274.
31. Becker CB, Bull S, Schaumberg K, Cauble A, Franco A: **Effectiveness of peer-led eating disorders prevention: a replication trial.** *J Consult Clin Psychol* 2008, **76**:347–354.
32. Knauss C, Paxton SJ, Alsaker FD: **Body dissatisfaction in adolescent boys and girls: objectified body consciousness, internalization of the media body ideal and perceived pressure from the media.** *Sex Roles* 2008, **59**:633–643.
33. Kroon Van Diest AM, Perez M: **Exploring the integration of thin-ideal internalization and self-objectification in the prevention of eating disorders.** *Body Image* 2012, http://dx.doi.org/10.1016/j.bodyim.2012.10.004.
34. Calogero RM: **Operationalizing self-objectification: Assessment and related methodological issues.** In *Self-objectification in women: Causes, consequences, and counteractions.* 1st edition. Edited by Calogero RM, Tantleff-Dunn S, Thompson JK. Washington, D. C: American Psychological Association; 2011:23–50.
35. Becker CB, Stice E: *Sorority Body Image Program: Group Leader Guide.* New York: Oxford University Press; 2008.
36. Lindberg SM, Hyde SJ, McKinley NM: **A measure of objectified body consciousness for preadolescent and adolescent youth.** *Psychol Women Q* 2006, **30**:65–76.
37. Stice E, Ziemba C, Margolis J, Flick P: **The dual pathway model differentiates bulimics, subclinical bulimics, and controls: Testing the continuity hypothesis.** *Behav Ther* 1996, **27**:531–549.
38. Stice E: **A prospective test of the dual-pathway model of bulimic pathology: mediating effects of dieting and negative affect.** *J Abnorm Psychol* 2001, **110**:124–135.
39. Stice E, Agras WS: **Predicting onset and cessation bulimic behaviors during adolescence: a longitudinal grouping analysis.** *Behav Ther* 1998, **29**:257–276.
40. Berscheid E, Walster E, Bohrnstedt G: **The happy American body: a survey report.** *Psychology Today* 1973, **7**(6):119–131.
41. Stice E, Fisher M, Martinez E: **Eating disorder diagnostic scale: additional evidence of reliability and validity.** *Psychol Assess* 2004, **16**:60–71.
42. Fairburn CG, Beglin SJ: **Assessment of eating disorders: interview or self-report questionnaire?** *Int J Eat Disord* 1994, **16**:363–370.
43. Fairburn CG, Cooper Z: **The eating disorder examination.** In *Binge Eating: Nature, Assessment, and Treatment.* 12th edition. Edited by Fairburn CG, Wilson G. NY: Guilford; 1993:317–360.
44. Luce KH, Crowther JH: **The reliability of the eating disorder examination—self-report questionnaire version (EDE-Q).** *Int J Eat Disord* 1999, **25**:349–351.
45. Mond JM, Hay PJ, Rodgers B, Beaumont PJV, Owen C: **Temporal stability of the eating disorder examination questionnaire.** *Int J Eat Disord* 2004, **36**:195–203.
46. Peterson CB, Crosby RD, Wonderlich SA, Crow SJ, Mitchell JE, Bardone-Cone A, Klein M, le Grange D: **Psychometric properties of the eating disorder examination-questionnaire: Factor structure and internal consistency.** *Int J Eat Disord* 2007, **40**:386–389.
47. Watson D, Clark LA: **Affects separable and inseparable: on the hierarchical arrangement of the negative affects.** *J Pers Soc Psychol* 1992, **62**:489–505.
48. Cohen J: *Statistical power analysis for the behavioral sciences.* 2nd edition. Hillsdale, NJ: Lawrence Earlbaum Associates; 1988.
49. Baron RM, Kenny DA: **The moderator-mediator variable distinction in social psychological research: conceptual, strategic, and statistical considerations.** *J Pers Soc Psychol* 1986, **51**:1173–1182.
50. Preacher KJ, Hayes AF: **Asymptotic and resampling strategies for assessing and comparing indirect effects in multiple mediator models.** *Behav Res Methods* 2008, **40**:879–891.
51. Hu L, Bentler PM: **Cutoff criteria for fit indexes in covariance structure analysis: conventional criteria versus new alternatives.** *Struct Equ Modeling* 1999, **6**:1–55.
52. Greif R, Farris S, You C, Becker C, Wilson GT: *Reducing eating disorder risk factors in members of a national sorority: 5-month follow-up.* Toronto, Canada: Poster presented at the 45th Annual Meeting of the Association of Behavioral and Cognitive Therapies; 2011.
53. Tiggeman M: **Mental health risks of self-objectification: A review of the empirical evidence for disordered eating, depressed mood and sexual dysfunction.** In *Self-Objectification in Women: Causes, Consequences, and Counteractions.* 1st edition. Edited by Calogero RM, Tantleff-Dunn S, Thompson JK. Washington, D. C: American Psychological Association; 2011:139–160.
54. Slater A, Tiggemann M: **Time since menarche and sport participation as predictors of self-objectification: a longitudinal study of adolescent girls.** *Sex Roles* 2012, **67**:571–581.

12

Clinical characteristics and distinctiveness of DSM-5 eating disorder diagnoses: findings from a large naturalistic clinical database

Kerstin Ekeroth[1*], David Clinton[1], Claes Norring[1,2] and Andreas Birgegård[1]

Abstract

Background: DSM-IV eating disorder (ED) diagnoses have been criticized for lack of clinical utility, diagnostic instability, and over-inclusiveness of the residual category "ED not otherwise specified" (EDNOS). Revisions made in DSM-5 attempt to generate a more scientifically valid and clinically relevant system of ED classification. The aim with the present study was to examine clinical characteristics and distinctiveness of the new DSM-5 ED diagnoses, especially concerning purging disorder (PD).

Methods: Using a large naturalistic Swedish ED database, 2233 adult women were diagnosed using DSM-5. Initial and 1-year follow-up psychopathology data were analyzed. Measures included the Eating Disorder Examination Questionnaire, Structural Eating Disorder Interview, Clinical Impairment Assessment, Structural Analysis of Social Behavior, Comprehensive Psychiatric Rating Scale, and Structured Clinical Interview for DSM-IV Axis I Disorders.

Results: Few meaningful differences emerged between anorexia nervosa binge/purge subtype (ANB/P), PD, and bulimia nervosa (BN). Unspecified Feeding and Eating Disorders (UFED) showed significantly less severity compared to other groups.

Conclusions: PD does not appear to constitute a distinct diagnosis, the distinction between atypical AN and PD requires clarification, and minimum inclusion criteria for UFED are needed. Further sub-classification is unlikely to improve clinical utility. Instead, better delineation of commonalities is important.

Keywords: Eating disorders, DSM-5, Clinical distinctiveness, Purging disorder

Background

Compared to its predecessor DSM-5 [1] attempts to generate a more scientifically robust and clinically relevant system of classification for eating disorders (ED). Although DSM-IV was fraught with problems and changes were necessary, the consequences of the revisions remain unclear. Since DSM-5 will have considerable impact on the future of both scientific and clinical work, research on the clinical characteristics and distinctiveness of the now finalized changes will inform about the utility and consequences of these amendments. DSM-IV has been criticized for lack of clinical utility, diagnostic instability, general irrelevance, and the over-inclusiveness of the residual category of "ED not otherwise specified" (EDNOS), a group that may encompass 50 to 70% of patients in tertiary care and outpatient settings [2,3], but which has been the subject of little research. In order to better define and limit EDNOS, DSM-5 lowers thresholds for AN and BN, and establishes binge eating disorder (BED) as a separate diagnosis. These changes are supported by research [4-6] and will likely decrease EDNOS to some extent [7-9]. However, many patients will still be classified under a "residual" or unspecified diagnostic category. Temporal instability is another major problem for DSM-IV [10-12], with many patients migrating to a diagnosis other than their initial one over time [13]. What's more, knowledge about the stability of EDNOS is limited [14], and many patients develop other EDs [12,15]. While some studies suggest that EDNOS represents a transitional stage of progression into or out of full ED, other

* Correspondence: kerstin.ekeroth@ki.se
[1]Resource Center for Eating Disorders/Center for Psychiatry Research Stockholm, Department of Clinical Neuroscience, Karolinska Institutet, Stockholm, Sweden
Full list of author information is available at the end of the article

work suggests that these patients constitute a mixed group, as seriously ill as AN or BN [2].

DSM-5 [1] renames EDNOS as Other Specified Feeding and Eating Disorders (OSFED) and includes subcategories for atypical AN (AAN), subthreshold BN (SubBN), purging disorder (PD), and night eating syndrome (NES). Although potentially a step forward, these OSFED "subtypes" are problematic. AAN includes the unspecified criterion "significant weight loss" (in normal weight or overweight individuals), which makes reliable research and clinical evaluation difficult. Also, since SubBN seems to be uncommon in clinical samples, its utility may be limited [7]. Additionally, DSM-5 includes a totally undefined category called Unspecified Feeding or Eating Disorder (UFED).

Perhaps the most researched of the new OSFED subcategories is PD. However, empirical support for PD is equivocal at best and studies have often found contradictory or no differences between PD and other EDs [16-20]. PD does not appear to differ in remission rates compared to other diagnoses [20-22], and studies of the persistence of symptoms present a varied picture [21-23]. Most work has compared PD to BN, and a few to AN and BED, but no comparisons have been made to other EDNOS categories, which is imperative if PD is to be considered meaningfully different from these, and expected to emerge in the future as a distinct diagnosis of its own [24].

Research on clinical characteristics, co-morbidity, outcome and diagnostic stability from large samples is needed to inform on the relevance and validity of the DSM-5. The aim of the present study was to examine the clinical characteristics and distinctiveness of DSM-5 ED diagnoses in general and PD specifically. It concerned ED-related and general psychopathology, co-morbidity, and outcome[a].

Methods

Participants

Data was drawn from the Stepwise quality assurance database, a large-scale internet-based data collection system for specialized ED care in Sweden. The database has been in use since 2005, and data for the present study came from 34 treatment units. Inclusion criteria were medical or self-referral to one of the participating treatment units, a diagnosed DSM-IV ED, plus intention to treat the patient at the unit in question. Baseline data from 2233 adult women registered after February 2008 (when a change in methodology was made), were available for the present study. Age ranged between 18 and 67 years ($M = 25.7$; $S.D. = 7.84$). DSM-IV ED diagnoses were: 16.4% AN (61.9% restrictive subtype, RAN), 31.7% BN (70.4% purging subtype), and 51.9% EDNOS (20.4% subthreshold AN, 14.2% subthreshold BN, 30.5% purging/compensatory behavior, 10.4% binge eating, and 24.5% other symptoms or variants). Of the complete sample 937 (42%) patients had not yet reached the 12-month follow-up point at the time of data extraction, thus only 1296 participants were considered eligible. From this group, 55% (530) had complete 12-month data and were considered representative of the complete sample after several comparative analyses were conducted. The first analysis compared patients with and without follow-up data on the initial assessments, and found no other differences besides those with follow-up data scoring somewhat higher on SASB 'self-emancipation' and 'self-control' than those without follow-up data[b]. The second analysis compared mean differences between the complete sample and the group with follow-up data within each respective diagnosis and no or only small effects ($d < 0.27$; $p < 0.01$) were found. Finally, we conducted the main analyses separately for the group of patients with follow-up data ($N = 530$) and results did not differ significantly compared to analyses on the entire sample (if anything, differences were fewer and smaller, and thereby in the direction of our conclusions).

In this clinical, naturalistic database, attrition was due to the following: patients moving to another treatment unit (15% of those without follow-up data), not having been eligible for treatment (for example due to having no full-syndrome ED; 31%), being abroad or otherwise indisposed during the eight-week time window for follow-up (33%), or having declined further follow-up (21%).

Procedure

Patients were assessed by ED specialists prior to treatment, usually within the first three visits. Individuals in need of inpatient care generally completed assessment during the first week of treatment. Assessment took about 80 minutes and included demographic information, psychiatric history, clinical ratings and interviews, as well as questionnaires. All patients approved using their data for research purposes.

Measures

Eating Disorder Examination Questionnaire (EDE-Q)

A 36-item measure of general ED symptoms and features, comprising four sub-scales of Restraint, Eating Concern, Shape Concern, and Weight Concern, plus a global score [25]. The EDE-Q has shown good psychometric properties [26]. Global score was used as a measure of overall eating psychopathology, while single items were used for operationalization of DSM-5 diagnoses (see below). In the present study, Cronbach's alphas were 0.82 for Restraint, 0.70 for Eating Concern, 0.89 for Shape Concern, and 0.74 for the Weight Concern scale.

Structured Eating Disorder Interview (SEDI)

A semi-structured clinical interview developed specifically for Stepwise. It is based directly on the DSM-IV ED criteria and consists of 20–30 questions, depending on what follow-up questions need to be asked. SEDI was used for operationalization of ED-diagnoses. Preliminary validation against the EDE-interview has shown a good concordance of 81% concerning specific ED diagnoses (including EDNOS and BED) and Kendall's Tau-b of $\tau = 0.69$ ($p < 0.001$)[27].

Structured Clinical Interview for DSM-IV Axis I Disorders (SCID-I)

A semi-structured diagnostic interview for assessing DSM-IV Axis I disorders. The present study used data on mood, anxiety, and substance abuse disorders [28]. SCID-I has shown fair to good psychometric properties [29-31].

Comprehensive Psychiatric Rating Scale - Self-rating Scale for Affective Syndromes (CPRS-S-A)

Consisting of 19 items measuring anxiety, depression and compulsiveness [32] which are common problems related to ED [33,34]. Because of the high intercorrelation between the scales ($r = 0.78 - 0.86$), a total/global symptom index ranging from 0 (no distress) to 3 (high distress) was used. In the present sample, Cronbach's alphas were 0.88, 0.81, and 0.85 for the Depression, Anxiety and Compulsiveness scales respectively. CPRS-S-A has shown good psychometric properties [32,35].

Clinical Impairment Assessment (CIA; version 3.0)

Is a 16-item questionnaire assessing the severity of psychosocial impairment caused by ED behaviors and attitudes covering mood, self-perception, cognitive functioning, interpersonal functioning, and work performance during the last 28 days [36,37]. Cronbach's alpha for the present sample was 0.92. The CIA has shown good psychometric properties in clinical [36,37], high risk [38] and community samples [39].

Structural Analysis of Social Behavior (SASB), intrex questionnaire

A 36-item questionnaire based on two orthogonal dimensions (affiliation and interdependence) that measures eight aspects of self-image [40]. The present study used the SASB variables of Self-emancipation (letting oneself go, not having strong principles) and Self-control (monitoring and restraining self), along with the Affiliation vector (i.e. the balance between positive and negative self-image, calculated by weighting and combining six affiliation-related scale scores), which corresponds to a measure of general self-esteem. SASB has previously been found to have relevance with respect to EDs [41,42], and has shown good psychometric properties [40,43,44]. Cronbach's alpha for the clusters Self-emancipation and Self-control were 0.55 and 0.68 respectively, and 0.90 for the Affiliation vector using the relevant scales as items.

Definition of purging disorder and operationalization of DSM-5 ED

A more detailed description of the operationalization of previously proposed DSM-5 ED diagnoses has been presented previously [7], and details are available upon request. "EDNOS other", not independently demarcated in the SEDI interview, was defined as at least one psychological symptom (weight phobia, self-esteem unduly affected by weight or body shape, disturbed body experience, or denial of seriousness of low weight), in addition to at least one behavioral symptom (binge eating, loss of control during eating, purging, or fasting/exercise) or physical (anorexic weight or amenorrhea) symptom. Since the study was designed prior to final publication of DSM-5 operationalization of DSM-5 ED diagnoses was based on information from http://www.dsm5.org as of October 2012. Applying SPSS syntax, diagnoses were based on SEDI and EDE-Q variables. Since the SEDI only assesses whether behaviors have been present at least twice a week for at least three months and the EDE-Q only asks about frequency of bingeing and compensation for the last month, it was not possible to be certain about the fulfillment of the DSM-5 criteria specifying frequency and duration of binge eating and compensatory behavior for once a week for at least three months. EDE-Q frequency items (for example concerning OBE) were only used to establish the lower DSM-5 criteria in cases where patients did not already meet DSM-IV criteria. Since DSM-5 criteria for PD lack specification of both frequency and duration the SEDI item assessing "regular purging" was used, which implies that it is not an occasional behavior. To avoid including underweight patients who could otherwise fulfill criteria for AN, only individuals with a BMI over 18.5 were included in PD.

A problem with DSM-5 criteria is the overlap between PD and AAN. Since the present database lacked data on "significant weight loss", which characterizes AAN, patients who only purged and fulfilled the psychological criteria could be diagnosed with either PD or AAN (most PD patients fulfilled the psychological criteria for AAN, however these do not apply to PD). This meant that it was possible to determine whether patients fulfilled PD criteria, but not whether they also fulfilled AAN criteria. It should be borne in mind that PD criteria do not require weight loss and there is no specification of what constitutes significant weight loss (within normal weight) for AAN. Using SPSS syntax to generate diagnoses, the PD and AAN groups exchanged patients depending on which diagnosis was defined first. By changing the order of definition, the PD group decreased from 184 to 4 patients. In the present study, the syntax solution that generated the most PD cases was used, since this definition of PD was true to DSM-5 whereas the AAN definition was incomplete.

Definition of remission

Within the group lacking a formal DSM-IV diagnosis according to the SEDI interview at follow-up, several patients had some remaining symptoms and fulfilled criteria for 'EDNOS Other'. Twenty one percent of all follow-ups, or about one third of the patients with no DSM-IV ED-diagnosis, still had some ED symptoms. Patients were judged to be in remission if they neither fulfilled criteria for a DSM-IV ED nor 'EDNOS Other'.

Analyses

Diagnostic groups were compared on the dependent variables using univariate ANOVAs. Alpha levels were set to $p < 0.01$ for both omnibus and *post hoc* tests, and η_p^2 (≥0.01 = small effect, ≥0.06 = medium effect, and ≥0.14 = large effect) and Cohen's d (≥0.2 = small effect, ≥0.5 = medium effect, and ≥0.8 = large effect) were used to assess effect sizes [45]. To check for differences between groups, *post hoc* Scheffé tests were used. To avoid inclusion of statistically significant results with no practical or clinical significance, pairwise *post hoc* contrasts required both a $p < 0.01$ and a Cohen's d ≥0.50. Welch's ANOVA and Games-Howell's *post hoc* were used with unequal and small group sizes in combination with unequal variances. ANOVA on residual gain scores was used to analyze differences in change from initial assessment to follow-up. χ^2 and Fisher's exact test were used on categorical data, and alpha was set to $p < 0.01$. *Post hoc* analyses of larger contingency tables were conducted through multiple pairwise tests and inspection of standardized residuals; alpha was set to $p < 0.001$. Cramer's V/Phi coefficients were used for measuring strength of associations with Rea and Parkers' [46] magnitude criteria: <0.10 = negligible, 0.10 - < .20 = weak, 0.20 - < 0.40 = moderate, 0.40 - < 0.60 relatively strong, 0.60 - < 0.80 = strong, ≥ 0.80 = very strong.

BED was omitted from analyses of purging behavior and inappropriate compensatory behavior since these behaviors should not be present in the diagnosis. For the same reasons RAN was omitted from analyses of OBE and purging behavior and PD from the analyses of OBE. For all statistical analyses, SPSS v. 19 was used.

Outliers

Inspection of data found outliers in EDE-Q questions concerning frequency of symptom behavior, such as vomiting, use of laxatives, diuretics, and excessive exercise. To deal with problematic outliers extreme values were first adjusted to a pre-defined reasonable maximum value. All values were subsequently z-transformed for each diagnostic group, and values/groups of values more than 1 *S. D.* from the next highest score were deleted.

Results

Since the present study was carried out prior to DSM-5 publication, we initially included the previously proposed, but later removed, subcategory of subthreshold BED. The decision to remove this subgroup from DSM-5 appears reasonable given our data since we found only 11 such cases (i.e. only 0.5% of the sample); these patients are not considered further in the analysis. Table 1 shows the distribution of diagnoses, BMI, and age when applying DSM-5 criteria. PD was found in 8.2% of patients, which was 32% of the OSFED group. In the OSFED group PD, AAN and Sub-BED together made up 88% (there were no SubBN patients), while the remaining patients were diagnosed with UFED.

Are DSM-5 diagnoses statistically and clinically distinct at presentation?

ED variables

To be significant, all pairwise *post hoc* contrasts required both $p < 0.01$ and Cohen's d ≥0.50. For categorical data, $p < 0.001$ was required. Significant ANOVAs were obtained for both the EDE-Q and the CIA with η_p^2 showing a large and a medium effect, respectively (Table 2). Post-hoc tests showed that the UFED group had less severe ED pathology and impairment compared to all other groups. On EDE-Q global scale, ANB/P, BN and PD reported greater severity of ED psychopathology and differed significantly from RAN, with medium effects. BN also differed from AAN and BED. Besides the lesser impairment reported in the UFED group, ANB/P patients experienced more impairment on the CIA than AAN and PD patients.

***Objective Binge Episodes* (*OBE*)[c]** Table 3 shows frequency and percent of patients reporting OBE. Based on the EDE-Q, 56% of all patients reported OBE. In BN and BED, 74 and 84% respectively reported OBE compared to about half of the patients with ANB/P and AAN. Among RAN and PD, 25 and 38% respectively reported

Table 1 Distribution of DSM-5 diagnoses, BMI, and age according to diagnosis

DSM-5 diagnosis	N	%	BMI *M (SD)*	Age *M (SD)*	12-month N
RAN	364	16.3	16.1 (1.6)	23.2 (6.6)	102
ANB/P	295	13.2	16.8 (1.4)	24.3 (7.1)	67
BN	874	39.1	23.6 (4.3)	26.4 (8.0)	219
BED	124	5.6	31.4 (7.7)	30.2 (10.2)	22
AAN	310	13.9	22.7 (4.5)	26.0 (7.0)	69
Sub BED	11	0.5	30.2 (7.6)	34.4 (13.2)	-
PD	184	8.2	21.9 (3.5)	25.4 (7.9)	39
UFED	71	3.2	19.9 (6.7)	26.1 (9.1)	12

RAN Restrictive Anorexia nervosa, *ANB/P* Anorexia Nervosa Bingeing/Purging type, *BN* Bulimia Nervosa, *BED* Binge Eating Disorder, *AAN* Atypical Anorexia Nervosa, *Sub BED* Subthreshold Binge Eating Disorder, *PD* Purging Disorder, *UFED* Unspecified Feeding and Eating Disorder, *BMI* Body Mass Index.

Table 2 Means, standard deviations, and significant differences (ANOVA) on measures of ED and general psychopathology according to DSM-5 diagnoses[a]

Dependent variable	RAN	ANB/P	BN	BED	AAN	PD	UFED		
	Mean (SD)	Mean (SD)	Mean (SD)	Mean (SD)	Mean (SD)	Mean (SD)	Mean (SD)	F	η_p^2
EDE-Q Global[1]	3.38 (1.36)	4.18 (1.18)	4.20 (0.95)	3.67 (1.08)	3.64 (1.16)	4.09 (0.97)	1.72 (1.22)	77.64***	.174
CIA[2]	29.07 (11.4)	33.61 (9.9)	30.51 (9.3)	29.82 (9.2)	26.39 (10.5)	28.41 (9.5)	19.19 (11.6)	24.27***	.070
CPRS [3]	1.14 (.51)	1.34 (0.52)	1.14 (.47)	1.14 (.39)	1.08 (.49)	1.14 (.49)	0.76 (.50)	16.22***	.042
SASB Affiliation[4]	-10.98 (37.2)	-28.3 (31.4)	-16.9 (33.0)	-21.4 (33.4)	-11.1 (35.2)	-16.0 (34.5)	17.3 (41.6)	20.48***	.053
SASB Self-emancipation	30.4 (15.6)	31.2 (17.0)	32.0 (15.4)	35.1 (17.1)	31.2 (15.3)	30.6 (14.2)	38.6 (18.6)	3.95***	.011
SASB Self-control[5]	62.1 (18.3)	59.8 (17.2)	54.8 (18.5)	49.5 (20.8)	57.0 (17.9)	53.7 (18.9)	52.5 (19.7)	12.72***	.033

RAN Restrictive Anorexia nervosa, *ANB/P* Anorexia Nervosa Bingeing/Purging type, *BN* Bulimia Nervosa, *BED* Binge Eating Disorder, *AAN* Atypical Anorexia Nervosa, *PD* Purging Disorder, *UFED* Unspecified Feeding and Eating Disorder, *EDE-Q Global* Eating Disorder Examination Questionnaire Global score, *CIA* Clinical Impairment Assessment, *CPRS* Comprehensive Psychiatric Rating Scale, *SASB* Structural Analysis of Social Behavior.
[a]For a significant post hoc difference both $p < 0.01$ and Cohen's $d \geq 0.50$ were required; *** $p < 0.001$.
[1]UFED < all; RAN < ANB/P, BN, PD; BN > BED, AAN.
[2]UFED < all; ANB/P > AAN, PD.
[3]UFED < all; ANB/P > AAN.
[4]UFED < all; ANB/P < RAN, AAN.
[5] BED < RAN, ANB/P.

OBE even though this should not be present regularly in these diagnoses. χ^2 indicated an overall significant difference ($p < 0.001$) between groups and pairwise tests showed that OBE was more frequent among BN and BED compared to the other groups, with effects ranging from weak to moderate for BN: i.e. phi = 0.18 (BN vs. ANB/P) to 0.25 (BN vs. AAN); and from moderate to relatively strong for BED i.e. phi = 0.26 (BED vs. AN/BP) to 0.50 (BED vs. UFED). More patients with ANB/P reported OBE compared to UFED (phi = 0.17). Welch's ANOVA showed a significant overall difference ($p < 0.001$) in mean frequency during the last month (Table 4), and Games-Howell showed that ANB/P, BN, and BED reported more OBE than AAN and UFED (excluding RAN and PD), with medium/large Cohen's d for all comparisons, except for ANB/P vs. AAN which almost reached a medium effect ($d = 0.49$).

Subjective Binge Episodes (SBE) Based on the EDE-Q, 59% reported SBE. Among RAN, ANB/P, BN, AAN and PD between 58% and 70% of the patients reported SBE, whereas the corresponding percentages in BED and UFED were 36% and 23%, respectively (Table 3). χ^2 indicated significant differences between groups, and pairwise tests suggested that SBE was less frequent among BED and UFED compared to the other diagnoses showing moderate effects (phi = 0.20 to 0.39), except for BED vs. BN, which was weak (phi = 0.16). Welch's ANOVA

Table 3 Number, percent and overall χ^2 for eating disorder behaviors on the EDE-Q according to DSM-5 diagnoses[a]

EDE-Q symptom	RAN	ANB/P	BN	BED	AAN	PD	UFED	Total	χ^2 (df, N)
	N (%)	N (%)	N (%)	N (%)	N (%)	N (%)	N (%)	N (%)	
OBE[1]	93 (25)	163 (55)	646 (74)	103 (83)	146 (47)	70 (38)	24 (34)	1245 (56)	133,94*** (4, 1674)
SBE[2]	216 (59)	205 (70)	524 (60)	44 (36)	179 (58)	122 (66)	16 (23)	1306 (59)	85,27*** (6, 2221)
Vomiting[3]	27 (7)	230 (78)	621 (71)	8 (6)	67 (22)	150 (82)	21 (30)	1124 (51)	340,79*** (4, 1734)
Laxatives[4]	8 (2)	60 (20)	138 (16)	2 (2)	5 (2)	33 (18)	1 (1)	247 (11)	64,52*** (4, 1734)
Diuretics[5]	4 (1)	29 (10)	46 (5)	1 (1)	9 (3)	12 (7)	1 (1)	102 (5)	17,11** (4, 1734)
Exercise[6]	155 (43)	150 (51)	473 (54)	13 (11)	153 (49)	102 (55)	13 (18)	1059 (48)	45,35*** (5, 2098)
Extreme fasting[7]	210 (58)	227 (77)	576 (66)	45 (36)	180 (58)	128 (70)	13 (18)	1379 (62)	99,75*** (5, 2097)

RAN Restrictive Anorexia nervosa, *ANB/P* Anorexia Nervosa Bingeing/Purging type, *BN* Bulimia Nervosa, *BED* Binge Eating Disorder, *AAN* Atypical Anorexia Nervosa, *PD* Purging Disorder, *UFED* Unspecified Feeding and Eating Disorder, *OBE* Objective Binge Episodes, *SBE* Subjective Binge Episodes.
[a]BED was omitted from all analyses except for OBE and SBE since purging behavior and inappropriate compensatory behavior should not be present in the diagnosis. For the same reason RAN was omitted from the analyses of OBE and purging behavior, and PD from the analyses of OBE. *** $p < 0.001$; ** $p < 0.01$.
[1]BN, BED > all; ANB/P > UFED.
[2]BED, UFED < all.
[3]AAN, UFED < all.
[4]ANB/P, BN, PD > all.
[5]ANB/P > AAN.
[6]UFED < all; RAN < BN.
[7]ANB/P > RAN, BN, AAN; UFED < all.

Table 4 Mean frequency, standard deviation and significant differences of eating disorder psychopathology during last four weeks according to DSM-5 diagnoses[a,b]

Dependent variable	RAN	ANB/P	BN	BED	AAN	PD	UFED	*F*	η_p^{2c}
OBE[1]	7.8 (7.9)	14.0 (15.5)	12.7 (9.9)	14.6 (7.9)	8.1 (7.1)	8.8 (7.2)	5.3 (3.4)	11.06***	.040
SBE[2]	11.3 (8.9)	12.0 (8.0)	10.9 (8.0)	11.3 (8.8)	9.8 (7.2)	9.8 (7.6)	6.1 (3.4)	6.27***	.012
Vomiting[3]	3.0 (2.6)	23.8 (24.9)	20.0 (21.2)	3.3 (1.6)	15.1 (19.7)	14.0 (13.2)	12.2 (10.1)	9.55***	.023
Laxatives[4]	2.0 (1.1)	9.6 (8.3)	11.5 (10.2)	1.0 (0)	4.8 (3.4)	8.3 (8.6)	4.0		
Diuretics[5]	2.5 (2.1)	11.2 (9.8)	12.7 (9.5)	2.0	4.6 (3.3)	10.4 (4.4)	—		
Exercise	15.9 (9.0)	15.7 (7.8)	13.2 (7.0)	6.7 (3.6)	15.5 (8.3)	14.8 (7.9)	14.3 (9.5)	4.74***	.023
Extreme fasting [d; 6]	1.79 (2.1)	2.69 (2.2)	1.76 (1.9)	0.69 (1.2)	1.68 (2.0)	2.10 (2.1)	0.38 (1.1)	35.30***	.046

RAN Restrictive Anorexia nervosa, *ANB/P* Anorexia Nervosa Bingeing/Purging type, *BN* Bulimia Nervosa, *BED* Binge Eating Disorder, *AAN* Atypical Anorexia Nervosa, *PD* Purging Disorder, *UFED* Unspecified Feeding and Eating Disorder, *OBE* Objective Binge Episodes, *SBE* Subjective Binge Episodes.

[a]For a significant post hoc difference both $p < 0.01$ and a Cohen's $d \geq 0.50$ were required.

[b]BED was omitted from all analyses except for OBE and SBE since purging behavior and inappropriate compensatory behavior should not be present in the diagnosis. For the same reason RAN was omitted from the analyses of OBE and purging behavior and PD from the analyses of OBE. Also, groups with n < 10 were omitted.

[c]η_p^2 has been calculated through a regular ANOVA, since it was not a possible option in the Welch analysis.

[d]Answers for 'extreme fasting' is 0 = no days, 1 = 1-2 days, 2 = 3-6 days, 3 = 7 days, 4 = 8-10 days, 5 = 12-13 days, 6 = every day.

***$p < .001$;

[1]ANB/P, BN, BED > AAN, UFED.

[2]UFED < RAN, ANB/P, BN.

[3]UFED < ANB/P.

[4]ANB/P, BN and PD included in the analysis. AAN and UFED not included due to small *n*.

[5]ANB/P, BN and PD included in the analysis. AAN and UFED not included due to small *n*.

[6]UFED < all; ANB/P > RAN, BN, AAN.

showed a significant overall difference ($p < 0.001$) in mean frequency during the last month (Table 4), and Games-Howell showed that UFED reported fewer SBE than RAN, ANB/P and BN with medium/large Cohen's *d* for all comparisons.

Compensatory behaviors Table 3 shows number, percent and χ^2 of patients reporting compensatory behaviors on EDE-Q[d]. Table 4 shows mean frequencies/last 28 days and significant differences for the same behaviors. χ^2 suggested significant differences on all compensatory behaviors.

Regular vomiting was reported by 82% of the PD group compared to 78% and 71% in the ANB/P and BN group, respectively. In the UFED and AAN groups, the percentages were 30% and 22%, respectively, which was significantly less compared to the other groups (excluding RAN and BED). Effects were relatively strong for AAN (phi = 0.44 to 0.58) and moderate to relatively strong for UFED (phi = 0.23 to 0.50). Welch analysis on mean frequencies/28 days was significant, and Games-Howell post-hoc showed that PD reported less vomiting compared to ANB/P and BN. However, Cohen's *d* showed only small effects for both comparisons. Also, UFED reported less vomiting compared to ANB/P with a medium effect.

Laxative use was reported significantly more often in ANB/P, BN, and PD than in other groups, with moderate effects for ANB/P and PD (phi = 0.20 to 0.30) and weak to moderate effects for BN (phi = 0.11 to 0.20). There were no significant differences between these groups in mean frequency/28 days (omitting AAN and UFED due to small *n*'s).

Use of *diuretics* was relatively uncommon, but was reported by 5% to 10% of patients with BN, PD and ANB/P. In AAN 3% reported the use of diuretics which was significantly less compared to ANB/P, however the effect was weak (phi = 0.14). Only ANB/P, BN and PD were included in the ANOVA of mean frequency/28 days, which suggested no significant difference.

Strenuous exercise for the purpose of weight control was reported to the same extent in PD, BN, ANB/P, and AAN, and to a much lesser degree in UFED (phi = 0.19 to 0.33). Strenuous exercise was also reported by fewer patients with RAN compared to BN, although with a weak effect (phi = 0.12). ANOVA/Welch was significant overall for mean frequency/28 days, and Games-Howell suggested a significantly higher frequency in ANB/P than in BN ($p < 0.01$), but Cohen's *d* showed only a weak effect.

Extreme fasting/dieting was most commonly reported in the ANB/P group followed by PD and BN. In the AAN and RAN groups close to 60% reported this behavior. It was significantly more often reported in ANB/P compared to RAN, BN, and AAN (phi = 0.20/0.10/0.20 respectively), and significantly less often in UFED compared to the other groups, with moderate effects for RAN, BN and AAN (phi = 0.26 to 0.31) and relatively strong effects for ANB/P and PD (phi = 0.49 and 0.46 respectively (excluding BED)). Additionally, UFED reported a significantly lower frequency/28 days compared to other groups. ANB/P frequency was significantly higher than RAN, BN and AAN, but Cohen's *d* showed small effects.

Psychiatric and personality variables

Means for the CPRS and SASB 'Affiliation', 'Self-emancipation', and 'Self-control' are shown in Table 2. On the CPRS, the UFED group reported fewer problems than the other groups, and ANB/P reported more problems compared to AAN. Likewise, on SASB 'Affiliation', UFED reported significantly better self-image compared to the other groups, and ANB/P reported more negative self-image compared to AAN and RAN. BED patients scored significantly lower on SASB 'Self-control' compared to RAN and ANB/P patients. All η_p^2 on the omnibus tests showed small effects.

Psychiatric co-morbidity

Table 5 presents numbers, percentages and overall significance (χ^2) for mood, anxiety, and alcohol/substance abuse or dependency disorders for each diagnostic group.

Mood disorders

UFED had a significantly lower rate of mood disorders compared to all other groups except RAN, ranging from weak (BN, AAN) to moderate/relatively strong (PD, ANB/P, BED) effects (phi = 0.17 to 0.41). There were medium effects between BED and RAN ($p < 0.001$; phi = 0.26), and BED and PD ($p < 0.001$; phi = 0.21), and a weak effect for BED vs. AAN ($p < 0.001$; phi = 0.18). RAN also differed significantly from BN and ANB/P, but with weak effects ($p < 0.001$; phi = 0.18 and 0.19 respectively).

Anxiety disorders

19% of the PD group had an anxiety disorder compared to only 8% of the UFED group. For other EDs, percentages varied between 13 and 18. However, the overall test did not reach significance.

Substance use disorders

RAN had a significantly lower rate of substance use disorders compared to all other groups ($p < 0.001$), except UFED. However, all effects were weak (phi = 0.13 - 0.15), apart from the RAN-BED difference, which was moderate (phi = 0.21).

Do DSM-5 diagnoses predict outcome after one year?

ANOVA on residual gain scores for the 12-month follow-up assessments did not show any significant differences between diagnoses on either the ED (EDE-Q and CIA) or the psychiatric/personality (CPRS and SASB) variables.

Remission rates and diagnostic stability

Table 6 presents remission rates and diagnostic cross-over/stability at 12-months. UFED had the highest remission rate (but a very low N) and BED and AN the lowest, but there were no significant differences in remission rates between diagnoses. Among PD patients, 44% were in remission at 12-months and 41% had crossed over to other diagnoses, which was very similar to BN. On average, 39% (range 17 to 55%) of all patients fulfilled criteria for an ED diagnosis other than their initial one at follow-up. If, however, migration to UFED, which was the only diagnosis that had increased at follow-up, and AAN (which only decreased slightly) was not included, migration to other diagnoses was on average 14% (i.e. from 4% for RAN to 25% for ANB/P).

Discussion

The present study examined the clinical characteristics and distinctiveness of the new DSM-5 ED diagnoses in general and PD in particular. To our knowledge this is the most comprehensive study to date, including PD and other OSFED subtypes, as well as UFED, assessed on general psychopathology, ED variables, psychiatric co-morbidity and outcome.

Strengths of the study include its large-scale naturalistic setting and the inclusion of the full range of EDs, ensuring good generalizability to clinical settings. However, some limitations should be noted. First, it is possible that a treatment-seeking sample may differ from a community sample in severity and psychiatric co-morbidity. Second, there was considerable attrition at follow-up. Statistical analyses, however, suggested that this did not impact on results. Third, both clinical interview and questionnaire data were used to match DSM-5 criteria

Table 5 Frequency, percent and overall significance (χ2) for Axis I co-morbidity according to DSM-5 diagnoses

	RAN	ANB/P	BN	BED	AAN	PD	UFED	Total	
	N = 364	N = 295	N = 874	N = 124	N = 310	N = 184	N = 71	N = 2222	χ^2(df, N)
Axis I disorders	N (%)	N (%)	N (%)	N (%)	N (%)	N (%)	N (%)	N (%)	
Mood disorders[1]	104 (29)	138 (47)	417 (48)	71 (57)	116 (37)	66 (36)	11 (15)	923 (42)	79,31***(6, 2222)
Anxiety disorders	47 (13)	53 (18)	143 (16)	21 (17)	51 (16)	35 (19)	6 (8)	365 (16)	7,90 (6, 2222)
Substance use disorders[2]	13 (4)	31 (11)	120 (14)	19 (15)	32 (10)	21 (11)	6 (8)	242 (11)	30,50***(6, 2222)

RAN Restrictive Anorexia nervosa, *ANB/P* Anorexia Nervosa Bingeing/Purging type, *BN* Bulimia Nervosa, *BED* Binge Eating Disorder, *AAN* Atypical Anorexia Nervosa, *PD* Purging Disorder, *UFED* Unspecified Feeding and Eating Disorder.

***$p < 0.001$.

[1]UFED < all except RAN; BED > RAN, AAN, PD; RAN < ANB/P, BN.

[2]RAN < all except UFED.

Table 6 Diagnostic stability/cross-over and remission rates at 12-month follow-up

	DSM-5 diagnoses at 12-month follow-up								
DSM-5 diagnoses at start	**RAN**	**ANB/P**	**BN**	**BED**	**AAN**	**PD**	**UFED**	**No diagnosis/ remission**	**Total**
RAN	29 (28%)	2 (2%)	2 (%)	0	17 (17%)	0	18 (18%)	34 (33%)	102 (19%)
ANB/P	6 (9%)	13 (19%)	6 (9%)	0	7 (10%)	5 (7%)	11 (16%)	19 (28%)	67 (13%)
BN	1(0.5%)	3 (1%)	42 (19%)	2 (1%)	20 (9%)	5 (2%)	54 (25%)	92 (42%)	219 (41%)
BED	0	0	4 (18%)	3 (14%)	2 (9%)	0	6 (27%)	7 (32%)	22 (4%)
AAN	0	1 (1%)	6 (9%)	0	13 (19%)	4 (6%)	14 (20%)	31 (45%)	69 (13%)
PD	1 (3%)	1(3%)	2 (5%)	0	4 (10%)	6 (15%)	8 (21%)	17 (44%)	39 (7%)
UFED	1 (8%)	0	1 (8%)	0	0	0	4 (33%)	6 (50%)	12 (2%)
Total	38 (7%)	20 (4%)	63 (12%)	5 (1%)	63 (12%)	20 (4%)	115 (22%)	206 (39%)	530

RAN Restrictive Anorexia nervosa, *ANB/P* Anorexia Nervosa Bingeing/Purging type, *BN* Bulimia Nervosa, *BED* Binge Eating Disorder, *AAN* Atypical Anorexia Nervosa, *PD* Purging Disorder, *UFED* Unspecified Feeding and Eating Disorder.

as closely as possible. However, due to lack of data the match was not perfect for duration and frequency, and there were no data on the unspecified criterion of "significant weight loss" necessary for AAN. Finally, it is possible that the more lenient DSM-5 criteria for AN and BN used here might have led to inclusion of patients with milder symptoms, potentially decreasing levels of psychopathology and affecting the comparability of the present study and other PD-studies using DSM-IV criteria. However, means for all psychopathology variables for AN and BN using DSM-IV definitions were only marginally elevated compared to those for the DSM-5 definitions.

A main finding was that there were no statistically significant or clinically meaningful differences between PD and BN, and the only difference between PD and ANB/P was on the CIA. Also, PD did not differ from any other diagnosis concerning change in psychopathology or remission rates from start to follow-up, which supports studies finding no differences in treatment outcome between PD, AN and BN [20,21]. SBE has been suggested to be of special importance in defining PD [47], but in the present sample it was common in several diagnoses and not distinctive for PD. Taken together, the present results suggest no grounds for considering PD as a distinct ED.

On the contrary, PD, AN and BN seem to be more similar to each other than distinct. Patients with PD, ANB/P and BN scored higher on the EDE-Q compared to RAN, which is in line with Tasca *et al.* [20] and studies finding fewer problems in RAN than ANB/P and BN despite a very serious medical condition [48]. In a meta-analysis, Keel [17] found no meaningful difference between PD and BN concerning ED severity. Keel suggested that a higher 'eating concern' in BN could distinguish the two disorders; however, the argument risks becoming circular. If one ED includes binge eating, which is associated with considerable distress, and the other does not, then higher eating concern in the former is to be expected. PD did not differ significantly from BED on measures of psychopathology, but more patients with PD reported SBE. The only significant difference between PD and AAN was more purging behavior in PD. This could partly be explained by the fact that 'purging only' patients who could have been categorized as AAN were included in the PD group. The conceptual overlap between conditions due to the absence of operationalization of "significant weight loss" in DSM-5 makes this question difficult to evaluate.

OBE measured through the EDE-Q was reported to a relatively high degree among patients with RAN and PD even though the behavior should not be present "regularly" in these diagnoses. Moreover, not all patients with BN or BED reported the behavior through self-report. The fact that self-reports and interview data might differ in various directions has been noted earlier [49-52] and especially the tendency to under-diagnose BN using self-report questionnaires [50]. Moreover, the SEDI has only been validated against the EDE interview [27], and no study has so far investigated the concordance between SEDI and EDE-Q. In the present study, self-reported OBE (EDE-Q), was counted as present if the patient reported the behavior at least once over a period of 28 days. This might not count as "regularly" according to the DSM criterion, which may help to explain the presence of OBE in RAN and PD. However, it was the interview data (SEDI) that formed the basis for the DSM-5 diagnoses, and EDE-Q frequency data were only used to establish the lower DSM-5 criteria in cases where patients did not already meet DSM-IV criteria.

Significant differences between ED diagnostic categories on important variables that are not criteria-related (e.g. ED psychopathology, distress, co-morbidity etc.) would support the distinctiveness of these categories [18,19]. However, when such differences are lacking and the distinctiveness of the categories is only supported by differences in variables that are used to define the categories, evidence for the scientific validity and clinical utility of these categories is weakened. Our failure to find differences on variables that are not criteria-related undermines the case for DSM-based diagnostic distinctions and supports a more transdiagnostic and synthetic view of ED. Nevertheless such differences may remain to be uncovered by future research. It will therefore be important to examine ED categories in regard to pivotal factors such as prognosis and outcome.

Psychiatric co-morbidity

UFED had significantly fewer mood disorders compared to the other groups, with moderately/relatively strong differences compared to PD, ANB/P and BED. PD had a lower rate of mood disorders than BED (just reaching the criteria for a moderate effect). In contrast to Keel *et al.* [18,21] we did not find PD to differ meaningfully from BN on any Axis I disorders. Keel and co-workers' suggestion that PD patients may be protected from developing considerable problems with OBEs because they have fewer problems with affect regulation, was therefore not supported by the present data. Except for fewer mood disorders in UFED, the only differences showing at least moderate effects were a higher rate of mood disorders in BED compared to RAN and PD, and a higher rate of substance abuse disorders compared to RAN. These latter differences are well in line with studies linking binge eating to substance abuse, and problems with impulse control and affect regulation [53-55]. In sum, few meaningful differences were found concerning psychiatric co-morbidity between the ED groups.

Remission and diagnostic stability

About one third of patients with AN or BED no longer had an ED at follow-up compared to almost 60% of UFED. This striking difference was not significant though, probably due to a very small UFED group. In accordance with other studies, we found no difference in remission rates between PD and other ED groups. Comparable to BN, about 40% of the PD group was in remission at follow-up, which is similar to other studies [13]. At follow-up, 41% of patients with PD met criteria for another ED, a figure comparable to BN. The large migration, especially to UFED but also to AAN, may reflect a partial remission of illness rather than a "true" change of diagnosis.

The observed diagnostic instability is troublesome for DSM, and suggests that many symptoms vary over time and are not merely an effect of recovery [10-12]. Many patients who are in partial remission or improved will fulfill criteria for a new diagnosis (i.e. EDNOS/OSFED/UFED) in both DSM-IV and DSM-5. According to Agras and coworkers [15], EDNOS may be a way-station between full syndromes and non-ED. It is probable that many EDs vary in both severity and type of symptoms over time, while causal and maintaining psychopathological processes remain largely the same. A diagnostic system capable of accounting for such symptom fluctuations would not only better capture the general patterns found in diagnostic research, but also be more valuable in clinical practice. One suggestion in this direction is the transdiagnostic model proposed by Fairburn and Bohn [56], which emphasizes the similarities among the diagnoses rather than the often transient differences in symptom presentations. An important challenge facing future revisions of DSM will be to integrate ideas about temporal changes in symptoms. Other possible approaches for defining ED could examine personality characteristics [57] or empirically derived clusters/dimensions [58-60]. Research suggests that dimensional measures of psychopathology generally increase both reliability and validity by 15% to 37%, especially in clinical samples [61]. Such a dimensional approach may better capture symptom fluctuations.

UFED

The UFED group had considerably less severe problems compared to other groups, which raises the question of where to draw the line between normal and pathological eating behavior. In the absence of a clear definition of what constitutes an ED, this delineation relies on clinical judgment [14]. In the present study, UFED mostly consisted of patients who did not receive a formal DSM-IV ED diagnosis, but still fulfilled inclusion criteria for "EDNOS Other". One possible interpretation of the milder psychopathology observed in this group could be that somewhere in the interval covered by the UFED the boundary between ED and "normal" eating behavior should be drawn.

DSM-5 definition of PD and AAN

The DSM-5 definitions of AAN and PD are problematic because of their overlapping descriptions combined with the absence of a definition of "significant weight loss" for AAN. However, nothing is mentioned about weight loss in the description of PD (earlier studies of PD have not determined the absence of significant weight loss, and perhaps they have partly studied AAN patients). As a consequence, it is difficult to determine the presence of PD without having first excluded AAN. Nevertheless, the suggestion that PD might constitute a distinct disorder requires a less ambiguous AAN definition. A definition would have to consider amount of weight, rate or time period of weight loss, and possibly initial and end weight. Keel and Striegel-Moore [24] stated that a candidate DSM-5 syndrome should be reliably differentiated from other similar syndromes, and believe this to be true of PD. However, our results find no convincing evidence that PD is a distinct ED diagnosis.

Conclusions

There appears to be few meaningful differences between AN binge/purge type, PD and BN, and PD does not appear to constitute a distinct diagnosis. In addition, the DSM-5 distinction between atypical AN and PD requires clarification, and there is a need to stipulate a minimal level of psychopathology for UFED. Given the general instability of ED symptoms and diagnoses, along with their highly problematic operationalization and the limited clinical relevance of DSM-5, it is highly doubtful whether further sub-classification will lead to greater clinical utility. Instead, attention should be focused on delineating what is and is not ED.

Consent

Written informed consent was obtained from the patient for the publication of research reports and any accompanying images based on the collected information.

Endnotes

[a]Note that the present study does not concern itself with the so called feeding disorders, i.e. the three diagnoses Pica, Rumination Disorder, and Avoidant/Restrictive Food Intake Disorder which has been moved from the category Disorders Usually First Diagnosed in Infancy, Childhood, or Adolescence in DSM-IV to the Feeding and Eating Disorders category in DSM-5. The reason for this is that the study uses a database that is developed for DSM-IV EDs, and thus does not contain the data necessary for studying the feeding disorders. Also, we did not have data for Night Eating Syndrome (NES).

[b]For 'self-emancipation' the difference did not reach a small effect, and for 'self-control' the effect was small ($\eta_p^2 = .015$).

[c]OBE is a diagnostic criterion for BN and BED and should not be present (regularly) for the diagnoses RAN and PD. There can however be differences between self-report questionnaires and clinical interviews, the latter being the basis for those diagnoses.

[d]Purging behavior is a diagnostic criterion and should not be present (regularly) for a diagnosis of RAN or BED, which explains the low frequencies of these behaviors in those groups. Also, other inappropriate compensatory behaviors such as excessive exercise and extreme dieting should not be (regularly) present in BED. There can however be differences between self-report questionnaires and clinical interviews, the latter being the basis for those diagnoses.

Abbreviations

AAN: Atypical anorexia nervosa; AN: Anorexia nervosa; ANB/P: Anorexia nervosa bingeing/purging type; BED: Binge eating disorder; BMI: Body mass index; BN: Bulimia nervosa; CIA: Clinical impairment assessment; CPRS-S-A: Comprehensive psychiatric rating scale - self-rating scale for affective syndromes; EDE-Q: Eating disorder examination questionnaire; OSFED: Other specified feeding and eating disorders; OBE: Objective binge episodes; UFED: Unspecified feeding and eating disorder; PD: Purging disorder; RAN: Restrictive anorexia nervosa; SASB: Structural analysis of social behavior; SBE: Subjective binge episodes; SCID-I: Structured clinical interview for DSM-IV Axis I disorders; SEDI: Structured eating disorder interview.

Competing interests

One author (Norring, C.) is a member of the ICD-11 revision workgroup. No other conflicts of interest, financial or other, exist.

Authors' contributions

All authors planned and designed the study, and discussed and analyzed the results. KE conducted the literature searches, the main statistical analyses, and wrote the first draft of the manuscript. AB, CN, and DC assisted in manuscript revisions and all authors have contributed to and have approved the final manuscript. We had full access to all of the data in the study and take responsibility for the integrity of the data and the accuracy of the data analysis. All authors read and approved the final manuscript.

Acknowledgements

The authors would like to thank the staff at the ED units for the data collection, and the patients for their essential cooperation.

Author details

[1]Resource Center for Eating Disorders/Center for Psychiatry Research Stockholm, Department of Clinical Neuroscience, Karolinska Institutet, Stockholm, Sweden. [2]Stockholm Centre for Eating Disorders, Stockholm County Council, Stockholm, Sweden.

References

1. American Psychiatric Association: *Diagnostic and Statistical Manual of Mental Disorders, Fifth Edition (DSM-5™)*. Arlington, VA: American Psychiatric Association; 2013.
2. Fairburn CG, Cooper Z, Bohn K, O'Connor ME, Doll HA, Palmer RL: **The severity and status of eating disorder NOS: implications for DSM-V.** *Behav Res Ther* 2007, **45:**1705–1715.
3. Helverskov JL, Lyng B, Clausen L, Mors O, Frydenberg M, Thomsen PH, Rokkedal K: **Empirical support for a reclassification of eating disorders NOS.** *Eur Eat Disord Rev* 2011, **19:**303–315.
4. Attia E, Roberto CA: **Should amenorrhea be a diagnostic criterion for anorexia nervosa?** *Int J Eat Disord* 2009, **42:**581–589.
5. Wilson GT, Sysko R: **Frequency of binge eating episodes in bulimia nervosa and binge eating disorder: Diagnostic considerations.** *Int J Eat Disord* 2009, **42:**603–610.
6. Wonderlich SA, Gordon KH, Mitchell JE, Crosby RD, Engel SG: **The validity and clinical utility of binge eating disorder.** *Int J Eat Disord* 2009, **42:**687–705.
7. Birgegard A, Clinton D, Norring C: **DSM-IV vs DSM-5: Implementation of proposed DSM-5 cirteria in a large naturalistic database.** *Int J Eat Disord* 2012, **45:**353–361.
8. Fairburn CG, Cooper Z: **Eating disorders, DSM-5 and clinical reality.** *Br J Psychiatry* 2011, **198:**8–10.
9. Keel PK, Brown TA, Holm-Denoma J, Bodell LP: **Comparison of DSM-IV versus proposed DSM-5 diagnostic criteria for eating disorders: reduction of eating disorder not otherwise specified and validity.** *Int J Eat Disord* 2011, **44:**553–560.
10. Castellini G, Lo Sauro C, Mannucci E, Ravaldi C, Rotella CM, Faravelli C, Ricca V: **Diagnostic crossover and outcome predictors in eating disorders according to DSM-IV and DSM-V proposed criteria: a 6-year follow-up study.** *Psychosom Med* 2011, **73:**270–279.
11. Eddy KT, Dorer DJ, Franko DL, Tahilani K, Thompson-Brenner H, Herzog DB: **Diagnostic crossover in anorexia nervosa and bulimia nervosa: implications for DSM-V.** *Am J Psychiatry* 2008, **165:**245–250.
12. Milos G, Spindler A, Schnyder U, Fairburn CG: **Instability of eating disorder diagnoses: prospective study.** *Br J Psychiatry* 2005, **187:**573–578.
13. Helverskov JL, Clausen L, Mors O, Frydenberg M, Thomsen PH, Rokkedal K: **Trans-diagnostic outcome of eating disorders: A 30-month follow-up study of 629 patients.** *Eur Eat Disord Rev* 2010, **18:**453–463.
14. Thomas JJ, Vartanian LR, Brownell KD: **The relationship between eating disorder not otherwise specified (EDNOS) and officially recognized eating disorders: meta-analysis and implications for DSM.** *Psychol Bull* 2009, **135:**407–433.

15. Agras WS, Crow S, Mitchell JE, Halmi KA, Bryson S: **A 4-year prospective study of eating disorder NOS compared with full eating disorder syndromes.** *Int J Eat Disord* 2009, **42:**565–570.
16. Fink EL, Smith AR, Gordon KH, Holm-Denoma JM, Joiner TE Jr: **Psychological correlates of purging disorder as compared with other eating disorders: an exploratory investigation.** *Int J Eat Disord* 2009, **42:**31–39.
17. Keel PK: **Purging disorder: subthreshold variant or full-threshold eating disorder?** *Int J Eat Disord* 2007, **40**(Suppl):S89–S94.
18. Keel PK, Wolfe BE, Gravener JA, Jimerson DC: **Co-morbidity and disorder-related distress and impairment in purging disorder.** *Psycholog Med* 2008, **38:**1435–1442.
19. Roberto CA, Grilo CM, Masheb RM, White MA: **Binge eating, purging, or both: eating disorder psychopathology findings from an internet community survey.** *Int J Eat Disord* 2010, **43:**724–731.
20. Tasca GA, Maxwell H, Bone M, Trinneer A, Balfour L, Bissada H: **Purging disorder: psychopathology and treatment outcomes.** *Int J Eat Disord* 2012, **45:**36–42.
21. Keel PK, Haedt A, Edler C: **Purging disorder: an ominous variant of bulimia nervosa?** *Int J Eat Disord* 2005, **38:**191–199.
22. Stice E, Marti CN, Shaw H, Jaconis M: **An 8-year longitudinal study of the natural history of threshold, subthreshold, and partial eating disorders from a community sample of adolescents.** *J Abnorm Psychol* 2009, **118:**587–597.
23. Eddy KT, Swanson SA, Crosby RD, Franko DL, Engel S, Herzog DB: **How should DSM-V classify eating disorder not otherwise specified (EDNOS) presentations in women with lifetime anorexia or bulimia nervosa?** *Psycholog Med* 2010, **40:**1735–1744.
24. Keel PK, Striegel-Moore RH: **The validity and clinical utility of purging disorder.** *Int J Eat Disord* 2009, **42:**706–719.
25. Fairburn CG, Beglin SJ: **Assessment of eating disorders: interview or self-report questionnaire?** *Int J Eat Disord* 1994, **16:**363–370.
26. Berg KC, Peterson CB, Frazier P, Crow SJ: **Psychometric evaluation of the eating disorder examination and eating disorder examination-questionnaire: A systematic review of the literature.** *Int J Eat Disord* 2012, **45:**428–438.
27. De Man Lapidoth J, Birgegård A: *Validation of the Structured Eating Disorder Interview (SEDI) against the Eating Disorder Examination (EDE). (Swedish).* Stockholm: Socialstyrelsen Dnr 21–4549; 2009.
28. First M, Gibbon M, Spitzer R, Williams J: *Structured Clinicical Interview for DSM-IV Axis I Disorders (SCID-I). Clinician version. Administration Booklet.* Washington, D.C.: American Psychiatric Press; 1995.
29. Lobbestael J, Leurgans M, Arntz A: **Inter-rater reliability of the Structured Clinical Interview for DSM-IV Axis I Disorders (SCID I) and Axis II Disorders (SCID II).** *Clin Psychol Psychother* 2011, **18:**75–79.
30. Ramirez Basco M, Bostic JQ, Davies D, Rush AJ, Witte B, Hendrickse W, Barnett V: **Methods to improve diagnostic accuracy in a community mental health setting.** *Am J Psychiatry* 2000, **157:**1599–1605.
31. Zanarini MC, Skodol AE, Bender D, Dolan R, Sanislow C, Schaefer E, Morey LC, Grilo CM, Shea MT, McGlashan TH, Gunderson JG: **The collaborative longitudinal personality disorders study: reliability of axis I and II diagnoses.** *J Pers Disord* 2000, **14:**291–299.
32. Svanborg P, Asberg M: **A new self-rating scale for depression and anxiety states based on the Comprehensive Psychopathological Rating Scale.** *Acta Psychiatr Scand* 1994, **89:**21–28.
33. Hudson JI, Hiripi E, Pope HG Jr, Kessler RC: **The prevalence and correlates of eating disorders in the National Comorbidity Survey Replication.** *Biol Psychiatry* 2007, **61:**348–358.
34. Swinbourne JM, Touyz SW: **The co-morbidity of eating disorders and anxiety disorders: a review.** *Eur Eat Disord Rev* 2007, **15:**253–274.
35. Mattila-Evenden M, Svanborg P, Gustavsson P, Asberg M: **Determinants of self-rating and expert rating concordance in psychiatric out-patients, using the affective subscales of the CPRS.** *Acta Psychiatr Scand* 1996, **94:**386–396.
36. Bohn K, Doll HA, Cooper Z, O'Connor M, Palmer RL, Fairburn CG: **The measurement of impairment due to eating disorder psychopathology.** *Behav Res Ther* 2008, **46:**1105–1110.
37. Bohn K, Fariburn C: *The Clinical Impairment Assessment Questionnaire (CIA3.0).* New York: Guilford Press; 2008.
38. Vannucci A, Kass AE, Sinton MM, Aspen V, Weisman H, Bailey JO, Wilfley DE, Taylor CB: **An examination of the clinical impairment assessment among women at high risk for eating disorder onset.** *Behav Res Ther* 2012, **50:**407–414.
39. Reas DL, Ro O, Kapstad H, Lask B: **Psychometric properties of the clinical impairment assessment: norms for young adult women.** *Int J Eat Disord* 2010, **43:**72–76.
40. Benjamin L: **SASB Intrex user's manual.** In *Book SASB Intrex user's manual.* City: Univeristy of Utah; 2000.
41. Bjorck C, Clinton D, Sohlberg S, Hallstrom T, Norring C: **Interpersonal profiles in eating disorders: ratings of SASB self-image.** *Psychol Psychother* 2003, **76:**337–349.
42. Bjorck C, Clinton D, Sohlberg S, Norring C: **Negative self-image and outcome in eating disorders: results at 3-year follow-up.** *Eat Behav* 2007, **8:**398–406.
43. Monsen JT, von der Lippe AL, Havik OE, Halvorsen MS, Eilertsen DE: **Validation of the SASB Introject Surface in a Norwegian clinical and nonclinical sample.** *J Pers Assess* 2007, **88:**235–245.
44. Erickson TM, Pincus AL: **Using Structural Analysis of Social Behavior (SASB) measures of self- and social perception to give interpersonal meaning to symptoms: anxiety as an exemplar.** *Assessment* 2005, **12:**243–254.
45. Cohen J: *Statistical power analysis for the behavioral sciences.* 2nd edition. New York: Academic Press; 1988.
46. Rea L, Parker R: *Designing and conducting survey research.* San Fransisco: Jossey-Boss; 1992.
47. Brown TA, Haedt-Matt AA, Keel PK: **Personality pathology in purging disorder and bulimia nervosa.** *Int J Eat Disord* 2011, **44:**735–740.
48. Garner DM, Garner MV, Rosen LW: **Anorexia nervosa "restricters" who purge: Implications for subtyping anorexia nervosa.** *Int J Eat Disord* 1993, **13:**171–185.
49. Mond JM, Hay PJ, Rodgers B, Owen C: **Self-report versus interview assessment of purging in a community sample of women.** *Eur Eat Disord Rev* 2007, **15:**403–409.
50. Allen KL, Fursland A, Watson H, Byrne SM: **Eating disorder diagnoses in general practice settings: comparison with structured clinical interview and self-report questionnaires.** *J Ment Health* 2011, **20:**270–280.
51. Berg KC, Peterson CB, Frazier P, Crow SJ: **Convergence of scores on the interview and questionnaire versions of the Eating Disorder Examination: a meta-analytic review.** *Psychol Assess* 2011, **23:**714–724.
52. Reas DL, Wisting L, Kapstad H, Lask B: **Convergent validity of the eating disorder examination and the eating disorder examination-questionnaire among university women in Norway.** *Eur Eat Disord Rev* 2011, **19:**357–361.
53. Burton E, Stice E, Bearman SK, Rohde P: **Experimental test of the affect-regulation theory of bulimic symptoms and substance use: a randomized trial.** *Int J Eat Disord* 2007, **40:**27–36.
54. Dawe S, Loxton NJ: **The role of impulsivity in the development of substance use and eating disorders.** *Neurosci Biobehav Rev* 2004, **28:**343–351.
55. Grilo CM, White MA, Masheb RM: **DSM-IV psychiatric disorder comorbidity and its correlates in binge eating disorder.** *Int J Eat Disord* 2009, **42:**228–234.
56. Fairburn CG, Bohn K: **Eating disorder NOS (EDNOS): an example of the troublesome "not otherwise specified" (NOS) category in DSM-IV.** *Behav Res Ther* 2005, **43:**691–701.
57. Krug I, Root T, Bulik C, Granero R, Penelo E, Jimenez-Murcia S, Fernandez-Aranda F: **Redefining phenotypes in eating disorders based on personality: a latent profile analysis.** *Psychiatry Res* 2011, **188:**439–445.
58. *National Institute of Mental Health Research Domain Criteria Project (RDoC).* http://www.nimh.nih.gov/research-funding/rdoc/nimh-research-domain-criteria-rdoc.shtml.
59. Clinton D, Norring C: **The comparative utility of statistically derived eating disorder clusters and DSM-IV diagnoses: relationship to symptomatology and psychiatric comorbidity at intake and follow-up.** *Eat Behav* 2005, **6:**403–418.
60. Castellini G, Fioravanti G, Lo Sauro C, Rotella F, Lelli L, Ventura L, Faravelli C, Ricca V: **Latent profile and latent transition analyses of eating disorder phenotypes in a clinical sample: A 6 year follow-up study.** *Psychiatry Res* 2013, **15:**92–99.
61. Markon KE, Chmielewski M, Miller CJ: **The reliability and validity of discrete and continuous measures of psychopathology: a quantitative review.** *Psychol Bull* 2011, **137:**856–879.

Prevalence and correlates of unhealthy weight control behaviors: findings from the national longitudinal study of adolescent health

Eric M Stephen[1], Jennifer S Rose[1*], Lindsay Kenney[1], Francine Rosselli-Navarra[2] and Ruth Striegel Weissman[1]

Abstract

Background: A recent study examined the prevalence, clinical correlates, age trends, and stability of unhealthy weight control behaviors (UWCB; purging and diet pill use) in a nationally representative sample of Norwegian boys and girls. The purpose of this study was to provide similar, comparative analyses for a nationally representative sample of American youth.

Methods: Data were extracted from the restricted use data files of survey Waves I, II, and III of the National Longitudinal Study of Adolescent Health (Add Health), selecting all participants who at Wave I had provided information on age, sex, and UWCB. Using UWCB information, three groups were created (purging, diet pill use, and no recent UWCB "controls") and compared on indicators of adverse health or mental health.

Results: Girls consistently were more likely than boys to report UWCB. UWCB were significantly associated with higher body mass index, self-perception of being overweight, low self-esteem, depression, and delinquency. Prevalence estimates for purging remained relatively constant across the three survey waves; in contrast, diet pill use was especially common at Wave III.

Conclusions: Age trends, gender differences, and clinical correlates of change in the likelihood of UWCB between Waves I-III were all identified in analyses comparing purging and diet pill use in American adolescents. Females and older adolescents were specifically more likely to engage in pill use than purging, and individuals with increased weight dissatisfaction, a history of delinquent behaviors, more depression symptoms, or lower self-esteem were more likely to engage in an unhealthy weight control behavior over time. While the Norwegian study found that prevalence of purging was lower among young adult participants, our results suggested that there were no significant differences in prevalence between age groups.

Keywords: Eating disorders, Purging behavior, Adolescent, Diet pill use, Weight control behavior

Background

Various community surveys have shown that disordered eating behaviors are prevalent in adolescents, correlated with indicators of psychosocial impairment, and predictive of unfavorable physical or mental health outcomes [1-3]. Although disordered eating symptoms such as binge eating, purging, or non-purging compensatory behaviors (for example fasting, excessive exercise, or diet pill use) have often been studied in adolescence as early symptoms of or as proxy variables for full syndrome eating disorders (e.g., anorexia nervosa or bulimia nervosa) [4], investigators have more recently begun to examine disordered eating as a clinically relevant phenomena even in the absence of a diagnostic eating disorder, determined by criteria in the DSM-5 (or DSM-IV).

For example, purging behaviors have received increasing scientific attention as symptoms of clinical relevance in their own right. Studies have shown that vomiting or misusing laxatives or diuretics to manage weight is associated with low self-esteem, depressive symptoms, substance use, and impaired psychosocial adjustment [5-10] and also predict excess weight gain [11]. Results

* Correspondence: jrose01@wesleyan.edu
[1]Department of Psychology, Wesleyan University, 207 High Street, Middletown, CT 06459, USA
Full list of author information is available at the end of the article

from a large community-based study indicated that women who used extreme weight control behaviors, regardless of whether or not these behaviors occurred in the context of binge eating, reported higher levels of psychopathology and psychosocial impairment [12]. Moreover, several genetic studies have found that, notwithstanding some overlap between latent risk factors for binge eating and purging, there may be distinct risk factors for purging versus binge eating, which warrants further investigation of compensatory behaviors [13,14].

Non-purging forms of weight control behavior have been studied less extensively, yet the limited available evidence indicates that these behaviors also are associated with measures of psychological distress such as anxiety or depressive symptoms [15]. Currently, there is some inconsistency as to whether diet pill use should be classified as a "purging" or "non-purging" weight control behavior [1,15]. Furthermore, research has rarely examined diet pill use outside of these grouped categories, and consequently little is known about the behavior itself.

Two longitudinal studies have reported on changes in purging and non-purging weight control behaviors from adolescence to young adulthood. Project EAT, a longitudinal study of high school students in Minneapolis/St. Paul (United States, US), found an age effect in that, over a 10-year period, the prevalence of diet pill use increased in girls and boys, laxative use increased in girls, and vomiting decreased in girls and boys [1]. New data from Project EAT also suggest a cohort effect: comparisons of two cohorts revealed that fewer students in a cohort recruited in 2010 reported extreme weight control behaviors than in the (original) 1999 sample [16]. The second study ("Young in Norway") was conducted among a nationally representative sample of Norwegian school children (ages 12 to 20 years at study entry), contrasting purging and non-purging weight control behaviors. In this study, diet pill use was classified as a non-purging behavior. Age differences in rates of purging and non-purging weight control behaviors were examined by grouping participants into four age categories: 14–16, 17–19, 20–22, and ≥ 23 years at each wave. In both boys and girls, prevalence estimates of purging and non-purging weight control behaviors gradually declined with the transition from adolescence to adulthood [15].

The purpose of the present study was to determine whether age trends and predictors of purging and non-purging weight control behaviors observed in Norwegian adolescents [15] could be replicated in a large, nationally representative sample of US youth from the National Longitudinal Study of Adolescent Health (Add Health) where non-purging behavior were limited to diet pill use. First, we tested age trends from adolescence into adulthood in two types of extreme weight control behaviors in boys and girls: vomiting or laxative use as one group, and diet pill use only as a separate group. Consistent with trends observed in the Young in Norway study, we hypothesized decreasing prevalence estimates with increasing age. Second, we examined correlates of these extreme weight control behaviors in boys and girls by comparing them to participants with no recent extreme weight control behaviors. Consistent with previous findings, we hypothesized that more girls than boys would report these extreme weight control behaviors. We further hypothesized that students who reported purging (vomiting or laxative use) or diet pill use for weight control would differ significantly (reflecting greater disturbance) from students who did not engage in any UWCB on measures of body weight, self-esteem, and self-reported depression.

Methods

Data source

The present study extracted data from the restricted-use National Longitudinal Study of Adolescent Health (Add Health) survey Waves I (1994–1995), II (1996), and III (2001–2002). Add Health has been following over 20,000 American adolescents over the course of fourteen years, with four waves of data collection since the study's inception when participants were in grades 7–12. (Wave IV did not collect data about purging and, therefore, was not used for the present study).

Wave I was conducted between 1994 and 1995, with sampling from 132 schools in the United States, representative for region, urbanicity, size, and ethnicity. Initially, 80 high schools were recruited, and each participating school identified a feeder middle school in the community, with the requirement of the inclusion of 7th graders. A total of 20,074 adolescents in grades 7–12 were tested using self-administered, in-school questionnaires given during a 60-minute class period. Wave II was conducted in 1996, and included over 15,000 of the participants originally tested in Wave I. In-home interviews were conducted with participants at Wave III (August of 2001 to April of 2002), with participants now in early adulthood. Further details about the study design can be found elsewhere [17].

Only participants, who provided consistent data across survey waves on birth date and gender, and completed questions concerning vomiting or use of laxatives or diet pills for weight control purposes in Wave I, were included in the present study. A total of 168 participants were dropped due to missing weight control behaviors at Wave I or inconsistent age and gender data across waves.

Instruments and procedures

Add Health surveys included a wide range of questions pertaining to psychological and physical health issues and behaviors. The variables used in this study are described below.

Demographic information was extracted from the Wave I dataset. *Age* was recorded in Waves II and III as age at last birthday. Age at Wave I was calculated by subtracting birth date from the date of interview.

Unhealthy weight control behaviors (UWCB). A two-part question measured whether participants engaged in a number of weight control behaviors. Participants were asked whether, in the past 7 days, they had been trying to lose or maintain weight (yes/no). Participants who answered "no" were instructed to skip the follow-up items; those answering "yes" were asked follow-up questions regarding what specific behaviors were used to do so (response choices included: vomiting; laxative use; diet pill use; dieting; exercising; other; none). Frequency of occurrence was not measured in the Add Health surveys.

Classification of participants based on unhealthy weight control behaviors. At each wave, participants were classified into one of three mutually exclusive groups. The *purging group* included those indicating vomiting or using laxatives (regardless of whether they also reported diet pill use) as their means of trying to lose or maintain weight; the *diet pill only group* included those reporting diet pill use but not purging behaviors for weight control purposes. Purging and diet pill use were coded as mutually exclusive in order to analyze diet pill use as a unique behavior and compare pill use with more commonly studied UWCB. Finally, a third group (*no recent UWCB*) comprised all remaining participants, i.e., participants who were not trying to control their weight or participants who reported that they had dieted or exercised (because these behaviors, unless taken to an extreme, are recommended as healthy weight management strategies). Participants reporting "other" behaviors to manage their weight were also classified into the comparison group.

Consistent with the Center for Disease Control (CDC), *Body Mass Index* (BMI) was calculated by dividing weight (in pounds) by the product of height (in inches) squared times the value 703 [18]. *Weight Self-Perception* was measured using a single item ("How do you think of yourself in terms of weight?"). Five responses were available using a Likert scale: "overweight", "slightly overweight", "about the right weight", "slightly underweight", and "very underweight".

Self-esteem was measured using four questions based on Rosenberg's Self-Esteem Scale [19] that were asked at each wave ("you have many good qualities"; "you have much to be proud of"; "you like yourself just the way you are"; and "you feel you are doing things just right"). Participants rated each item on a scale from 1 to 5, and a total score was calculated by summing the items [20]. (Cronbach's alpha =0.79 at Wave I, 0.80 at Wave II, and 0.78 at Wave III).

Depressive symptoms. At each wave, participants completed a modified version of the Center for Epidemiologic Studies-Depression (CES-D) scale. Participants rated symptom frequency in the past week on a scale from 0 (never or rarely) to 3 (most of the time). Using the 9 items that were asked at all three waves, we created a total score by adding across all items for each wave. [21] Cronbach's alpha was 0.81 at Wave I, 0.82 at Wave II, and 0.80 at Wave III. Because of its skewed distribution in our sample, the scale was then natural log transformed.

Delinquency. Consistent with other studies that have utilized Add Health data, [22] seven questions concerning delinquent behavior available in all three study waves were used to create a binary delinquency variable. Specifically, participants were asked "In the past 12 months, how often did you: (1) Damage property that didn't belong to you; (2) Steal something worth more than $50; (3) Go into a house or building to steal something; (4) Use or threaten to use a weapon to get something from someone; (5) sell marijuana or other drugs; (6) steal something worth less than $50; (7) Take part in a fight where a group of your friends was against another group". Responses to each individual question were dichotomized by recoding the original 4-point Likert format (never, one or two times, three or four times, five times or more) into never versus one or more. The recoded items were then summed. Because the delinquency summary score was extremely skewed with most participants reporting no delinquent behaviors (greater than or equal to 59.0% at all waves), and the majority of the rest reporting just one delinquent behavior (greater than or equal to 20.7% at all waves), we recoded it into a binary categorical variable with a meaningful cut point (0 = no instances, 1 = one or more instances of delinquent behavior).

Statistical analyses

All analyses were performed using Stata 13.1. Chi-square tests were used first to analyze the differences in prevalence for purging and diet pill use at each wave as well as between boys and girls. Mixed effects logistic regression models were tested to identify changes in these behaviors over the three waves for boys and girls. Mixed effects logistic regression analysis was next used to test for age and gender trends in purging and diet pill use. Finally, mixed effects logistic regression models adjusting for age and gender as covariates were performed to examine differences in the UWCB groups on all measures of psychosocial factors.

Results

Sample description

At Wave I, data were available for 10,173 boys and 10,437 girls (mean age = 15.66, SD = 1.75); at Wave II, our sample included 7,108 male and 7,510 female participants (mean age = 16.22, SD = 1.64); and at Wave III, 7,104 male participants and 7,927 female participants (mean age = 21.96, SD = 1.77) were included. In all, 55.99% participants included in our study had data for all three study waves. Efforts to change (gain or lose) weight or maintain weight were reported by a majority of participants. At each wave, about one-third of the participants reported that they were trying to lose weight (34.32%, 33.38%, 33.69% at waves I, II, and III, respectively). Trying to maintain weight also was reported by a substantial subset of participants at Wave I (34.28%) and Wave II (33.11%) but was less common at wave III (15.10%). Fewer participants reported efforts to gain weight than trying to lose or maintain weight at each of the waves (Wave I: 19.66%; Wave II: 18.88%; Wave III: 15.62%). Only a minority of participants at Wave I (11.74%) and Wave II (14.63%) reported that they were not trying to do anything to change or maintain their current weight; at Wave III, about one-third of the sample (35.59%) reported that they made no efforts to change or maintain their weight.

It should also be noted that some attrition bias was found in this sample, such that men were more likely to drop out (OR = 0.90, p < 0.001, CI = 0.85-0.96 at Wave II and OR = 0.71, p < 0.000, CI = 0.67-0.76 at Wave III) as were older participants (OR = 1.56, p < 0.000, CI = 1.53-1.60 at Wave II and OR = 1.09, p < 0.000, CI = 1.08-1.11 at Wave III). However, neither purging nor laxative use at Wave I was associated with attrition at Wave II, and neither purging nor laxative use at Waves I or II was associated with attrition at Wave III.

Gender and age trends for UWCB prevalence

Table 1 summarizes the prevalence of purging and diet pill use at each wave by gender. As shown in Table 1, significantly more girls than boys reported vomiting, laxative misuse, or using diet pills to lose or maintain weight at each of the three waves. Additionally, because of the small numbers of individuals reporting purging by means of vomiting or laxative misuse, the two groups were combined into one "purging" category, which similarly showed higher rates of purging for girls than boys at all three waves. Mixed effects logistic regression analyses were run to evaluate change in each outcome across the three waves. The results indicated diet pill use increased significantly for men, and both diet pill and laxative use increased significantly for women.

Furthermore, because of the range of ages found in each study wave and the desire to analyze changes both over time and across ages, mixed logistic regression models were also tested with age as a predictor variable, broken into four age categories (14–16, 17–19, 20–22, and 23 or above) to ensure a sufficient sample size in each group. Similar analyses were also performed to test for gender effects overall. Figure 1 illustrates the changes in prevalence of purging and diet pill use from adolescence into early adulthood, and Table 2 shows these age group and gender effects for both the purging (vomiting or laxative misuse) and diet pill only groups against the current UWCB group. As shown in this table, significant gender differences were found for both purging and diet pill use. However, age effects were found only for diet pill use; there was no significant difference for purging across age groups. Further, Table 3 breaks down the prevalence of purging and pill use in each age group by wave, given the possibility for individuals to be classified in the same age group over multiple waves. Age-adjusted prevalence rates were also calculated using population data from the 2000 United States Census due to the higher number of observations in older age groups [23]. In multivariate modeling, however, these repeat observations are also accounted for through the use of mixed models.

Table 1 Prevalence and change in UWCB among male and female participants, Waves I-III

	Wave I		Wave II		Wave III		Mixed model		
	N	%	N	%	N	%	Coefficient	Standard error	p
Males									
Purging[abc]	24	0.24%	14	0.20%	9	0.13%	0.00	0.00	0.11
Vomiting[abc]	16	0.16%	12	0.17%	4	0.06%	0.00	0.00	0.09
Laxative Use[abc]	8	0.08%	3	0.04%	6	0.08%	0.00	0.00	0.97
Pill Use Only[abc]	17	0.17%	15	0.21%	109	1.54%	0.01	0.00	0.00
No UWCB	10132	99.60%	7077	99.59%	6977	98.34%	–	–	–
Females									
Purging	62	0.59%	73	0.97%	57	0.72%	0.00	0.00	0.25
Vomiting	32	0.31%	50	0.67%	23	0.29%	0.00	0.00	0.90
Laxative Use	32	0.31%	29	0.39%	39	0.49%	0.00	0.00	0.048
Pill Use Only	112	1.07%	106	1.41%	409	5.14%	0.02	0.00	0.00
No UWCB	10259	98.33%	7327	97.62%	7489	94.14%	–	–	–

[a]Significant gender differences at T1 ($p < 0.05$), [b]Significant gender differences at T2 ($p < 0.05$), [c]Significant gender differences at T3 ($p < 0.05$).

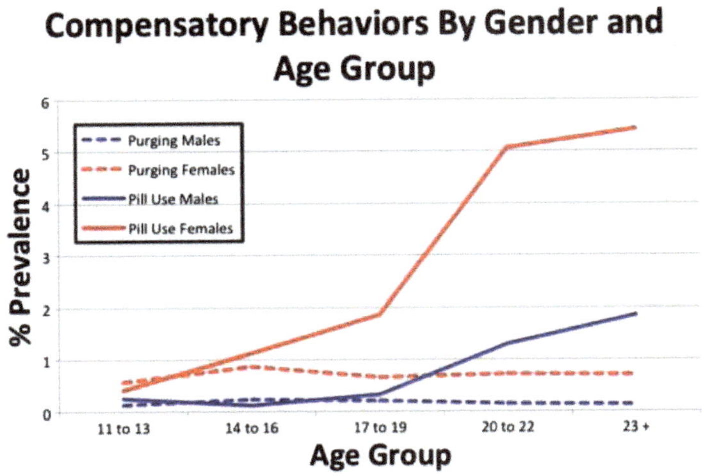

Figure 1 Prevalence for purging and diet pill use from adolescence to young adulthood.

Clinical correlates for UWCB

Mixed effects logistic regression analysis was then used to examine a range of clinical correlates separately for purging and diet pill use. In each model, age and gender were used as control variables, and each variable of interest was interacted with time in order to ascertain the main effect of the variable as well as its effect over time. Because of the high correlation between perceived weight image and BMI, these variables and their interaction with time were tested together in a model to determine whether they were independently associated with purging and pill use. Results are shown in Table 4.

Significant overall group differences were found for each of the clinical correlates examined in this study, with the exception of BMI. Participants who either purged or used diet pills as a form of UWCB perceived themselves as more overweight, reported higher depression symptom scores, reported lower self-esteem, and were more likely to have engaged in delinquent behaviors. After adjusting for weight image, BMI was not significantly associated with either the purging or diet pill group. Significant interactions with time were found in diet pill use for depression scores and self-esteem. Participants with higher levels of depression and lower self-esteem at Wave I showed a smaller increase in diet pill use over time. None of the clinical correlates were associated with changes in the likelihood of purging over time.

Table 2 Mixed logistic regression model results for age and gender differences in UWCB groups

	Purging	Pill use only
	Coefficient (95% CI)	Coefficient (95% CI)
Age	0.94 (0.83-1.06)	2.01 (1.87-2.16)*
Gender	4.20 (2.95-5.98)*	4.40 (3.62-5.35)*

* - p < 0.001.

Discussion

This study examined prevalence and correlates of UWCB as well as trends over time in these behaviors in a large, nationally representative sample of males and females. Consistent with prior research, UWCB were reported by far more female participants than male participants [1,15]. The prevalence estimates obtained in our sample for vomiting or laxative misuse for weight control reasons are lower than estimates reported in other studies [15], most likely due to the short time frame used in Add Health for measuring UWCB (past 7 days). Regardless of how many adolescents engage in purging, experts uniformly agree that vomiting or laxative abuse is a health risk behavior and should be addressed via therapeutic or preventive interventions [15].

Individuals who acknowledged purging had greater weight dissatisfaction than those in the no recent UWCB group. These results are noteworthy because the no recent UWCB group included participants who reported using various behaviors to try and lose or maintain weight that were not considered to be UWCB as defined in this study. This makes our comparisons more conservative than had we used a comparison group comprised of individuals who did not report any efforts to manage their weight.

Prior studies have shown that UWCB actually are associated concurrently and prospectively with increased weight [1]. Moreover, also in keeping with prior studies, compared to the no recent UWCB group, the purging group scored lower on self-esteem and higher on depression [4]. At Wave I, the purging group was more likely

Table 3 Overall and age-adjusted prevalence of purging and pill use in each age group by Wave

		Purging				Diet pill use			
Age group	Wave	Cases (n)	Population (N)	Rate per 100,000	Age-adjusted rate per 100,000	Cases (n)	Population (N)	Rate per 100,000	Age-adjusted rate per 100,000
11-13	1	13	2846	456.78	89.56	9	2846	316.23	62.01
	2	0	675	0.00	0.00	3	675	444.44	87.15
	3	–	–	–	–	–	–	–	–
	Total:	**13**	**3521**	**369.21**	**72.39**	**12**	**3521**	**340.81**	**66.83**
14-16	1	50	10460	478.01	92.52	59	10460	564.05	109.18
	2	50	7259	688.80	133.33	54	7259	743.90	143.99
	3	–	–	–	–	–	–	–	–
	Total:	**100**	**17719**	**564.37**	**109.24**	**113**	**17719**	**637.73**	**123.44**
17-19	1	22	7223	304.58	60.33	61	7223	844.52	167.28
	2	35	6502	538.30	106.62	61	6502	938.17	185.82
	3	9	1568	573.98	113.69	45	1568	2869.90	568.44
	Total:	**66**	**15293**	**431.57**	**85.48**	**167**	**15293**	**1092.00**	**216.29**
20-22	1	1	77	1298.70	243.20	0	77	0.00	0.00
	2	2	176	1136.36	212.80	3	176	1704.55	319.20
	3	31	7266	426.64	79.90	246	7266	3385.63	634.01
	Total:	**34**	**7519**	**452.19**	**84.68**	**249**	**7519**	**3311.61**	**620.15**
23+	1	–	–	–	–	–	–	–	–
	2	–	–	–	–	–	–	–	–
	3	26	6216	418.28	94.12	277	6216	4456.24	1002.77
	Total:	**26**	**6216**	**418.28**	**94.12**	**277**	**6216**	**4456.24**	**1002.77**

Those cells where there are no observations are indicated by –. Data used for the weighted rates comes from the 2000 United States Census.

than the no recent UWCB group to report having engaged in delinquent behaviors; however, there was no significant difference in the likelihood of purging or diet pill use over time for those engaged in delinquent behavior compared to those who did not. Both purging and delinquent behaviors fall in the spectrum of disinhibited or impulsive behavior. Reports of delinquent behavior declined with each successive wave in all three groups, possibly reflecting increasing maturity and self-control, although rates of purging showed no evidence of declining over time. Additional studies are needed to further explore the relationship between delinquent behavior and purging.

It is important to note that the models testing both BMI and weight dissatisfaction showed significant associations between weight dissatisfaction for both UWCB outcomes, but there were no significant associations for BMI. This may be due to the fact that a significant number of individuals in this sample who did not show any recent UWCB were also trying to lose or maintain weight. Future research may wish to investigate how these purging and pill use groups differ specifically from those who were not trying to lose or maintain weight as opposed to the no recent UWCB group more broadly in order to more fully understand the differences between weight dissatisfaction and BMI as clinical correlates.

Overall, our findings suggest that purging and diet pill use are associated with a less favorable profile on the clinical correlates examined in this study. Among those who reported purging or diet pill use only to manage their weight, these correlates suggest more pathology compared to the no recent UWCB group, including higher weight dissatisfaction, greater prevalence of delinquent behaviors, lower self-esteem, and increased depression. However, only depression and self-esteem were associated with change in the likelihood of pill use over time, and none of the clinical correlates were related to changes in the likelihood of purging. Research is needed to determine whether educating individuals about the lack of efficacy of purging as a long-term weight management strategy would reduce the prevalence or incidence of these behaviors.

To our knowledge, ours is the first study to examine the prevalence of diet pill use in the absence of purging behaviors [24]. Diet pill use was considerably more prevalent than purging, and unlike purging, showed a considerable increase with age. At Wave I, diet pill users were significantly older than purgers. More importantly, the diet pill group differed significantly from the no recent UWCB group on all clinical correlates with the exception of BMI. Diet pill use was associated with greater weight

Table 4 Mixed logistic regression results for differences in clinical correlates for each UWCB group

	Purging				Pill use			
	Coefficient	SE	p	95% CI	Coefficient	SE	p	95% CI
Females dompared to males	1.21	0.17	0.00	0.87-1.55	1.51	0.10	0.00	1.30-1.71
Age difference	−0.06	0.03	0.07	−0.12-0.01	0.15	0.02	0.00	0.11-0.19
CESD (log trans) Difference	0.72	0.16	0.00	0.41-1.03	0.42	0.10	0.00	0.23-0.63
Linear change across waves	0.12	0.28	0.67	−0.42-0.66	0.76	0.14	0.00	0.23-0.63
CESD Difference over time	0.11	0.12	0.39	−0.14-0.35	−0.13	0.06	0.02	−0.24-0.02
Females compared to males	1.26	0.18	0.00	0.92-1.61	1.47	0.10	0.00	1.27-1.67
Age difference	−0.07	0.03	0.05	−0.13-0.00	0.14	0.02	0.00	0.10-0.19
Self-esteem difference	−0.16	0.04	0.00	−0.23- -0.09	−0.24	0.03	0.00	−0.30- -0.19
Linear change across waves	1.10	0.46	0.02	0.20-2.00	−0.32	0.28	0.26	−0.87-0.23
Self-esteem difference over time	−0.05	0.03	0.08	−0.11-0.01	0.06	0.02	0.00	0.03-0.09
Females compared to males	1.51	0.18	0.00	1.16-1.86	1.68	0.11	0.00	0.12-0.20
Age difference	−0.04	0.03	0.20	−0.11-0.02	0.16	0.02	0.00	0.12-0.20
Delinquency difference	0.63	0.21	0.00	−0.22-1.04	0.66	0.17	0.00	0.32-1.00
Linear change across waves	0.21	0.15	0.17	−0.09-0.51	0.55	0.10	0.00	0.35-0.76
Delinquency difference over time	0.07	0.18	0.70	−0.28-0.41	−0.06	0.11	0.59	−0.28-0.16
Females compared to males	1.13	0.18	0.00	0.77-1.49	1.25	0.11	0.00	1.03-1.46
Age difference	−0.08	0.04	0.02	−0.15- -0.01	0.11	0.02	0.00	0.07-0.15
Weight image difference	0.93	0.18	0.00	0.59-1.28	0.99	0.15	0.00	0.70-1.28
Linear change across waves	1.05	0.47	0.03	0.13-1.96	0.42	0.30	0.17	−0.18-1.01
Weight image difference over time	−0.02	0.15	0.88	−0.31-2.66	0.06	0.09	0.54	−0.12-0.28
BMI Difference	0.03	0.02	0.14	−0.01-0.08	0.04	0.02	0.06	0.00-0.07
BMI Difference over time	−0.03	0.02	0.09	−0.06-0.00	−0.01	0.01	0.52	−0.03-0.01

Note: CESD = Center forEpidemiologic Studies Depression scale; SE = standard error; p = significance level; CI = confidence interval.

dissatisfaction, more delinquent behaviors, and less favorable scores on measures of psychological adjustment such as self-reported depression or self-esteem at Wave I. In addition, higher levels of depression and lower self-esteem were associated with an increased likelihood of diet pill use over time.

In contrast to findings from a Norwegian study where the prevalence of purging was found to be lower among late adolescent or young adult participants [15], our findings from the Add Health sample suggest that purging prevalence remained relatively unchanged across the age groups, and diet pill use was far more prevalent among participants in the age groups of 17 years and older. Thus, the development of these behaviors may be different for American youth, and more research on predictors of purging—particularly diet pill use in the absence of purging—is warranted to further identify how these behaviors develop in American youth.

Several limitations need to be acknowledged. The Add Health measures used in our analyses relied on self-report, which is subject to recall errors or biased reporting. The time frame used for measuring presence of UWCB was shorter (past 7 days) than is typical in most epidemiological studies of disordered eating. Therefore, it is unclear the extent to which individuals in the comparison group (no recent UWCB) may have also engaged in diet pill use, laxative misuse, or vomiting for weight control purposes during the longer time frame covered in some of the psychosocial measures. For example, no time frame was specified for measuring self-esteem, and delinquency was based on the past 12 months. Inadvertent inclusion in the no recent UWCB group of individuals who might have reported "yes" to the question about purging or diet pill use had the time frame been broader renders our group comparisons more conservative. Similarly, those who reported "other" mechanisms with which to lose or maintain weight were not asked about what those mechanisms were, and therefore it is possible that these could be classified as UWCB.

Limitations are also associated with several of the variables used in this study. For example, Add Health did not collect information on the type of diet pills used. Similarly, data on binge eating, a symptom often associated with purging or diet pill use, were not collected. In addition, because frequency information was not available for UWCB, we were unable to study the severity of these behaviors. Finally, low frequency of engagement in delinquent behaviors limited us to defining delinquency more broadly as a binary yes/no for engagement in delinquent behaviors and precluded an examination of each behavior separately.

Another potential limitation arises from our classification of purging and diet pill use. Specifically, despite the fact that this was a large, nationally representative, epidemiological study, the low prevalence of UWCB required that we group individuals who vomited and those who abused laxatives into one group. Larger samples are needed to determine whether these two types of purging behavior should be classified into distinct groups. This may require oversampling on these behaviors given their low prevalence rate in the population. Moreover, we prioritized purging over diet pill use, allowing into our purging group individuals who also used diet pills but not vice versa (i.e., the diet pill group only reported diet pill use and not purging).

Finally, concerns arise regarding the analyses in Tables 2 and 3 given that not every subject has an equal probability of contributing to the various age-specific prevalences. While the use of the mixed modeling helps to deal with this issue, such unequal opportunities may present a problem. This concern is also compounded by the fact that men and individuals who were older were significantly more likely to drop out of the study at a follow up point, and thus the results of this study must be interpreted with caution.

Nonetheless, these limitations were offset by several strengths. The study involved a nationally representative sample, and therefore did not contain the limitations inherent in studies of patient samples. Furthermore, the large sample size afforded us the opportunity to analyze both men and women, and the longitudinal design allowed us to gain information on our sample over a considerable period of time (8 years) from adolescence into early adulthood. Finally, the classification system allowed an opportunity to study diet pill use, a previously understudied behavior, as a unique UWCB.

Conclusion

This study examined the prevalence of vomiting, laxative misuse, and diet pill use among adolescents, as well as the age trends of these behaviors from adolescence into adulthood and the clinical correlates that predict diet pill use and purging UWCB. Results suggest that girls or women are more likely than boys or men to engage in each of these behaviors and that diet pill use, but not vomiting or laxative misuse, increases over time. Furthermore, results have shown significant differences between diet pill use, purging UWCB, and the control group for a variety of clinical correlates, supporting research indicating that it is important to prevent, identify, and treat nonclinical levels of disordered eating. Our results differed from the Norwegian study in that we did not find that purging prevalence was lower in young adults. Whether these differences between our and the Norwegian study reflect cultural differences or are a function of methodological differences awaits further investigation.

Competing interests

The authors have no conflicts of interest to report.

Authors' contributions

EMS conducted all statistical analyses, contributed to Methods selection, provided data interpretation, and wrote the Results and Discussion sections of the manuscript. JR contributed to interpretation of data and revisions to drafts of the manuscript. LK contributed to the conception of the study as well as the drafting of introduction and discussion sections of the manuscript. FR made significant revisions to the original manuscript for intellectual content. RS made substantial contributions to the original manuscript and supervised all data analysis and interpretation. All authors read and approved the final manuscript.

Acknowledgements

This research was supported by Academic Research Enhancement Award DK092768-01A1 (Striegel Weissman) from the National Institute of Diabetes, Digestive, and Kidney Disease. The Add Health study is directed by Kathleen Mullan Harris and designed by J. Richard Udry, Peter S. Bearman, and Kathleen Mullan Harris at the University of North Carolina at Chapel Hill. It is funded by grant P01-HD31921 from the Eunice Kennedy Shriver National Institute of Child Health and Human Development, along with funding from 23 other federal agencies and foundations. Data were collected under protocols approved by the Institutional Review Boards of the University of North Carolina at Chapel Hill, and the Miriam Hospital.

Author details

[1]Department of Psychology, Wesleyan University, 207 High Street, Middletown, CT 06459, USA. [2]Department of Psychology, Manchester Community College, Great Path MS#4, PO Box 1046, Manchester, CT 06040, USA.

References

1. Neumark-Sztainer D, Wall M, Larson NI, Eisenberg ME, Loth K: **Dieting and disordered eating behaviors from adolescence to young adulthood: findings from a 10-year longitudinal study.** *J Am Diet Assoc* 2011, **111**(7):1004–1011.
2. Talamayan KS, Springer AE, Kelder SH, Gorospe EC, Joye KA: **Prevalence of overweight misperception and weight control behaviors among normal weight adolescents in the United States.** *Sci World J* 2006, **6**:365–373.
3. Alm ME, Neumark-Sztainer D, Story M, Boutelle KN: **Self-weighing and weight control behaviors among adolescents with a history of overweight.** *J Adolesc Health* 2009, **44**(5):424–430.
4. Steinhausen HC, Gavez S, Winkler Metzke C: **Psychosocial correlates, outcome, and stability of abnormal adolescent eating behavior in community samples of young people.** *Int J Eat Disord* 2005, **37**(2):119–126.
5. Piran N, Robinson SR: **Patterns of associations between eating disordered behaviors and substance use in two non-clinical samples: a university and a community based sample.** *J Health Psychol* 2011, **16**(7):1027–1037.
6. Keel PK, Striegel-Moore RH: **The validity and clinical utility of purging disorder.** *Int J Eat Disord* 2009, **42**(8):706–719.
7. Ackard DM, Fulkerson JA, Neumark-Sztainer D: **Psychological and behavioral risk profiles as they relate to eating disorder diagnoses and symptomatology among a school-based sample of youth.** *Int J Eat Disord* 2011, **44**(5):440–446.
8. Pisetsky EM, Chao YM, Dierker LC, May AM, Striegel-Moore RH: **Disordered eating and substance use in high-school students: results from the**

Youth Risk Behavior Surveillance System. *Int J Eat Disord* 2008, **41**(5):464–470.
9. Haedt AA, Edler C, Heatherton TF, Keel PK: **Importance of multiple purging methods in the classification of eating disorder subtypes.** *Int J Eat Disord* 2006, **39**(8):648–654.
10. Haedt AA, Keel PK: **Comparing definitions of purging disorder on point prevalence and associations with external validators.** *Int J Eat Disord* 2010, **43**(5):433–439.
11. Neumark-Sztainer D, Wall M, Story M, Standish AR: **Dieting and unhealthy weight control behaviors during adolescence: associations with 10-year changes in body mass index.** *J Adolesc Health* 2012, **50**(1):80–86.
12. Mond J, Hay P, Rodgers B, Owen C, Crosby R, Mitchell J: **Use of extreme weight control behaviors with and without binge eating in a community sample: implications for the classification of bulimic-type eating disorders.** *Int J Eat Disord* 2006, **39**(4):294–302.
13. Wade TD, Treloar S, Martin NG: **Shared and unique risk factors between lifetime purging and objective binge eating: a twin study.** *Psychol Med* 2008, **38**(10):1455–1464.
14. Sullivan PF, Bulik CM, Kendler KS: **Genetic epidemiology of binging and vomiting.** *Ber J Psychiatry* 1998, **173:**75–79.
15. Abebe DS, Lien L, Torgersen L, von Soest T: **Binge eating, purging and non-purging compensatory behaviours decrease from adolescence to adulthood: a population-based, longitudinal study.** *BMC Public Health* 2012, **12:**32.
16. Neumark-Sztainer D, Wall MM, Larson N, Story M, Fulkerson JA, Eisenberg ME, Hannan PJ: **Secular trends in weight status and weight-related attitudes and behaviors in adolescents from 1999 to 2010.** *Prev Med* 2012, **54**(1):77–81.
17. Udry JR, Bearman JS, Harris KM: *The Longitudinal Study of Adolescent Health: Research Design*; [cited 2013 July 11]; Available from: http://www.cpc.unc.edu/projects/addhealth/design/.
18. Centers for Disease Control and Prevention: *About BMI for Adults*; 2011. [cited 2013 July 28]. Available from http://www.cdc.gov/healthyweight/assessing/bmi/adult_bmi/index.html?s_cid=tw_ob064.
19. Rosenberg A: *Society and the Adolescent Self-Image*. Princeton, New Jersey: Princeton University Press; 1965.
20. Kort-Butler LA: **Experienced and vicarious victimization: do social support and self-esteem prevent delinquent responses?** *J Crim Justice* 2010, **38:**496–505.
21. Adkins DE, Wang V, Elder GH Jr: **Structure and Stress: Trajectories of Depressive Symptoms across Adolescence and Young Adulthood.** *Soc Forces* 2009, **88**(1):31.
22. Aalsma MC, Tong Y, Wiehe SE, Tu W: **The impact of delinquency on young adult sexual risk behaviors and sexually transmitted infections.** *J Adolesc Health* 2010, **46**(1):17–24.
23. United States Census Bureau: *United States Census 2000: General Demographic Characteristics;* 2000. [cited 2014 April 15]; Available from: http://www.census.gov/census2000/states/us.html.
24. Austin SB, Nelson LA, Birkett MA, Calzo JP, Everett B: **Eating Disorder Symptoms and Obesity at the Intersections of Gender, Ethnicity, and Sexual Orientation in US High School Students.** *Am J Public Health* 2013, **103**(2):e16–e22.

The HOPE (Helping to Outline Paediatric Eating Disorders) Project: development and debut of a paediatric clinical eating disorder registry

Hunna J Watson[1,2,3,4*], Julie McCormack[1], Kimberley J Hoiles[1,4], David Forbes[1,3] and Julie Potts[1]

Abstract

Background: The HOPE (Helping to Outline Paediatric Eating Disorders) Project is an ongoing registry study made up of a sequential cross-sectional sample prospectively recruited over 17 years, and is designed to answer empirical questions about paediatric eating disorders. This paper introduces the HOPE Project, describes the registry sample to-date, and discusses future directions and challenges and accomplishments. The project and clinical service were established in a tertiary academic hospital in Western Australia in 1996 with a service development grant. Research processes were inbuilt into the initial protocols and data collection was maintained in the following years. Recognisable progress with the research agenda accelerated only when dedicated research resources were obtained. The registry sample consists of consecutive children and adolescents assessed at the eating disorder program from 1996 onward. Standardised multidisciplinary data collected from family intake interview, parent and child clinical interviews, medical review, parent, child and teacher psychometric assessments, and inpatient admission records populate the HOPE Project database.

Results: The registry database to-date contains 941 assessments, of whom 685 met DSM-IV diagnostic criteria for an eating disorder at admission. The majority of the sample were females (91%) from metropolitan Perth (83%). The cases with eating disorders consist of eating disorders not otherwise specified (68%), anorexia nervosa (25%) and bulimia nervosa (7%). Among those with eating disorders, a history of weight loss since illness onset was almost universal (96%) with fear of weight gain (71%) common, and the median duration of illness was 8 months.

Conclusions: Over the next five years and more, we expect that the HOPE Project will make a strong scientific contribution to paediatric eating disorders research and will have important real-world applications to clinical practice and policy as the research unfolds.

Keywords: Adolescent, Child, Cohort, Eating disorder, Paediatric, Registry

Background

Eating disorders are serious mental illnesses involving extreme disturbances in eating attitudes and behaviour. The lifetime prevalence of paediatric eating disorders is 0.3% for anorexia nervosa (AN) and 0.9% for bulimia nervosa (BN) [1], though overall prevalence is higher, given >50% present with "eating disorders not otherwise specified" (EDNOS) [2]. Approximately 1.1 in 100,000 children are admitted annually to inpatient eating disorder services, where life-preserving medical intervention is the focus [3]. Among consecutively admitted paediatric eating disorder inpatients, 61% had life-threatening complications of malnutrition, 58% required nasogastric feeding to preserve life, 67% met the psychological diagnostic criteria for AN, and 34% received psychotropic medications [3]. The extreme physical and psychological toll of these illnesses is reflected in the heightened risk of mortality [4] and medical consequences such as impaired vertical growth, cardiac complications (i.e., arrhythmias), gastrointestinal problems, and poor bone health (i.e., osteoporosis) [5,6]. Socioeconomic impact is high but not widely quantified; in Australia eating disorders are estimated to account for $69 billion per year [7].

* Correspondence: Hunna.watson@health.wa.gov.au
[1]Eating Disorders Program, Princess Margaret Hospital for Children, Perth, Australia
[2]Centre for Clinical Interventions, Perth, Australia
Full list of author information is available at the end of the article

Despite the serious nature of eating disorders, they are not well understood. In the past century many myths have flourished [8,9], characterising eating disorders as; "a lifestyle choice", a "phase", "about vanity", diseases of "white upperclass females", prevalent only in Western cultural environments, not posing medical risk, not occurring in people who are normal weight or overweight, a consequence of parenting, and incurable. Scientific evidence has been instrumental in overturning myths and generating break-throughs in prevention, health care, and public health policy, yet research still lags behind patient, family, health care, and public needs [10,11].

Novel investigations using a range of research methods are required to advance knowledge and registry and cohort studies based upon clinic populations and medical records are perhaps an underutilised source of information. Grey areas, within diagnosis and assessment, risk and etiological candidates, medical issues, patient and family needs, can conceivably be brought to light through these research designs. At project inception in 1996, eating disorders in children and adolescents were barely described and no evidence-based treatments were available, so the broad aim of the "HOPE Project" was to systematically describe and understand paediatric eating disorders. Nearly 20 years later, the scientific environment has progressed, however the original aims still apply; to cultivate discovery of new knowledge about paediatric eating disorders that will be of interest to the general community, health professionals, policy-makers, and individuals affected by eating disorders.

Currently few large (case $N > 100$) paediatric eating disorder registry or cohort studies exist; a review on outcomes which contained a systematic search of studies between 1980 to 2005 with observational designs, either cohort or case series, identified only one; the International Collaborative Outcome Study of Eating Disorders in Adolescence (ICOSEDA) [12-14]. Expert sites that conduct observational studies on naturalistic clinic samples are rare. Stanford University [15-17], which has a large retrospective cohort (~1,400 patients) and a prospective cohort (~160 patients) and the University of Chicago (UoC), [2,18,19] which has a retrospective cohort (~400 patients) and a prospective cohort (~200 patients) are recent exceptions. The Children's Hospital at Westmead and the Royal Children's Hospital in Australia are collecting prospective data and will emerge as other nuclei. The contributions these research sites have made are varied, as reflected in the citations, to summarise would prove unwieldy. On the basis of published outputs, peers have deemed the findings significant, and the registries have been complementary in knowledge generation rather than duplicative.

In other clinical areas, registry studies have been more utilised than they have in mental health and behavioural science, cancer and heart and blood diseases are examples [20]. Challenges of registry research are that the registry population is not randomly sampled, and patients who do not present for treatment or who visit service providers not participating in the registry are missed. The time and effort required to record information on standardised research forms, and obtain and archive written informed consent, can be onerous for busy clinicians. Compellingly, the samples are typically heterogenous and recruited without strict inclusion criteria. The typically wide array of data allows for flexibility in addressing evolving empirical questions and sample size is usually large compared with stand-alone studies. Finally, the design offers flexibility in the clinical research setting, where sometimes meeting the deadlines of stand-alone studies funded by granting bodies that require unique data collections and entirely new ethics approvals is difficult. We chose a registry design because of the possibilities and flexibility - registry studies offer the opportunity to answer large numbers of questions efficiently and cost effectively and offer the best method to study the natural history of diseases, especially rare ones in real world clinical environments with heterogeneous patient groups [21]. There can be specific advantages when a priori hypotheses are difficult to define, as was the case when the HOPE Project team commenced this research.

This paper introduces the HOPE Project, a large cross-sectional registry containing data of sequential participants recruited over 17 years in a specialist paediatric tertiary eating disorder program. The HOPE Project registry is a newly available research resource for paediatric eating disorders, which aims to address evolving scientific questions. The main objective of this report is to outline the development and methodology of the HOPE Project registry, and to profile in brief the baseline psychosocial, clinical, and medical characteristics of the sample to-date. Secondary objectives are to communicate our research strategic plan and to describe the lessons learned developing this registry within a traditional clinical setting.

Methods

Registry sample

The registry ($N = 941$) comprises 194 children (< 13 years) and 747 adolescents (13–17 years) consecutively assessed by a specialist eating disorder program at a tertiary academic hospital from service inception (1996) to April 2013; though the registry is ongoing. We define children as < 13 years because the average age of menarche onset is 12.8 years [22]. Referrals inclusive to age 16 are currently accepted and prior to 2005 referrals to age 17 inclusive were accepted because of a public health service gap.

At the time of writing, the HOPE Project had an inclusion rate of 96.7%. All patients (and families) assessed by the Princess Margaret Hospital for Children Eating Disorders Program (PMH EDP) historically since inception to 2012 were included in this study; except for a small percentage ($n = 27$) who did not want their information used for quality and research purposes. Therefore, the inclusion rate from 1996–2012 was 97%. In 2013 a modified consent processes was introduced and 20/25 (80%) of invited patients and families participated.

Ethics approval for the current iteration of the HOPE Project was granted by PMH Human Research Ethics Committee (HREC). HREC support occurred over many years; leading toward approval for the iteration we now call the HOPE Project. Various consent procedures were used historically, due to different requirements for ethics over this time period and a registry specific waiver of new consent was granted for the recent iteration of the project, which gained approval in 2012. Currently we are trialling a new consent process with opt-in parental consent, patient assent, and patient reconsent at age 18 years, which may attenuate the inclusion rate going forward.

Clinical setting

PMH EDP is the clinical setting and operates the only public paediatric eating disorder program in the state. Referrals are accepted from general practitioners, paediatricians, psychiatrists, psychologists, school nurses and counsellors, other professionals, and the general public. There are no definitive service exclusion criteria, although there is initial diversion towards community services if no indicators for medical admission are present, weight loss is not sustained or rapid, and the family are able to engage with community services. Patients for whom community treatments do not avert decline can be re-referred. PMH EDP is multidisciplinary with staff spanning paediatric medicine, psychiatry, clinical psychology, nursing, dietetics, occupational therapy, physiotherapy, social work, and teaching staff. Historically, PMH EDP provided a small clinical service focused on outpatient care with short medical admissions. With expanded funding which saw a ten-fold increase in clinical staffing in 2007, the service evolved to offer an integrated and more comprehensive continuum of care ranging from outpatient to day patient and inpatient, with outreach support plus a statewide training and consultation program. Research also had the opportunity to flourish as detailed next.

Study background

PMH EDP clinical service was established initially with a service development grant, with a strong research ethos enabling data collection on all assessments from service inception. Despite minimal research resources and a commanding period of clinical expansion in the years following, a strong research culture continued; data collection remained unchanged, with the exception of adding or changing measures. The significant milestones in progressing the registry research agenda were the funding of part-time researchers through project grants in 2008- and 2010–2011 respectively, which enabled electronic input of hard copy data and introduction of a follow-up assessment clinic (2011-) in collecting 6-, 12-, and 24-month data. Currently, 65 participants (7.2%) have attended the 6 month follow-up clinic, whilst 28 participants (3.1%) have attended the 12 month follow-up clinic. The 24 month follow-up clinic will begin in 2013. During the period of funding expansion a permanent part-time research position was developed and recent grant acquisitions have secured ongoing research capacity. This has led to the completion of electronic data input, data cleaning, a research strategic plan, and capacity for research support to local universities. Historical inpatient records that date back to the beginning of the registry have also been acquired for the HOPE Project.

All data were collected prospectively on standardised research forms; thus none of the data were collected retrospectively (i.e., through chart reviews). From inception, data have been collected through two means, through standardised clinical and research instruments completed by the clinician, parents, child, and/or teacher. The second means is via research coding boxes (developed by clinical researchers) that appear on standard clinical forms completed during routine assessment. Hence, data for the cohort are prospective and standardised; the exceptions are the diagnostic, amenorrhoea, and EDE dissatisfaction variables that underwent cleaning (described later) and the body mass index (BMI) z score which underwent updating (described later), although based entirely on prospectively collected source data.

Procedure

Data were abstracted from a clinical audit database based on the data collection process described and from research forms stored in the medical and psychological records where data were found to be missing during audit. All intake data originated from routine intake assessment (see Figure 1) spanning two consecutive half-days. Sociodemographic and psychosocial characteristics were abstracted from the psychosocial interview record form and psychometric assessments, which measure issues related to the presentation (i.e., comorbid psychopathology) plus broader areas such as parental stress and family functioning. Clinical characteristics at intake and lifetime clinical characteristics (i.e., duration of illness, previous eating disorder treatment, current suicidal ideation) were abstracted from the record forms of the

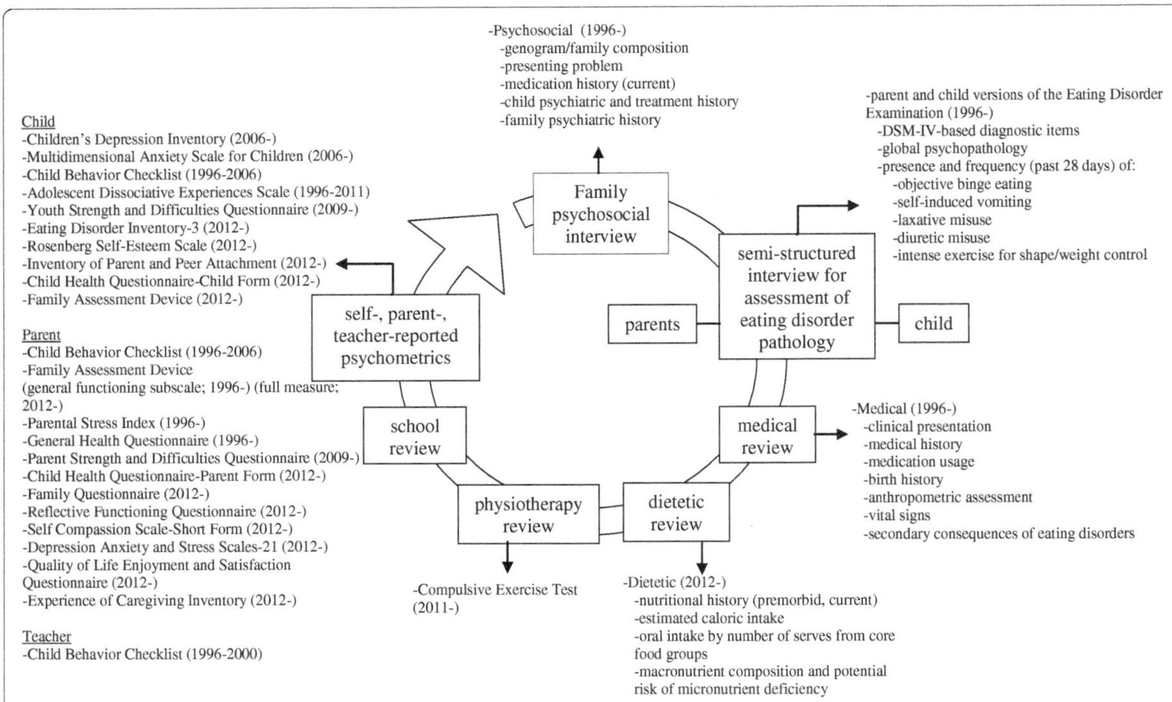

Figure 1 Routine intake assessment within the eating disorder service.

psychosocial interview, medical review, and the separate child and parent versions of the clinician-administered Eating Disorder Examination interviews [23], and psychometric instruments. Medical variables were abstracted from the medical review record form. Six and 12-month follow-up data has likewise been extracted from routine follow-up assessment, with 24-month data upcoming. All variables were inputted by research staff, trained students, or research assistants.

Eating disorder diagnostic status was established with two respective nomenclatures, the fourth edition of the Diagnostic and Statistical Manual (DSM-IV) [24] and the tenth revision of the International Classification of Diseases (ICD-10) [25]. Diagnostic status with respect to an eating disorder was originally inputted into the registry database based on the DSM-IV diagnosis assigned by the clinical team at a multidisciplinary assessment meeting, which is recorded for each patient on his/her psychosocial interview form along with other summary data, clinical formulation, and treatment plan. However, during audit where error and bias were noted, diagnoses for each case were re-assigned retrospectively (discussed later).

Quality assurance

To reduce bias in clinical diagnosis and account for changes in diagnostic criteria and systems over time, the diagnoses of all individuals in the HOPE Project registry were reviewed in 2012. To this end, the standardised medical questionnaire and child Eating Disorder Examination (EDE) [23] form, both administered at intake, were reviewed, and a research diagnosis was assigned. A hierarchical diagnostic scheme was applied whereby individuals were evaluated for AN, BN, and EDNOS/atypical eating disorders. Pertinent barriers to reliable archival diagnostic abstraction for the entire registry from clinical team assessment, and that led to the decision to re-assign intake diagnosis were: diagnostic status at intake was absent for some cases (sometimes clinicians confirmed diagnosis in the first three months as more information became available), ICD and DSM were interchangeably reported, and occasional errors in diagnostic records were apparent, for instance, a child who approximated but did not meet threshold diagnostic criteria for AN or BN may have been ascribed one of these diagnoses; while clinically some degree of flexibility is appropriate this does not satisfy the methodological rigour necessary for research.

Some systematic errors in measurement were identified and specific correction remedies followed. Amenorrhoea was extracted from the medical questionnaire but oral contraceptive (OC) use was not recorded on the medical research form. An audit of child and parent EDE records, which included an item pertaining to OC use, enabled restriction of amenorrhoea coding to the subpopulation of female patients without OC pill use. Some clinician coding errors became apparent during data entry of the EDEs, identifiable because detailed note-taking on the EDE record form by the administering clinician is positioned alongside the research coding boxes. Occasionally, administering clinicians counted intense exercise episodes/duration that was for reasons other than weight and shape control (i.e., social) within the scoring of the exercise variables. When rating dissatisfaction with shape and body weight, sometimes patients endorsed dissatisfaction in a healthy direction (i.e., dissatisfied "because I am still too bony and want to look healthier"), which instead of leading to a high score should be scored zero by the administering clinician. These issues prompted an audit of all child and parent EDEs by research assistants, and recoding of scores where necessary. We audited male records carefully during this process, checking that dissatisfaction items were scored in the appropriate direction, with discussions with a senior clinical staff member (J. M.) to establish consensus where necessary. All staff receive training on the EDE, prior to administration and we have also carried out sessions with staff on EDE scoring, and individualised staff feedback via an audit of EDE measure completion. Lastly, only one investigator (K. H.) familiar with these issues is permitted to enter EDE data.

To recover missing information, we exhaustively audited all patient files, searched all storage spaces, and searched for archived data on the hospital's electronic records management services.

The Centers for Disease Control and Prevention revised and updated their growth charts in 2000, thus all BMI *z* scores were later audited and updated.

Measures

The HOPE Project has involved the administration of several well-recognised psychometric instruments and other study-specific standardised research record forms over time (see Figure 1 for measures and time periods of data collection). For brevity, below we report on the psychometric instruments and measures that contributed data to the present report. Further general information about study-specific measures is deferred to Figure 1.

Sociodemographics

Sociodemographic data, including sex, age, rural residence, and parents at residence, were recorded by a clinician during the psychosocial intake interview with parents and child.

Eating disorder examination

Eating disorder symptoms were assessed via clinician-administered structured interviews; the child and parent-informant versions of the EDE [23], respectively. The EDE was originally designed for adults and is widely considered the gold standard for assessing eating disorder pathology and assisting to yield diagnosis. The EDE provides a global rating of eating disorder psychopathology and frequencies of disordered eating behaviours, including objective binge eating, self-induced vomiting, excessive exercise for shape and weight control, and laxative and diuretic misuse, over the previous 28 days. Cognitive symptoms, such as fear of weight gain, are measured by subscale items.

Percent expected BMI and BMI z score

Children were weighed wearing underwear and a hospital gown, using electronic scales accurate to 50 gm. Height was measured with the patient barefoot standing on a hard surface and using a Hardpenden stadiometer, accurate to 1 mm. Percent expected body mass index (BMI kg/m^2) based on Centers for Disease Control 2000 growth charts demarcated children with a BMI < 85% of expected. BMI *z*-scores were calculated via Epi Info 7 [26] by entering the patient's age, height, and weight into the program.

Depression, anxiety, and suicidal ideation

Depression symptoms were assessed with the Children's Depression Inventory (CDI; clinical cut-off: *T*-score ≥ 65) [27] and anxiety symptoms with the Multidimensional Anxiety Scale for Children (MASC; clinical cut-off: *T*-score ≥ 65) [28]. Current suicidal ideation was recorded if the child endorsed at least one of the two responses on item 9 on the CDI (i.e., "I think about killing myself but I would not do it", "I want to kill myself").

Other clinical information

Family history of an eating disorder was assessed during the psychosocial interview by asking parents whether a relative has had a past or current eating disorder. The response (yes/no) and type of disorder, if affirmative, were recorded by the clinician. This method is unvalidated and has unestablished reliability and validity. Duration of illness was recorded on the medical questionnaire by the physician at medical review and was obtained through discussion with the parents and child present. The physician recorded maximum previous weight to determine history of weight loss. Amenorrhoea was defined in accordance with DSM-IV anorexia nervosa criteria and was coded based on the physician's classification of the individual as amenorrhoeic, though later cleaned to exclude cases taking the OC pill (described earlier).

Results and discussion

At the time of this report, the HOPE Project registry database contains 941 youth referred and assessed. Of the 941, 685 met criteria for a DSM-IV eating disorder,

168 did not, and for 88, eating disorder status was unable to be determined due to missing height/weight data ($n = 3$) or child EDE interview records ($n = 85$). Only one critical item needed to be missing to render the case unsuitable for confirmation of research diagnosis.

The profile of the cohort is shown in Table 1. Most patients were female, adolescent, and had a diagnosable eating disorder. According to medical records and clinical observation, the cases without formal eating disorder diagnosis ($n = 168$) commonly had unusual food habits, related to other psychiatric diagnoses such as obsessive-compulsive disorder, other anxiety disorders, depression, problems such as picky or selective eating, or physical problems such as chronic fatigue syndrome, irritable bowel syndrome, Crohn's disease, celiac disease, or, in rare cases, a brain tumour. Ego-syntonicity and lack of endorsement of cognitive symptoms led to some not meeting diagnostic criteria, with ongoing engagement with PMH EDP suggesting eventual clinical diagnosis. Other assessed children were symptomatic (i.e., severe body image concerns) but missed the diagnostic thresholds; according to clinical literature [29] these children may have been prodromal, subclinical, at outer limits of normal parameters, or syndromal but casualties of the limitations of the DSM-IV taxonomic system especially as it applies to children. We plan to investigate these diagnostic issues further outside of this report.

The profile of the subset of the cohort with eating disorders is shown in Table 2. Most patients in the HOPE Project registry met the criteria for EDNOS. On average, patients presented at approximately 14 years of age with

Table 1 Sociodemographic characteristics of the entire cohort (*N* = 941) and eating disorder status

	N	Entire cohort
Sex (female)	941	852 (90.5%)
Age, *M* ± *SD* [range]	941	14.34 ± 2.02 [4.25,17.92]
<12 yrs		111 (11.8%)
12-14 yrs		207 (22.0%)
14- 16 yrs		455 (48.4%)
>16 yrs		168 (17.9%)
Rural residence	915	152 (16.6%)
Parents at residence	822	
Biological parents		531 (64.6%)
Mother and stepfather		149 (18.1%)
Single mother		112 (13.6%)
Other		30 (3.6%)
Eating disorder status	941	
No eating disorder		256 (27.2%)
DSM-IV eating disorder		685 (72.8%)

Estimates are *n* (%) unless otherwise indicated. *N* column is total number with valid (i.e., non-missing) data.

a recent history of weight loss. Intense exercise (45%), self-induced vomiting (28%), and objective binge eating (19%) were commonly reported disordered eating behaviours. Similar to observations in other paediatric studies [16], laxative and diuretic misuse among children and younger adolescents is rare, perhaps because these are harder to access for this age group and require financial resources. Also prevalence may be higher than self-report, with one previous study among adolescents with AN at our service finding that prevalence of laxative use increased almost two-fold relative to self-report when positive screens from biochemical tests were counted [30].

Although psychiatric comorbidities are not formally diagnosed in the HOPE Project sample, symptoms of depression and anxiety were judged on dimensional rating scales and found to be common, particularly depressive symptoms and current suicidal ideation. Comorbidity of mood and anxiety symptoms is well-established in adults with eating disorders [31] and there is recognition of these relationships among young people too, particularly depression [16,32].

The geographic spread of referrals was evident, with 17% (1 in 6) referred from rural Western Australia (up to four days drive away from PMH EDP). Rural-based referrals may be underrepresented at admission; compared to Western Australia population estimates, 27% of persons aged 5–19 years reside in rural Western Australia [33]. Alternatively in the absence of national or state epidemiological data, there may be an unknown difference in prevalence rates in rural and metropolitan Australia.

General comparability of the HOPE Project sample is evident with the UoC ($N = 401$) [18] and Stanford ($N = 1432$) [15] observational study samples. All contain children and adolescents consecutively referred to a specialist eating disorder program, Stanford and HOPE Project participants were drawn from outpatient to inpatient care, and UoC from outpatient. Like the other samples, ours contains mainly females (HOPE 94%; Stanford 91%; UoC 90%) in mid-adolescence (HOPE $M = 14$ years, UoC $M = 15$ years, Stanford $M = 15$ years), with predominantly EDNOS (HOPE 68%; UoC 60%; Stanford 63%) and an approximate one year duration of illness (HOPE median = 8 months; Stanford $M = 15$ months; UoC not reported). Difficulty lies in comparing the HOPE profile to other paediatric eating disorder samples in the scientific literature, for many well-characterised groups have been randomised controlled trial (RCT) samples or based on small retrospective studies that restrict diagnosis to certain eating disorders (i.e., [34]). There may be some systematic differences between RCT and clinic treatment seeking-youth samples [35]. A strength of the HOPE Project is that sampling is naturalistic and ecologically representative of a tertiary setting. Selection

Table 2 Sociodemographic, clinical, and medical characteristics of the eating disorder subset of the cohort ($n = 685$)

	N	Eating disorder clinic cohort ($N = 685$)
Sociodemographic characteristics, total sample		
Sex (female), *n* (%)	685	641 (93.6%)
Age, $M \pm SD$ [range]	685	14.7 ± 1.6 [8.7,17.9]
<12 yrs		45 (6.6%)
12-14 yrs		146 (21.3%)
14-16 yrs		374 (54.6%)
>16 yrs		120 (17.5%)
Rural residence, *n* (%)	663	115 (17.3%)
Family history, total sample		
Eating disorder history, *n* (%)	572	151 (26.4%)
Physical features, total sample		
BMI *z* score, $M \pm SD$ [range]	636	−1.41 ± 1.48 [−8.17,2.13]
Weight loss[1], *n* (%)	538	514 (95.5%)
< 85% of expected height/weight, *n* (%)	577	355 (61.5%)
Amenorrhoea, *n* (%)	659	280 (42.5%)
Primary		30 (4.6%)
Secondary		250 (37.9%)
Comorbid psychopathology, total sample		
CDI *T*-score ≥ 65, *n* (%)	262	127 (48.5%)
MASC *T*-score ≥ 65, *n* (%)	264	89 (33.7%)
Current suicidal ideation, *n* (%)	271	114 (42.1%)
Current self-harm, *n* (%)	493	134 (27.2%)
Eating disorder features, total sample		
Duration of illness (months), median ± IQR [range]	635	8 ± 5–12 [1,120]
Diagnosis, *n* (%)	685	
Anorexia nervosa		172 (25.2%)
Restricting		141 (20.6%)
Binge/purge		31 (4.5%)
Bulimia nervosa		48 (7.0%)
Purging		45 (6.6%)
Non-purging		3 (0.4%)
Eating disorders not otherwise specified		465 (67.9%)
Child version: EDE global, $M \pm SD$ [range]	675	3.07 ± 1.57 [0.0,5.95]
Parent version: EDE global, $M \pm SD$ [range]	598	2.94 ± 1.29 [0.0,6.93]
Objective binge eating, *n* (%)	685	129 (18.8%)
Purging, *n* (%)	685	237 (34.6%)
Self-induced vomiting, *n* (%)	685	195 (28.5%)
Laxative misuse, *n* (%)	685	49 (7.2%)
Diuretic misuse, *n* (%)	685	5 (0.7%)
Intense exercise to control shape/weight, *n* (%)	685	307 (44.8%)
Fear of weight gain (≥ 4 on EDE item), *n* (%)	673	479 (71.2%)
Eating disorder features, those with behaviour present		
Objective binge eating, median ± IQR [range]	129	10 ± 3–19 [1,168]
Purging	237	20.00 ± 5–33.5 [1,308]

Table 2 Sociodemographic, clinical, and medical characteristics of the eating disorder subset of the cohort ($n = 685$) *(Continued)*

Self-induced vomiting, *M* ± *SD* [range]	195	27.17 ± 32.07 [1,224]
Laxative misuse, *M* ± *SD* [range]	49	22.29 ± 47.13 [1,280]
Diuretic misuse, *M* ± *SD* [range]	5	50.40 ± 23.43 [28,84]

Discrepancies in available *N* on the CDI and MASC reflect the later introduction of these measures. Values are *n* (%) unless otherwise indicated. Median and IQR are presented for skewed variables. *BMI* body mass index, *CDI* Children's Depression Inventory, *EDE* Eating Disorder Examination, *MASC* Multidimensional Anxiety Scale for Children. [1]Lower weight at intake than parent- or self-reported maximum ever weight.

bias is likely low, given the sequential recruitment method, lack of exclusion criteria, variety of service referral methods, and large catchment area. The service is the only specialist public (free-of-charge) paediatric eating disorder service in Western Australia (which has a total population of 2.45 million) [36] and the primary port of tertiary referral for health professionals and other members of the community. The very high inclusion rate negates selection bias, though biases may become apparent in future studies when missing data patterns are evaluated.

The cohort would be expected to be dynamic over time, reflecting changing trends in epidemiology and state health system capacity, which will be explored in subsequent HOPE studies. During the lifespan of the HOPE Project, there has been some evidence that the prevalence of eating disorders has continued to increase [37] while the age of onset of eating disorders has decreased [1], and greater recognition of eating disorders and burden and severity [8]. Whether these trends hold true is impossible to know, accurate descriptions of epidemiology across nations and including EDNOS has only just recently been described and replication is necessary. The authors have observed that the phenomenology of eating disorders has followed the trends of eating and body concerns in society in general, for example with increasing emphasis on exercise and health, and changes in cognitive content from sugar, towards fat and more recently carbohydrates. Over the last two decades, anecdotally referrals to PMH EDP have increased with no equivalent growth in assessment numbers and greater diversion of cases to community settings, which may mean cohort patients in the latter years are a more physically or psychiatrically unwell group than for the early days of the program.

Looking forward, it is envisioned that the HOPE Project registry will produce valuable knowledge in specific areas of paediatric eating disorders, such as diagnosis and assessment, epidemiology, risk and etiological candidates, medical issues, and patient and family needs, and generate implications for policy, practice, and research. As well as enabling comparisons with findings from other cohorts, we anticipate that the large number of variables contained in the HOPE Project will significantly enable expansion of knowledge into new territories. A scoping project undertaken under the oversight of the HOPE Project steering committee has identified research priorities and possibilities for the next five years. Selection of projects follows a governance strategy that places precedence on clinically- and/or policy-relevant projects.

Three HOPE studies are underway. The first, examines parent–child concordance on the EDE, to highlight gaps and issues in parent and child reporting, which we expect to assist assessment procedures. The second, compares children and adolescents with eating disorders on cognitive, behavioural, diagnostic, and medical presentation and aims to inform health care professionals about developmental issues. The third study investigates rural health inequalities, and whether rurality translates to a more compromised clinical and medical status at presentation, and greater inpatient service use.

Several projects are in the planning phase. In the eating disorders field, there has been debate over the applicability of diagnostic systems to younger populations [38]. We plan to compare DSM-IV, proposed DSM-5 (which has also been coded in our registry), and ICD-10 diagnostic systems, to examine concordance and whether the preponderance of EDNOS diagnoses is reduced with the DSM revisions. We will also examine those who do not meet formal diagnostic criteria for an eating disorder at admission but go on to have subsequent treatment. Gender differences will be explored taking into account physical, psychological and diagnostic factors, with potentially one of the larger samples of young clinical males available, to investigate similarities and differences from females. Finally, efforts to describe and characterise patients on clinical features, such as severity dimensions or symptom clusters would assist the field to characterise the heterogeneity within eating disorder diagnoses. The cohort database may be utilised to explore, test or replicate taxonomic models of eating disorders such as the functional staging model of anorexia nervosa [39] due to its broad array of medical, behavioural, and psychological variables.

The HOPE Project is embedded within a five-year research strategic plan for the PMH EDP, which goes wider than traditional research outputs and focuses on building a dynamic, collaborative, and sustainable research team culture. Areas of emphasis include: the development of research capacity, data management infrastructure and processes, scholarly output, and partnerships, collaboration and leadership. Promoting knowledge-practice transfer both within and beyond the PMH EDP, including with consumer and carer groups, is a key goal. Other important outcomes include developing researchers and clinicians with dual expertise and commitment, increasing levels of staff participation, confidence and capacity, and developing internal mechanisms and structures for up-to-date dissemination and integration of scientific knowledge. Challenges to collaboration between clinical and research agendas include clinical pressures and a lack of confidence by clinicians in their research capabilities. Current strategies include whole-of-team research meetings that give visibility to research issues and enable sharing of knowledge and skills, joint project teams that partner researchers and clinicians, and the allocation of research time for clinicians. We have found that an agenda that balances clinical and research issues is helpful as well as prioritisation of research projects with high clinical utility and ensuring research protocols have obvious clinical relevance. We believe research questions and interpretation of findings becomes richer and more relevant when embedded in a clinical context, and whilst researchers and clinicians contribute differently to the research process, ultimately with time and mutual exchange of knowledge and skills, we anticipate the products of this collaboration will be synergistic. In the future, we plan to develop mechanisms for consumer participation in the HOPE Project that go beyond contributing personal data, and include consumers and carers in research processes such as determining study prioritisation, design, and discussion of implications.

Already we have learnt many lessons in undertaking registry research in a clinical setting, and some constant challenges remain including sourcing financial support for the ongoing registry when funders typically prefer time-limited and specific projects, and securing dedicated research roles and resources. Obtaining adequate financial support for the HOPE Project and/or follow-up protocols has so far remained elusive; however attaining distinct project funding has proved more achievable. Embedding larger data collection goals relevant to the HOPE Project within discrete projects has enabled the progression of the project, alongside the creation of dedicated research positions, creative use of student volunteers, and an arrangement with the local universities that students contribute time to data entry and cleaning in exchange for use of registry data.

Managing the potential for measurement bias (i.e., inaccuracies in data recording, missing data) is an ongoing challenge, attributed to staff flux (changeover, practicum students) and varying levels of awareness of the importance and uses of the data, and inadequate research resourcing to maintain data collation and entry activity. Using cohort data is essential in promoting the value of the database [40], and this alongside routine focus on data integrity will ensure longevity of the registry. Preventative action we have found helpful includes dedicated research roles, regular training and supervision, auditing of records and measures with confidential individualised feedback to clinicians, integration of quality and research goals, less rotation of assessment staff, and encouragement of good record-keeping skills. Quality assurance is an ongoing issue managed as part of the HOPE Project and we have found that prevention (and early intervention) is the best cure.

Resources exist for assisting eating disorder researchers to understand and avoid the pitfalls associated with controlled trials [41], yet fewer resources were identified to support ongoing observational research. HREC grant processes may need revision to ensure registry studies are not evaluated through the same lens as controlled treatment trials. There is a growing movement within epidemiology to educate HRECs about issues specific to observational studies (i.e., problem of selection bias), so that standards historically designed and applied for controlled trials (i.e., opt-in consent rather than opt-out consent) can be reconsidered in observational designs to achieve balance on research for the good of the public and the individual's right to privacy [42,43].

Conclusions

This paper has described and debuted the HOPE Project, an ongoing clinical registry of children and adolescents referred for eating disorder assessment at a specialist hospital-based program over a 17-year period. We believe the HOPE Project will offer a unique and ongoing opportunity to cultivate scientific knowledge about paediatric eating disorders. The trials and tribulations of establishing a research registry within an evolving clinical service have been described, and we have outlined that although challenging, research of this nature, in situ in a clinical setting, is both possible and extremely valuable. The potential for illuminating the nature of paediatric eating disorders, as they appear and evolve in an archetypal public health service, is immense. It is our aspiration that ultimately the knowledge generated from the HOPE Project will inform prevention, early intervention, assessment and treatment practices in real world clinical and policy environments.

Abbreviations

AN: Anorexia nervosa; BMI: Body mass index; BN: Bulimia nervosa; DSM: Diagnostic and Statistical Manual; EDE: Eating Disorder Examination; EDNOS: Eating disorders not otherwise specified; HOPE: Helping to Outline Paediatric Eating Disorders; ICD: International Classification of Diseases; PMH EDP: Princess Margaret Hospital for Children Eating Disorders Program.

Competing interests

The authors declare that they have no competing interests.

Authors' contributions

JM, JP, and DF enabled standardised data collection from the outset of PMH EDP inception. JM, JP, DF and HW conceived the cohort study. HW acquired ethical approval, established the cohort registry database, prepared the manuscript, and conducted data analysis. KH assists to manage the registry database and project and conducted data analysis. JM has managed the project since it was conceived, acquired research resourcing, conducted regular assessment training with staff, and prepared the manuscript. All authors reviewed and approved the final version of the manuscript.

Authors' information

HJW, PhD, MPsych(Clin). Senior Research Psychologist at PMH EDP, Senior Research Scientist at Centre for Clinical Interventions, Adjunct Research Fellow at the School of Paediatrics and Child Health, The University of Western Australia, and Adjunct Lecturer at the School of Psychology and Speech Therapy, Curtin University, Perth, Australia. JM, MPsych(Clin). Specialist Clinical Psychologist at PMH EDP, Perth, Australia. KH, BSc(Hons)Psych. Research assistant at PMH EDP and PhD Candidate at the School of Psychology and Speech Pathology, Curtin University, Perth, Australia. DF, MB BS. FRACP. Paediatrician at PMH EDP and Associate Professor at the School of Paediatrics and Child Health, The University of Western Australia, Perth, Australia. JP, BSc(Nurs). Manager at PMH EDP, Perth, Australia.

Acknowledgments

Firstly, we acknowledge Chris Harris, Karen Gullick and Professor Brett McDermott, former clinical staff who contributed to the conception of research endeavours within PMH EDP and the development of standardised data collection protocols. We are grateful for the contribution of many other past and present clinical staff who recorded clinical data and thank the many volunteer research assistants who assisted with the development of the cohort registry database, including Jabrulla Shakoor, Nicole Chang, Shalane Sadri, Shane Fernandez, Matthew Hamilton, Jeremy Alman, and Colette McKenna. We express our gratitude to Link Market Services for its sponsorship of part of the publication fee, and to WA Department of Health Targeted Research Fund for supporting our project.

Funding

Princess Margaret Hospital for Children Foundation. State Health Research and Advisory Council. Telethon Institute for Child Health Research.

Author details

[1]Eating Disorders Program, Princess Margaret Hospital for Children, Perth, Australia. [2]Centre for Clinical Interventions, Perth, Australia. [3]School of Paediatrics and Child Health, The University of Western Australia, Perth, Australia. [4]School of Psychology and Speech Pathology, Curtin University, Perth, Australia.

References

1. Swanson SA, Crow SJ, Le Grange D, Swendsen J, Merikangas KR: **Prevalence and correlates of eating disorders in adolescents. Results from the national comorbidity survey replication adolescent supplement.** *Arch Gen Psychiatry* 2011, **68:**714–723.
2. Eddy KT, Doyle AC, Hoste RR, Herzog D, le Grange D: **Eating disorder not otherwise specified in adolescents.** *J Am Acad Child Adolesc Psychiatry* 2008, **47:**156–164.
3. Madden S, Morris A, Zurynski YA, Kohn M, Elliot EJ: **Burden of eating disorders in 5-13-year-old children in Australia.** *Med J Aust* 2009, **190:**410–414.
4. Arcelus J, Mitchell AJ, Wales J, Nielsen S: **Mortality rates in patients with anorexia nervosa and other eating disorders. A meta-analysis of 36 studies.** *Arch Gen Psychiatry* 2011, **68:**724–731.
5. Birmingham CL, Treasure J: *Medical management of eating disorders.* 2nd edition. Cambridge: Cambridge University Press; 2010.
6. Katzman DK, Kanbur NO, Steinegger CM: **Medical screening and management of eating disorders in adolescents.** In *The Oxford Handbook of Eating Disorders.* Edited by Agras WS. New York: Oxford University Press; 2010:267–291.
7. The Butterfly Foundation/Deloitte Access Economics: *Paying the price: The economic and social impact of eating disorders in Australia.* Sydney: The Butterfly Foundation; 2012.
8. Treasure J, Smith G, Crane A: *Skills-based learning for caring for a loved one with an eating disorder: The New Maudsley Method.* London: Routledge; 2007.
9. Mond JM: **Eating disorders as "brain-based mental illnesses": an antidote to stigma?** *J Ment Health* 2013, **22:**1–3.
10. Klump KL, Bulik CM, Kaye WH, Treasure J, Tyson E: **Academy for eating disorders position paper: eating disorders are serious mental illnesses.** *Int J Eat Disord* 2009, **42:**97–103.
11. Vitiello B, Lederhendler I: **Research on eating disorders: current status and future prospects.** *Biol Psychiatry* 2000, **47:**777–786.
12. Berkman N, Bulik C, Brownley K, Lohr K, Sedway J, Rooks A, Gartlehner G: **Management of Eating Disorders. Evidence Report/Technology Assessment No. 135.** In *Management of Eating Disorders.* Rockville, MD: AHRQ Publication No. 06-E010; 2006. Prepared by the RTI International-University of North Carolina Evidence-Based Practice Center under Contract No. 290-02-0016.
13. Berkman ND, Lohr KN, Bulik CM: **Outcomes of eating disorders: a systematic review of the literature.** *Int J Eat Disord* 2007, **40:**293–309.
14. Steinhausen HC, Boyadjieva S, Griogoroiu-Serbanescu M, Neumarker KJ: **The outcome of adolescent eating disorders: findings from an international collaborative study.** *Eur Child Adolesc Psychiatry* 2003, **12**(Suppl 1):I91–I98.
15. Peebles R, Wilson JL, Lock JD: **Self-injury in adolescents with eating disorders: correlates and provider bias.** *J Adolesc Health* 2011, **48:**310–313.
16. Peebles R, Wilson J, Lock J: **How do children with eating disorders differ from adolescents with eating disorders at initial evaluation?** *J Adolesc Health* 2006, **39:**800–805.
17. Peebles R, Hardy KK, Wilson JL, Lock JD: **Are diagnostic criteria for eating disorders markers of medical severity?** *Pediatrics* 2010, **125:**e1193–e1201.
18. Eddy KT, Le Grange D, Crosby RD, Hoste RR, Doyle AC, Smyth A, Herzog DB: **Diagnostic classification of eating disorders in children and adolescents: how does DSM-IV-TR compare to empirically-derived categories?** *J Am Acad Child Adolesc Psychiatry* 2010, **49:**277–287. quiz 293.
19. Berg KC, Swanson SA, Stiles-Shields EC, Eddy KT, Peterson CB, Grange DL: **Response patterns on interview and questionnaire versions of the eating disorder examination and their impact on latent structure analyses.** *Compr Psychiatry* 2013.
20. Williams RJ, Tse T, Harlan WR, Zarin DA: **Registration of observational studies: is it time?** *CMAJ* 2010, **182:**1638–1642.
21. Mann CJ: **Observational research methods. Research design II: cohort, cross sectional, and case-control studies.** *Emerg Med J* 2003, **20:**54–60.
22. Parker MA, Sneddon AE, Arbon P: **The menstrual disorder of teenagers (MDOT) study: determining typical menstrual patterns and menstrual disturbance in a large population-based study of Australian teenagers.** *BJOG* 2010, **117:**185–192.
23. Fairburn C, Cooper Z: **The Eating Disorder Examination (12th Edition).** In *Binge-eating: Nature, assessment and treatment.* Edited by Fairburn C, Wilson G. New York: Guilford Press; 1993:317–360.
24. American Psychiatric Association: *Diagnostic and statistical manual of mental disorders.* 4th edition. Washington, DC: American Psychiatric Association; 2000.
25. World Health Organization: *International Classification of Diseases. 10th revised edn.* Geneva: World Health Organization; 1992.
26. Centers for Disease Control and Prevention: *Epi Info 7 (Version 7.1.0.6) [Computer Program].* 2012.
27. Kovacs M: **The Children's Depression Inventory (CDI).** *Psychopharmacol Bull* 1985, **21:**995–998.
28. March JS: *MASC - Multidimensional Anxiety Scale for Children: Technical manual.* Toronto: Multi-Health Systems Inc; 1997.
29. le Grange D, Loeb K: **Early identification and treatment of eating disorders: prodrome to syndrome.** *Early Interv Psychiatry* 2007, **1:**27–39.
30. Turner J, Batik M, Palmer LJ, Forbes D, McDermott BM: **Detection and importance of laxative use in adolescents with anorexia nervosa.** *J Am Acad Child Adolesc Psychiatry* 2000, **39:**378–385.
31. Bulik CM: **Anxiety and depression in eating disorders.** In *Eating Disorders and Obesity: A Comprehensive Handbook. Volume 2.* Edited by Brownell K. New York: Guilford Press; 2001:193–198.
32. McDermott B, Forbes D, Harris C, McCormack J, Gibbon P: **Non-eating disorders psychopathology in children and adolescents with eating disorders: implications for malnutrition and symptom severity.** *J Psychosom Res* 2006, **60:**257–261.
33. Australian Bureau of Statistics: *Population by age and sex, regions of Australia: Past and future releases.* 2012 [cited 2013 3rd April].

34. Fosson A, Knibbs J, Bryant-Waugh B, Lask B: **Early onset anorexia nervosa.** *Arch Dis Child* 1987, **62:**114–118.
35. Stiles-Shields C, Goldschmidt AB, Lock J, Le Grange D: **Are adolescent treatment studies of eating disorders utilizing clinically relevant samples? A comparison of RCT and clinic treatment-seeking youth with eating disorders.** *Eur Eat Disord Rev.* in press.
36. Australian Bureau of Statistics: *3101.0 - Australian demographic statistics, Sep 2012.* 2013 [cited 2013 3rd April].
37. Hay PJ, Mond J, Buttner P, Darby A: **Eating disorder behaviors are increasing: findings from two sequential community surveys in South Australia.** *PLoS One* 2008, **3:**e1541.
38. Bravender T, Bryant-Waugh R, Herzog D, Katzman D, Kriepe RD, Lask B, Le Grange D, Lock J, Loeb KL, Marcus MD, *et al*: **Classification of eating disturbance in children and adolescents: Proposed changes for the DSM-V.** *Eur Eat Disord Rev* 2010, **18:**79–89.
39. Thomson S, Marriott M, Telford K, Law H, McLaughlin J, Sayal K: **Adolescents with a diagnosis of anorexia nervosa: parents' experience of recognition and deciding to seek help.** *Clin Child Psychol Psychiatry.* in press.
40. Mitchell JE, Selzer F, Kalarchian MA, Devlin MJ, Strain GW, Elder KA, Marcus MD, Wonderlich S, Christian NJ, Yanovski SZ: **Psychopathology before surgery in the longitudinal assessment of bariatric surgery-3 (LABS-3) psychosocial study.** *Surg Obes Relat Dis* 2012, **8:**533–541.
41. Lock J, Brandt H, Woodside B, Agras WS, Halmi WK, Johnson C, Kaye W, Wilfley D: **Challenges in conducting a multi-site randomized clinical trial comparing treatments for adolescent anorexia nervosa.** *Int J Eat Disord* 2012, **45:**202–213.
42. The Council for International Organizations of Medical Sciences (CIOMS): *International Ethical Guidelines for Epidemiological Studies.* Geneva: Council for International Organizations of Medical Sciences (CIOMS) in collaboration with the World Health Organization (WHO); 2008.
43. Evans SM, Bohensky M, Cameron PA, McNeil J: **A survey of Australian clinical registries: can quality of care be measured?** *Intern Med J* 2011, **41:**42–48.

Meta analysis on the efficacy of pharmacotherapy versus placebo on anorexia nervosa

Jasmijn de Vos[1*], Laura Houtzager[1,2], Georgia Katsaragaki[1], Elske van de Berg[1], Pim Cuijpers[3] and Jack Dekker[1*]

Abstract

Background: Anorexia Nervosa (AN) has a devastating impact on the psychological and physical well being of affected individuals. There is an extensive body of literature on interventions in AN, however more studies are needed to establish which form of pharmacotherapy is effective. The few meta-analyses that have been done are based on one type of medication only. This article is the first to present data on three different, most commonly used, forms of pharmacotherapy. The primary objective of this meta-analysis was to create an overview and to determine the efficacy of three forms of pharmacotherapy (antidepressants, antipsychotics, hormonal therapy) compared to treatment with placebo in patients with AN.

Method: A systematic literature search was performed to identify all randomized controlled intervention trials investigating the effectiveness of pharmacotherapy for AN within the following databases: PubMed, PsycINFO, Embase and Cochrane Library. In addition, 32 relevant reviews and meta-analyses were screened for additional intervention studies. A meta-analysis was performed on a total of 18 included studies ($N = 869$). Efficacy was measured in terms of weight gain or weight restoration.

Results: The pooled effect sizes indicating the difference between antidepressants and placebo, and between antipsychotics and placebo on weight were not significant. Because of the small sample size no meta regression and subgroup analyses could be conducted. The pooled effect size indicating the difference between hormonal therapy and the placebo condition on weight (all weight measures) at post-treatment was 0.42 (95% CI: 0.11 ~ 0.73), which was significant. For hormonal therapy heterogeneity was high ($I^2 = 64.70$). No evidence for publication bias was found. Meta-regression analyses of the weeks of medication treatment ($slope = -0.008$) yielded a significant effect ($p = 0.04$).

Conclusions: In this study we found that hormonal therapy has a significantly larger effect on weight compared to placebo in the treatment of AN. However for these analyses heterogeneity was high, which means that these results have to be regarded with caution. We found that anti-depressants and antipsychotics had no significant effect on weight compared to placebo in the treatment of AN, although the power to detect significant effects was too low.

Keywords: Pharmacotherapy, Placebo, Treatment, Anorexia nervosa, Meta-analysis

* Correspondence: jasmijn.de.vos@arkin.nl; jack.dekker@arkin.nl
[1]Arkin Mental Health Institute, Klaprozenweg 111, PO Box 75848, 1070, AV, Amsterdam, the Netherlands
Full list of author information is available at the end of the article

Background

Anorexia nervosa

Anorexia Nervosa (AN) has a devastating impact on the psychological and physical wellbeing of affected individuals. The disorder is characterized by restricting intake of calories and energy which will lead to a low body weight, extreme fear of gaining weight and being preoccupied with behavior that will avoid gaining weight, and is usually accompanied by a significant disturbance in the perception of the shape and or size of a person's body. In addition, body shape and weight have an undue influence on the affected persons self-esteem and self-evaluation [1].

At least 90% of individuals with AN are female. The prevalence is 0,5% - 1,0%. The course and outcome of AN are highly variable. AN has a high comorbidity with depressive symptoms, anxiety and obsessive compulsive symptoms. For a great part the etiology remains to be discovered. However, it is clear that a combination of multiple factors, genetic, neurobiological as well as psychosocial, lead to the development of this disease [2].

Treatment goals in AN include restoration of normal body weight, treat physical complications, a normal and healthy eating pattern, improvement of body image and self-esteem. Equally important is the improvement of other co morbid psychological symptoms. Because AN is associated with other psychopathology the treatment is often long and may involve several stages and intervention types [2].

Treatment

Pharmacotherapy is often used in the treatment of AN. The fact that pharmacological interventions are established forms of treatment of several disorders that overlap with AN, has led many to conclude that pharmacotherapy may be useful in symptom reduction in AN [3]. According to Claudino et al. the rationale for pharmacological treatment of AN is based on neurobiological research into the control of appetite and food intake and on biological models of AN, on clinical observations and uncontrolled studies [4] The focus of pharmacological interventions in AN depends on the phase of illness. In the acute phase drugs are given to increase body weight and reduce AN symptoms (such as recurring thoughts about weight, caloric intake, depression, anxiety and obsessive/compulsive symptoms). In the second phase pharmacotherapy is expected to improve underlying psychopathology and prevent relapse [4,5].

Various types of medication have been studied in the treatment of AN; antidepressants, antipsychotics, nutritional supplementation and hormonal medication [3,5-7]. Agras and Robinson conclude in their review that there are no evidence-based psycho-pharmacological treatments available for either adolescent or adult patients with AN [8]. Two recent meta-analyses have reported on the effectivity of antipsychotics on anorexia nervosa [9,10]. Two other meta-analyses have been published on the efficacy of antidepressants and estrogens preparations [4,11]. In the described meta analyses different outcome measures were used, for example not only weight, but also bone health [11]. The overlapping conclusion of these articles is that more research needs to been done and they recommend the use of similar outcome measures. In this article we have set a step in that direction. This is the first study to present meta analyses on three different, most commonly used, forms of pharmacotherapy (antidepressants, antipsychotics, hormonal therapy) and report on the primary outcome measure for anorexia nervosa; weight.

Lack of evidence

Considering the abovementioned findings, the results of pharmacotherapy compared to placebo treatment are scarce. Despite a considerable number of trials performed to elucidate the efficacy of three different forms of pharmacotherapy on AN, it remains unclear how far the results can be attributed to placebo effects. This can be explained by a number of factors; many patients with AN are difficult to engage in medical treatment and are unwilling to participate in randomized controlled trials, and many of these patients are so ill that they require a multiplicity of interventions [5]. As Powers & Santana state surprisingly few studies have been undertaken for AN and more over few studies have actually evaluated medications know to cause weight gain [12].

Although there are several studies published on AN as a symptom of other diseases, for example cancer, we chose to focus on AN as an eating disorder and on randomized controlled trials with a placebo condition. There are various systematic reviews exploring pharmacotherapy for AN but as far as we know only four meta-analyses have been published on the subject; one meta-analysis by Claudino et al. [4] that examines the effectivity of antidepressants for AN, one that reports on the effects of estrogen preparations [11] and two on the efficacy on antipsychotics [9,10]. The present study adds to the available body of evidence by providing an overview of the three most commonly used medicament treatments for AN: antidepressants, antipsychotics and hormonal medication. The meta-analysis of Sim et al. [11] doesn't report on weight as a primary outcome measure, but on bone density loss. They also included cohort studies with "no medication" control groups instead of placebos. Thus, the present meta-analysis is the first one to report on the effects of hormonal medication on weight restoration. Furthermore, this meta-analysis contains an up to date search; the meta-analyses on antidepressants and estrogen preparations [4,11] performed their searches until April 2005 and march 2008 respectively. We chose to focus on pharmacotherapy versus placebo conditions only, while previous meta-analyses have also included studies comparing pharmacotherapy with treatment-as-usual [9] and studies comparing pharmacotherapy with pharmacotherapy [4,10]. Finally, subgroup analyses were performed where possible; only two previous meta-analyses have performed subgroup analyses [9,10].

Method

Search strategy

This meta-analysis is part of broader meta-analysis project on eating disorders. An extensive electronic database search for open and randomized controlled trial (RCTs) was conducted within the following databases: PubMed, PsycINFO, Embase and Cochrane Library. The search terms (both text words and MeSH terms) included a wide range of combined terms indicative of eating disorders (e.g. anorexia nervosa, bulimia nervosa, binge eating disorder, eating disturbance) and therapy (e.g. psychotherapy, nutrition therapy, counselling). The Additional file 1 "PubMed search string" contains an example of the search terms used. The complete search terms and filters used are available on request from the corresponding author. The screening process consisted of a number of steps. During all screening phases, the references were rated by three independent researchers (JdV, GK, LH). Disagreements were discussed and resolved in consensus and in cases of unresolved disagreement a senior reviewer (JD) was consulted. Studies were then either included or excluded from further analysis. The first step consisted of the application of the inclusion criteria to the 9722 abstracts and titles. Studies were selected if they (a) reported an author/ had an abstract, (b) were about treatment of eating disorders, (c) were written in English or Dutch. In the second phase the database was split into three eating disorder groups (Anorexia Nervosa, Bulimia Nervosa and Binge Eating Disorder). In the third phase we screened 32 earlier reviews and meta-analyses concerning treatment of eating disorders for additional relevant studies.

Selection of studies

The next step was to proceed with the anorexia nervosa studies. For this meta/analysis we focus on randomized controlled trials. A total of 139 potential anorexia RCTs remained for a subsequent full-text screening. The database was split into two forms of treatment, pharmacotherapy and psychotherapy. In this meta/analysis, we included studies if they were a (a) randomized controlled trial, and (b) comparing pharmacotherapy with an placebo controlled condition and reported on (c) patients with Anorexia Nervosa with an age minimum of 12 years. Outcome had to be measured in (d) terms of weight gain. Studies in the acute and maintenance phase of treatment were both included.

Meta-analysis

We conducted meta-analyses on a) antidepressants, b) antipsychotics and c) hormonal medication. Those were the most commonly used pharmacological treatments. For all three we conducted a separate meta-analysis on weight, the primary measure, comparing pharmacotherapy versus placebo.

Primary outcome measures

Most randomized controlled trials report some kind of weight measure as primary outcome measures. Only published data were used. The selection of primary outcome measures for this meta-analyses includes a range of weight related variables:

Efficacy at the end of treatment, measured in terms of weight gain or weight restoration as follows:

(a) post weight in kg: the kg of the experimental and control group at the end of treatment.
(b) post weight in BMI. This is an index for weight in relationship with height, as reported at the end of treatment for both experimental and control group.
(c) post weight in IBW. Weight measured in percentage of Ideal Body Weight.
(d) weight gain in kg and g. The difference in weight from pre-treatment to post treatment, as reported at the end of treatment.
(e) IBW gain. The difference in IBW from pre-treatment to post treatment, as reported at the end of treatment.
(f) post lean body mass. The fat free mass of the experimental and control group at the end of treatment.
(g) post % fat mass. The absolute amount of body fat of the experimental and control group at the end of treatment.

Effect sizes (Cohen's d) were computed for each of the primary studies. The post- to post-pharmacotherapy effect sizes were calculated by subtracting the average post-treatment score of the pharmacotherapy condition from the average post-treatment score of the placebo condition and dividing the result by the pooled standard deviations of both conditions Effect sizes of 0 – 0.32 are considered to be small, whereas effect sizes of 0.33 – 0.55 are moderate, and effect sizes of 0.56 – 1.2 are large [13].

To calculate the pooled mean effect size, we used the statistical (computer) program Comprehensive Meta Analysis (version 2.2.021; Biostat, Englewood, NJ, USA). Only measures explicitly describing weight at post treatment were used. When means and standard deviations were not presented, we used other statistics (e.g. t-value, p-value) to compute the effect size (n = 4). When neither the means and standard deviations nor a statistical test between the relevant scores was presented, the study was excluded because the data were not suitable for this meta-analysis.

As an indicator of homogeneity, we calculated Q-statistics. A significant Q-value rejects the null hypothesis of homogeneity. We also calculated the I^2 statistic, which is an indicator of heterogeneity in percentages. A low value of 0% indicates that there is no observed heterogeneity, higher percentages indicate increasing amounts of heterogeneity, of which the highest is a value of 75% which indicates a high amount of heterogeneity (31).

Publication bias was tested according to Duval and Tweedie's trim and fill procedure [14] using Comprehensive Meta-analysis. We ran the publication bias analyses on all primary outcome measures.

Subgroup analyses

Subgroup analyses were performed using the procedures implemented in Comprehensive Meta-analysis (version 2.2.021; Biostat, Englewood, NJ, USA). In this subgroup-analysis, studies were divided into two or more subgroups. For each subgroup the pooled mean effect size was calculated, and a test was conducted to examine whether the subgroups' effect sizes differ significantly from one another. We used the mixed effect model of subgroup-analyses, which pools studies within subgroups with the random effects model, but tests for significant differences between subgroups with the fixed effects model.

We conducted subgroup analyses for the following characteristics:

- Mono treatment (only pharmacotherapy or not)
- Setting: inpatient or outpatient or other (not reported or a combination of in-and outpatient)

The risk of bias quality assessments were based on the domains described by the Cochrane Collaboration [15]. The domains were evaluated for each study by two independent researchers. A code was given for each domain: yes (=the study reports correctly on this domain and there is no risk of bias), no (=the study reports on this domain but according to the description the domain could be biased) and unclear (=the study does not provide sufficient information to make an assessment). Disagreements were discussed and resolved in consensus and in cases of unresolved disagreement a senior reviewer (JD) was consulted. The domains that assessed the risk of bias are the following:

- Sequence generation: describes whether there was a random component in sequence generation
- Allocation concealment. describes whether assignment could be foreseen
- Blinding. Were participants and/or personal blind for the treatment condition
- Incomplete data. Did the study report on missing outcome data
- Selective outcome. Were all expected outcomes reported
- Risk of bias. Assesses total risk of bias

Meta regression analyses were performed in order to assess whether pre-treatment mean weight (kg and BMI), mean age, duration of illness (in months) and *n* weeks predicted the effect sizes. A significant positive or negative slope suggests that the variable is associated with the outcome.

Power calculation

Because we expected only a limited number of studies, we conducted a power calculation to examine how many studies would have to be included in order to have sufficient statistical power to identify relevant effects. We conducted a power calculation according to the procedures described by Borenstein and colleagues [16]. We hoped to find a sufficient number of studies to be able to identify a small effect size of 0.3. These calculations indicated that we would need to include at least 20 studies with a mean sample size of 30 (15 participants per condition), to be able to detect an effect size of $d = 0.30$ (conservatively assuming a medium level of between-study variance, $\tau 2$, a statistical power of 0.80, and a significance level, alpha, of 0.05). Alternatively, we would need 15 studies with 40 participants each to detect an effect size of $d = 0.30$, or 14 studies with 50 participants.

Results

Inclusion of studies

The search yielded 12.997 results: PubMed (3675), PsycINFO (3660), Embase.com (5382) and Cochrane Library (280). The latest search update was performed in October 2012. After the duplicates were removed, 9722 titles and abstracts remained. A flow-chart showing the progress of the study selection is provided in Figure 1. After the last screening of full-text articles the search resulted in a total of 18 studies [17-34], which compared antidepressants, antipsychotics or hormones with placebo (Table 1 shows the treatment conditions for each study).

Study characteristics

All 18 studies were randomized controlled trials, reporting on a total of 869 subjects. The control conditions included 438 subjects and the experimental conditions of 431 subjects. Table 1 presents the study characteristics of these studies.

The majority of the studies (N = 12) included adult patients, two reported on adolescents and three reported on both adults-adolescents. The number of patients in experimental conditions ranged from 7 to 55 per study.

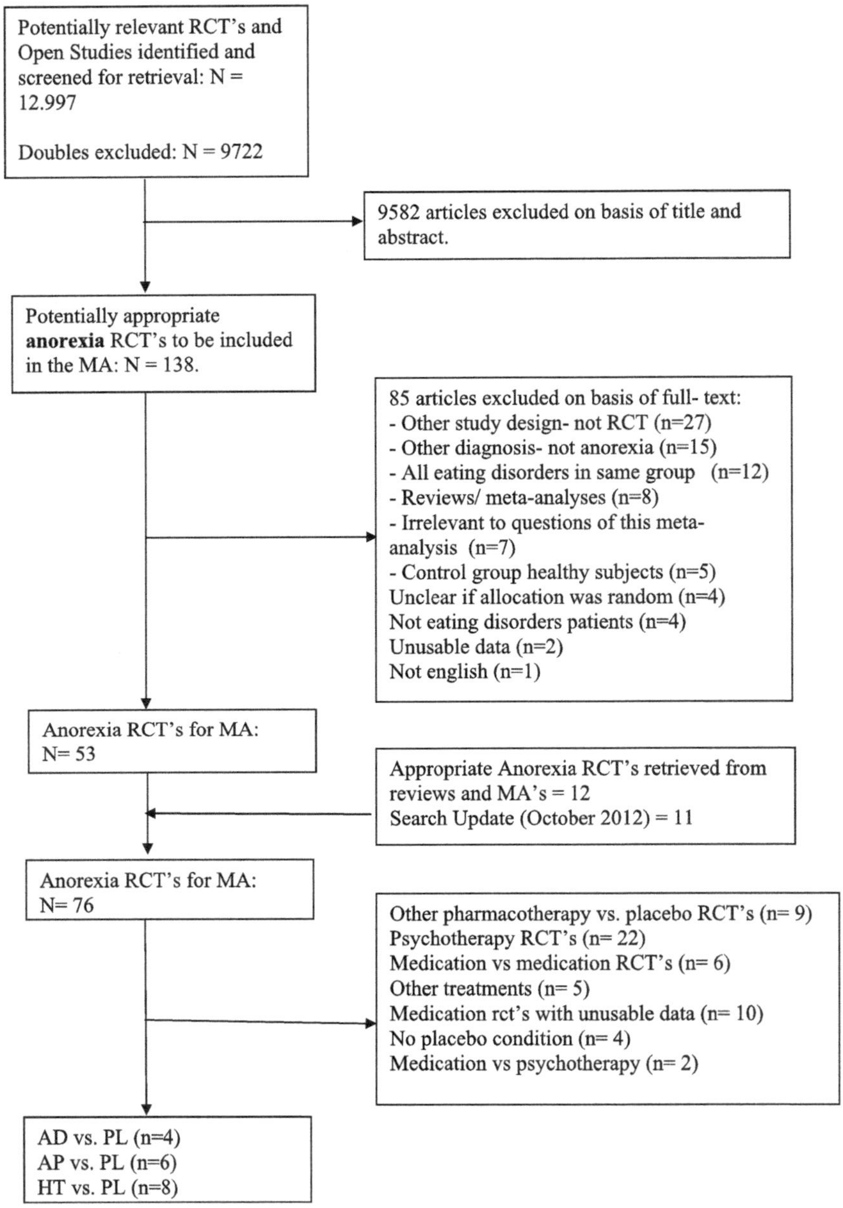

Figure 1 Flowchart of the search process.

Fourteen studies recruited participants from clinical populations. In the remaining four studies a combination of clinica l and community recruitment was used. The larger part of the studies included patients with restricted AN and the binging/purging variant (N = 16), one study reported on the restricting type only and for one study it was unknown. Mean pre-treatment weight score ranged from 14 to 18.1 (BMI). This indicates that patients were severely underweight. A normal, healthy BMI ranges from 20 to 25. Six studies reported on inpatients, ten over outpatients, one of patients in a day care program and one unknown. Only two studies had male patients.

The majority of studies reported on hormonal treatments (the comparisons were N = 10), six reported on antipsychotics and four reported on the use of antidepressants. A broad variety of adjunctive treatments were mentioned, such as individual therapy, group therapy, family therapy, behaviour therapy, caloric repletion, meal supervision, behavioural incentives and more.

Table 1 Characteristics of the included studies

1st Author, Year	Length of RCT	Recruitment	Anorexia type	Treatment conditions	Baseline mean weight[a]	N	Mean age	Type and dosage[b]	Setting	Adjunctive treatment	Weight outcome measures	Drop-out
Attia, 1998 [17]	7 weeks	Clinical	Restricting/ Binge-purge	1. AD 2. Placebo	73 (IBW) 72 (IBW)	15 16	26	Fluoxetine 60 mg	Inpatient	1. Individual therapy 2. Group therapy 3. Family therapy 4. Behavior therapy 5. Caloric repletion	1.% IBW 2. Change in % IBW/day	27% 25%
Attia, 2011 [18]	8 weeks	Clinical	Restricting/ Binge-purge	1. AP 2. Placebo	16.7 17.4	11 12 (1 male)	27.7	Olanzapine 2.5 mg 5 mg 10 mg	Outpatient		1. BMI	26% 25%
Bissada, 2008 [19]	10 weeks	Clinical	Restricting/ Binge-purge	1. AP 2. Placebo	16.39 15.93	18 16	29.7 23.6	Olanzapine 2.5 mg 5 mg 7.5 mg 10 mg	Day hospital	1. Meal supervision 2. Group therapy	1. BMI	14% 28%
Brambilla 2007a [20]	3 months	Clinical	Unknown	1. AP 2. Placebo	15.5 15.8	15 15	23.7 26.3	Olanzapine 2.5 mg 5 mg	Outpatient	1. CBT	1. BMI	14%
Brambilla 2007b [21]	3 months	Clinical	Restricting/ Binge-purge	1. AP 2. Placebo	15.7 16.3	10 10	23	Olanzapine 2.5 mg 5 mg	Outpatient	1. CBT 2. Nutritional rehabilitation	1. BMI	n.m.
Di Vasta 2012 [22]	18 months	Clinical	Restricting/ Binge-purge	1. H 2. Placebo	18.1	47 47	18.1	Dehydroepiandrosterone 50 mg	Outpatient	1. Routine care = medical, nutritional, psychological monitoring	1. Kg 2. BMI 3. Lean mass 4. Fat mass	34% 38%

1st Author, Year	Length of RCT	Recruitment	Anorexia type	Treatment conditions	Baseline mean weight[a]	N	Age	Type	Setting	Adjunctive treatments	Weight outcome measures	Drop-out
Fazeli 2010 [23]	12 weeks	Community and clinical	Restricting/ Binge-purge	1. GH 2. Placebo	17.4 17.2	10 11	28 29.2	Nutropin 15 mg	Outpatient		1. Kg ch. 2.%IBW ch. 3.% lean ch. 4. Lean ch. 5. Extremity lean ch.	10% 18%

Table 1 Characteristics of the included studies *(Continued)*

											6.% fat ch.	
											7. Fat mass ch.	
											8. Trunk fat ch.	
											9. Extremity fat ch.	
Grinspoon 1996 [24]	9 months	Clinical	Restricting/ Binge-purge	1. GH 30 mg	16.3	11	23	Insulin-like growth factor I	Inpatient		1.%IBW	0
				2. GH 100 mg	17	11		30 or 100 mg			2. BMI	19%
				3. Placebo	15.6	11						9%
Grinspoon 2002 [25]	6 days	Clinical	Restricting/ Binge-purge	1. GH + H	35 kg	16	24.2	Recombinant human IGF-I + Ovcon	Outpatient	1. Calcium	1.Kg	12%
				2. GH	35 kg	14	23	2x 30 mg		2. Multivitamins	2. Lean body mass (kg)	28%
				3. Placebo + GH	35.4 kg	15	27.6					0
				3. Placebo	32.3 kg	15	26.3					7%
Halmi 1986 [26]	32-45 days	Clinical	Restricting/ Binge-purge	1. AH	79 (IBW)	23	20.56	Amitryptyline	Inpatient		1. Days to target weight	n.m.
				2. AD	77 (IBW)	24		160 mg (max)			2. Average kg gain/day	
				3. Placebo	75 (IBW)	25						
Hill 2000 [27]	28 days	Clinical	Restricting/ Binge-purge	1.GH	14	7	14.5	Recombinant human growth hormone	Inpatient	1. Standard treatment	1. Average kg gain/day	n.m.
				2. Placebo	15	8 (1 male)	15	0.05 mg				
1st Author, Year	**Length of RCT**	**Recruitment**	**Anorexia type**	**Treatment conditions**	**Baseline mean weight[a]**	**N**	**Age**	**Type**	**Setting**	**Adjunctive treatments**	**Weight outcome measures**	**Drop-out**
Kafantaris 2011 [28]	10 weeks	Clinical	Restricting	1. AP	16.9	10	17.1	Olanzapine	Outpatient and inpatient	1. Individual medication	1. BMI	30%
				2. Placebo	16	10		2.5 mg		2. Psychotherapy	2.%MBW	20%
								5 mg		3. Family therapy		
								7.5 mg		4. Nutritional therapy		
								10 mg				
Lacey 1980 [29]	n.m.	Clinical	Restricting/ Binge-purge	1. AD	40.6 (kg)	8	n.m.	Clomipramine	Inpatient	1. Individual psychotherapy	1. Kg	25%
				2. Placebo	37.7 (kg)	8		50 mg		2. Caloric repletion	2. Mean kg gain	12%
											3. Rate kg gain/ day	

Table 1 Characteristics of the included studies *(Continued)*

Miller 2011 [30]	12 months	Community and clinical	Restricting/ Binge-purge	1. OM/ H	17.8	20	25.2	Risedronate/ Testosterone	Outpatient		1. Kg	23%
				2. OM	17.6	20	25.3	35 mg/ 150 mg			2. Lean body mass	
				3. H	17.5	19	27.1					
				4. Placebo	17.9	18	26.9					
Misra 2011 [31]	18 months	Community and clinical	Restricting/ Binge-purge	1. H	17.4	55	16.5	Fysiologic estrogen replacement	Outpatient	1. Behavior therapy	1. Kg	56%
				2. Placebo		55		100 mg			2. BMI	54%
											3. Fat mass	
											4. Lean mass	
Strokosch 2006 [32]	13x28 days	Clinical	Restricting/ Binge-purge	1. H	17.9	61	15.2	Norgestimate/ Ethinyl Estradiol	Outpatient		1. Kg	34%
				2. Placebo	17.6	62	15.1	180-250 mg/ 35 mg			2. BMI	21%
Vandereycken 1984 [33]	2x3 weeks	Clinical	Restricting/ Binge-purge	1. AP	40.4 (kg)	9	23.2	Sulpiride	Inpatient	1. "Uniform therapeutic programme"	1. Daily g change	n.m.
				2. Placebo	38.3 (kg)	9	23.7	300 or 400 mg				
Walsh 2006 [34]	1 year	Community and clinical	Restricting/ Binge-purge	1. AD	15.4	49	22.4	Fluoxetine	Outpatient	1. CBT	1. BMI	57%
				2. Placebo		44	24.2	20 mg to 60 mg		2. Family therapy		57%
										3. Medication monitoring		

Note. AD = Antidepressants; AH = Antihistamines; AP = Antipsychotics; ch. = change; CBT = Cognitive Behavioral Therapy; GH = Growth hormone; GI = Gastrointestinal; H = Hormones (other); n.m. = not mentioned; OM = Osteoporosis medication.

[a]Weight is BMI unless stated otherwise.

[b]More than one dosage mentioned means an increase of dosage after X weeks.

The quality of the 18 included studies was not optimal. Although all studies were randomized controlled trials, only five studies were assessed as having a low risk of bias based on the Cochrane domains [15]. The rest of the studies were assessed as having a high risk of bias. Sixteen trials reported blinding for the assessors and/or the patients and for two it was unknown. A random component in the sequence generation was reported in only nine studies; the rest of the studies used a non- random approach (N = 2) or did not report it (N = 7). Allocation concealment was done properly in only seven studies and with a high risk of bias in eleven studies. We also evaluated the use of incomplete data focusing on whether or not intention-to-treat analyses were performed. Incomplete data were adequately imputed in ten cases. Two studies performed completers- only analyses and six did not report it. Finally, fourteen studies reported all their outcomes, two studies reported only significant outcomes and for two studies it was unclear. Table 2 presents the quality assessment per study.

Weight was assessed in various ways. We reported on combined ES. To assure that this did not influence the results we performed the meta/analyses including for example only BMI or kg. This did not have an effect on the results, we therefore report on all weights. Some studies had weight measures such as weight gain and IBW gain [17,23,26,27,29,33]. To ensure that this was a valid approach we looked at the equivalence of weight measures of the groups at baseline. Almost all studies (except Halmi, 1986) mentioned explicitly that there were no significant differences in weight at time of randomization.

Pharmacotherapy versus placebo

Before performing the three meta-analyses of the most commonly used pharmacotherapy, we performed a meta-analysis comparing all three forms of pharmacotherapy with placebo. There were 20 studies that reported outcomes on weight. Figure 2 presents the outcomes of the meta-analysis.

The pooled effect size at post-treatment was 0.33, (95% CI: 0.14 ~ 0.52), indicating a significant effect. Heterogeneity was medium/ high ($I^2 = 40.08$). There was one outlier [25]; when removed the effect size decreased and became 0.25, still remaining significant. When the outlier was removed, heterogeneity became low ($I^2 = 0$). There was no evidence of publication bias. Subgroup analyses yielded no significant differences between subgroups. Meta regression analyses for mean age (slope = 0.014), duration of illness (slope = 0.014), mean weeks of

Table 2 Risk of bias assessments

Study	Sequence generation	Allocation concealment	Blinding	Incomplete data	Selective outcome	Total risk of bias assessment
Attia, 1998 [17]	No	No	Yes	Yes	Yes	High
Attia, 2011 [18]	Yes	Yes	Yes	Yes	Yes	Low
Bissada, 2008 [19]	Yes	Yes	Yes	No	Yes	Unclear
Brambilla, 2007a [20]	Unclear	Unclear	Yes	Unclear	Yes	Unclear
Brambilla, 2007b [21]	Unclear	Unclear	Yes	Yes	Yes	Unclear
Di Vasta 2012 [22]	Yes	Yes	Yes	Yes	Yes	Low
Fazeli 2010 [23]	Unclear	Unclear	Unclear	Unclear	Yes	Unclear
Grinspoon 1996a [24]	Unclear	Unclear	Yes	Unclear	Unclear	High
Grinspoon, 1996b [24]	Unclear	Unclear	Yes	Unclear	Unclear	High
Grinspoon, 2002a [25]	Yes	Unclear	Yes	Yes	Yes	Unclear
Grinspoon, 2002b [25]	Yes	Unclear	Yes	Yes	Yes	Unclear
Halmi 1986 [26]	Unclear	Unclear	Yes	Unclear	No	Unclear
Hill 2000 [27]	Yes	Unclear	Yes	Unclear	Unclear	Unclear
Kafantaris 2011 [28]	Yes	Yes	Yes	Yes	Yes	Low
Lacey 1980 [29]	No	Unclear	Yes	Yes	Yes	Unclear
Miller 2011 [30]	Unclear	Unclear	Yes	No	No	Unclear
Misra 2011 [31]	Yes	Unclear	Yes	Yes	Yes	Low
Strokosch 2006 [32]	Yes	Unclear	Yes	No	Yes	Unclear
Vandereycken 1984 [33]	Unclear	Unclear	Yes	Unclear	Yes	Unclear
Walsh 2006 [34]	Yes	Yes	Yes	Yes	Yes	Low

Note. yes (=the study reports correctly on this domain and there is no risk of bias); no (=the study reports on this domain but according to the description the domain could be biased); unclear (=the study does not provide sufficient information to make an assessment).

Study name	Outcome	Std diff in means	Lower limit	Upper limit	p-Value
Attia 11	BMI	0,11	-0,71	0,93	0,80
Attia 98	IBW	-0,14	-0,85	0,56	0,69
Bissada 08	BMI	0,56	-0,23	1,34	0,17
Brambilla 07 - PNE	BMI	-0,32	-1,20	0,57	0,48
Brambilla 07- ICP	BMI	0,18	-0,54	0,90	0,62
DiVasta 12	Combined	0,15	-0,25	0,56	0,46
Fazeli 10	Combined	-0,47	-1,33	0,40	0,29
Grinspoon 02a	Kg	1,41	0,85	1,98	0,00
Grinspoon 02b	Kg	0,27	-0,24	0,78	0,30
Grinspoon 96a	Combined	0,40	-0,44	1,25	0,35
Grinspoon 96b	Combined	1,05	0,16	1,94	0,02
Halmi 86b	Weight gain	0,43	-0,24	1,09	0,21
Hill 00	Weight gain	0,67	-0,37	1,71	0,21
Kafantaris 11	BMI	0,21	-0,81	1,23	0,68
Lacey 80	Combined	0,01	-0,98	0,99	0,99
Miller 11	lean body mass	0,71	0,05	1,38	0,04
Misra 11	Combined	-0,01	-0,38	0,37	0,96
Strokosch 06	Combined	0,29	-0,08	0,66	0,13
Vandereycken 84	Weight gain (g)	0,84	-0,13	1,80	0,09
Walsh 06	BMI	0,38	-0,03	0,79	0,07
		0,33	0,14	0,52	0,00

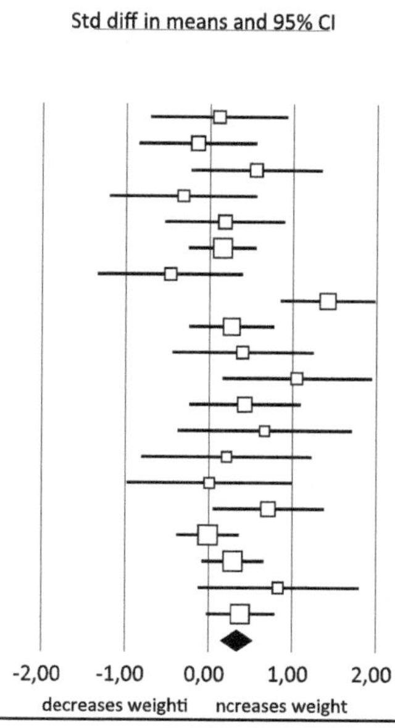

Figure 2 Effects of pharmacotherapy vs. placebo on weight.

treatment (slope = −0.0016) and mean BMI at the beginning of treatment (slope = 0.040) yielded no significant associations ($p = 0.36$; $p = 0.89$; $p = 0.54$; $p = 0.50$ respectively).

Antidepressants versus placebo

There were 4 studies that reported outcomes on weight (see Figure 3). The pooled effect size indicating the difference between antidepressants and the placebo condition on weight (all weight measures) at post-treatment was 0.26 (95% CI: −0.03 ~ 0.56), which was not significant (Table 3).

The heterogeneity for Antidepressants was low ($I^2 = 0$). The effect size comparing antidepressants with placebo at post-treatment was higher when adjusted for publication bias (d = 0.35; 95% CI: 0.06 ~ 0.64; number of trimmed studies = 1, right of mean), indicating a significant effect.

Because of the small sample size no meta regression or subgroup analyses could be conducted.

Antipsychotics versus placebo

Figure 4 shows that there were 6 studies that reported the effects of antipsychotics on weight. The pooled effect size indicating the difference between antipsychotics and the placebo condition on weight (all weight measures) at post-treatment was 0.25 (95% CI: −0.09 ~ 0.60), which was not significant (Table 3).

The heterogeneity for Antipsychotics was low ($I^2 = 0.00$). No evidence for publication bias was found. Because of the

Study name	Outcome	Std diff in means	Lower limit	Upper limit	p-Value
Attia 98	IBW	-0,14	-0,85	0,56	0,69
Halmi 86b	Weight gain	0,43	-0,24	1,09	0,21
Lacey 80	Combined	0,01	-0,98	0,99	0,99
Walsh 06	BMI	0,38	-0,03	0,79	0,07
		0,26	-0,03	0,56	0,08

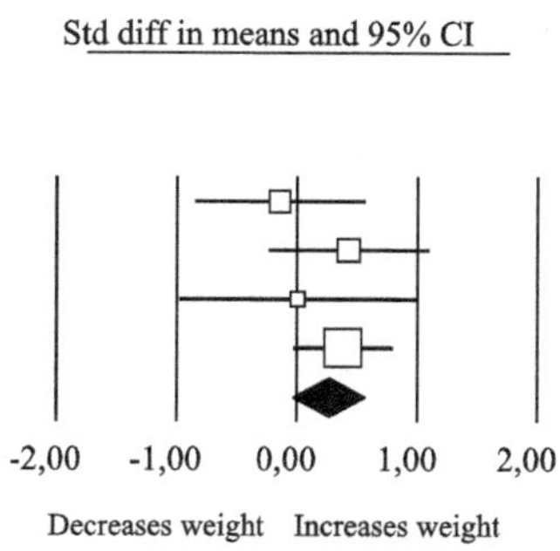

Figure 3 Effects of antidepressants vs. placebo on weight.

Table 3 Meta-analyses of studies examining the effects of pharmacotherapy versus placebo for anorexia nervosa

	N	*d*	95% CI	*Z*	*p*	*Q*	I^2
Pharmacotherapy vs. placebo	20	0.33	0.14 ~ 0.52	3.47	0.00	31.71	40.08
Outlier removed	19	0.25	0.11 ~ 0.39	3.45	0.00	16.28	0.00
Antidepressants vs. placebo	4	0.26	−0.04 ~ 0.56	1.73	0.08	2.11	0.00
Antipsychotics vs. placebo	6	0.25	−0.09 ~ 0.60	1.43	0.15	3.74	0.00
Hormonal treatment vs. placebo							
All studies	10	0.42	0.11 ~ 0.73	2.67	0.01	25.50	64.70
Outlier removed	9	0.26	0.04 ~ 0.47	2.37	0.02	10.41	23.15
One effect size per study (highest excluded)	8	0.21	0.02 ~ 0.39	2.19	0.03	7.09	1.26
One effect size per study (lowest excluded)	8	0.45	0.07 ~ 0.83	2.31	0.02	25.39	72.43

small sample size no meta regression and subgroup analyses could be done.

Hormonal pharmacotherapy versus placebo

There were 8 studies that reported on weight and 10 comparisons because of multiple conditions in some studies [24,25]; see Figure 5). Grinspoon et al. [24] administered 30 mg and 100 mg of recombinant human insulin-like growth factor I. In Grinspoon et al. [25] the therapeutic conditions consisted of recombinant human IGF-I and oral contraceptive administration. The pooled effect size indicating the difference between hormonal therapy and the placebo condition on weight (all weight measures) at post-treatment was 0.42 (95% CI: 0.11 ~ 0.73), which was significant (Table 3).

For hormonal therapy heterogeneity was high ($I^2 = 64.70$). No evidence for publication bias was found. There was one outlier [25]; when removed the effect size decreased and became 0.26, still remaining significant. When the outlier was removed, heterogeneity became a bit lower ($I^2 = 23.15$). Meta-regression analyses of the weeks of medication treatment (slope = −0.008) yielded a significant effect ($p = 0.04$). Meta regression analyses of BMI at the beginning of treatment (slope = −0.02326) and mean age (slope = 0.03932) yielded no significant effects ($p = 0.83$; $p = 0.05$ respectively). Subgroup analyses for hormonal therapy did not yield any significant results.

In this meta-analysis we included two studies in which two hormonal treatments were compared with the same control group [24,25], thus resulting in multiple comparisons in the same analysis. Because those comparisons are not independent from each other, this may have resulted in an artificial reduction of heterogeneity and have influenced the pooled effect size. We therefore performed a sensitivity analysis by including only one effect size per study. First, we conducted the analysis including only the comparison with the largest effect size from that study and then we did the same with the smallest effect size. As can be seen in Table 3, excluding the highest effect sizes resulted to a smaller (still significant) effect size and a large reduction in heterogeneity ($I^2 = 1.26$).

Discussion and conclusion

Main findings

To our knowledge this is the first meta analysis focusing on three forms of pharmacotherapy in the treatment of AN. By analyzing these data we aimed to provide an overview of more detailed information of the effectiveness of

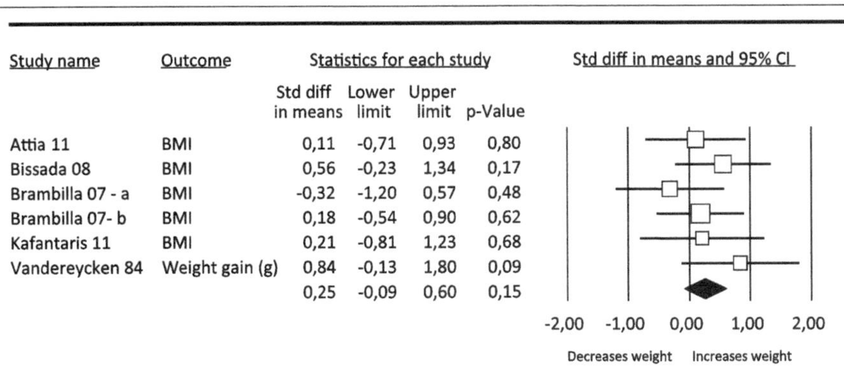

Figure 4 Effects of antipsychotics vs. placebo on weight.

Study name	Outcome	Statistics for each study				Std diff in means and 95% CI
		Std diff in means	Lower limit	Upper limit	p-Value	
DiVasta 12	Combined	0,15	-0,25	0,56	0,46	
Fazeli 10	Combined	-0,47	-1,33	0,40	0,29	
Grinspoon 02a	Kg	1,41	0,85	1,98	0,00	
Grinspoon 02b	Kg	0,27	-0,24	0,78	0,30	
Grinspoon 96a	Combined	0,40	-0,44	1,25	0,35	
Grinspoon 96b	Combined	1,05	0,16	1,94	0,02	
Hill 00	Weight gain	0,67	-0,37	1,71	0,21	
Miller 11	lean body mass	0,71	0,05	1,38	0,04	
Misra 11	Combined	-0,01	-0,38	0,37	0,96	
Strokosch 06	Combined	0,29	-0,08	0,66	0,13	
		0,42	0,11	0,73	0,01	

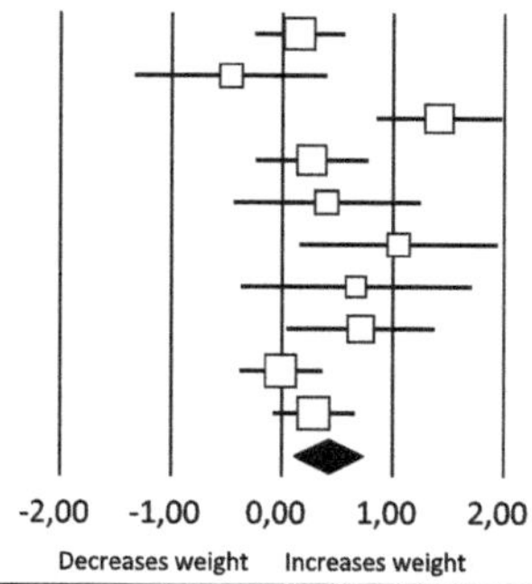

Figure 5 Effects of hormonal medication vs. placebo on weight.

pharmacological interventions on AN, compared to placebo.

When grouping all medication together, we found that pharmacotherapy is more effective than placebo. This grouping allowed an increase in power in order to perform subgroup and meta regression analyses. Unfortunately, they did not yield significant results. When performing meta-analyses for the three most common medicine apart, we found that hormonal therapy has a significantly larger effect on weight compared to placebo in the treatment of AN. This is a moderate effect size [13]. However for these analyses heterogeneity was high, which means that these significant results have to be regarded with caution. The sensitivity analyses support this conclusion. Meta regression analyses suggest that less weeks of hormonal treatment are associated with a better effect (a significant negative slope). It is possible that anorexia patients benefit on short term when it comes to (hormonal) medication, but fail to have a better recovery on long term. There are indications that for example alterations in the regulation of the hormone leptin may play a part in the persistence of anorexia nervosa. During recovery of anorexia patients, normalization of leptin levels seems to precede normalization of weight; this may be a contributing factor to the difficulties patients experience with maintaining normal weights, in this case for longer treatments [35]. Larger effect sizes for weight do not necessarily mean normalization of weight. Furthermore, weight goals differ depending on the treatment phase (acute phase or maintenance phase). In the acute phase the aim of treatment is mostly weight gain. However, weight gain alone cannot be considered a successful treatment of AN as other symptoms may continue to exist (e.g. absence of menstruation, preoccupation with body weight). Most trials focus on weight restoration; unfortunately this is only one aspect of the complex pathology of AN.

We found that antidepressants had no significant effect on weight compared to placebo in the treatment of AN. [4] found that antidepressants did not only fail to improve weight when compared to placebo, but also eating related psychopathology. However when we adjusted for publication bias the effect became higher, and significant favouring antidepressants over placebo treatment. Claudino et al. however only included subjects in the acute underweight phase, while this meta-analysis had broader criteria (acute and maintenance phase).

This meta-analysis also suggests that antipsychotics had no significant effect on weight compared to placebo in the treatment of AN. This latter is in line with the findings of Kishi et al. [9] and Lebow [10]. Kishi concludes on basis of their results that "taken together, the currently available evidence seems to tilt the risk-benefit balance against antipsychotics in patients with anorexia nervosa".

Considering the grave consequences of AN all small steps that are helpful in treatment should be taken into consideration. However the results of this study should be interpreted within the study's limitations.

Antidepressants and antipsychotics are the most commonly used medicamental treatments for anorexia nervosa in the Netherlands. Yet in both cases we failed to reveal efficacy when compared to placebo. There has been a lot of research trying to explain the placebo response, focusing on non/specific factors, expectancy and conditioning. Some studies have tried to identify "placebo prone personality types" with no consistent conclusions. There are some indications that use others as a healing resource and build positive relationships tend to benefit more from placebos, a hypothesis that supports continuity of care and effective interpersonal relationships to produce those placebo effects [36].

The limited findings of antidepressant and antipsychotic trials also raise an ethical dilemma: should those medications be used to treat anorexia nervosa in the acute phase? Clinicians should consider whether it is more beneficial to treat anorexia nervosa patients with pharmacotherapy in the stabilisation or prevention relapse phase, not aiming only at weight but also secondary symptoms as depression (see also the conclusion of Claudino et al. [4]). The design of the studies included also raise moral dilemmas. For example, how ethical is it to withhold treatment from anorexic patients and offer them a placebo instead? Furthermore, not all studies reported funding information. This aspect is essential when medication trials are published.

Limitations and recommendations

Several limitations of our meta analysis caution against over-interpretation of the results. One methodological shortcoming is that the quality of the 18 included studies was not optimal and some of the studies had very small sample sizes. Six out of eight studies of hormonal therapy for example had an unclear or high risk of bias. Yet those studies yielded positive findings. The power was an important problem, we could not include the number of studies that were necessary according to power calculations, which unfortunately made it impossible to run subgroup analyses for antidepressants and antipsychotics.

The studies contain relatively small patient samples, lending the results to a narrow foundation. In addition there is major variety in treatment and patient groups. The heterogeneity in the comparison between hormonal therapy and placebo was large. Furthermore some patients in the experimental as well as control conditions received various forms of adjunctive treatment, varying from very intensive clinical treatment to weekly outpatient sessions, making it difficult to draw conclusions. Some studies included adolescents as young as 12 years old. Changes in weight could be attributed to growth and not medication, especially in longer RCT's.

Other methodological shortcomings of the studies involve the outcome measures and reporting of outcomes. Although we've tried to report on many outcome measures and subgroups, this on the one hand reduced our sample sizes considerably, making it very hard to draw conclusions. On the other hand it lead to a lot of irrelevant results. Furthermore, the primary outcome measure was improvement of weight, as this is considered the first step in recovering from AN. Most of the trials therefore reported on weight, but unfortunately did so in various ways, making aggregation of the results very difficult, if not impossible. More over a number of studies only reported significant results, leaving out non significant but possibly relevant data and information. Because we inserted published data only, this may have caused a bias in our analyses.

Some evidence of heterogeneity was found between studies. Two main reasons for this could be that studies were found to be pursuing similar objectives (improvement in the treatment of AN) but with differences in goals and in expected actions of the pharmacological interventions.

Recommendations

Although considerable research had been devoted to AN evidence considering treatment efficacy is scarce. As demonstrated in this MA, trials reporting on pharmacotherapy compared to placebo had major limitations. Therefore it is of extreme importance that researchers would systematically use the same outcome measures. Furthermore the use of dichotomous data or the use of categories of levels of improvement in symptoms would facilitate research in the future. There is an urgent need for more and better quality studies with a better operationalization of the terms of improvement for AN. RCT's need to focus not only on weight restoration but on a broader definition of improvement. In these future studies, researchers must also attend to issues of statistical power and research design.

Additional file

Additional file 1: PubMedSearchString.

Abbreviations

AN: Anorexia nervosa; BMI: Body mass index; IBW: Ideal body Weight; RCT: Randomized controlled trial; AD: Antidepressants; AH: Antihistamines; AP: Antipsychotics; CBT: Cognitive Behavioral Therapy; ch.: Change; GH: Growth hormone; GI: Gastrointestinal; H: Hormones (other); n.m.: Not mentioned; OM: Osteoporosis medication.

Competing interests

The authors declare that they have no competing interests.

Authors' contributions

JdV, LH, GK, PC and JD participated in the design of the study. PC addressed important methodological issues. JdV, LH and GK screened and assessed the studies. JD and GK were involved in the statistical analysis. PC and EvdB provided a critical revision of the article. JdV, LH and JD approved the final manuscript. All authors read and approved the final manuscript.

Acknowledgements

We would especially like to thank Ellen Driessen for providing statistical and content advice on this meta-analysis. Ruth de Kraker and Tim Ziermans have also been a big help in getting this meta-analysis started. Finally, we would like to thank Joost de Wit, Margo de Jonge, Damelis Martina, Suzanne Schut, Nick Lommerse, Laura Bakker, Isabel Alvarez-Perez for assisting in the screening of almost 13.000 articles.

Author details

[1]Arkin Mental Health Institute, Klaprozenweg 111, PO Box 75848, 1070, AV, Amsterdam, the Netherlands. [2]De Viersprong Mental Health Institute, Bergen op Zoom, the Netherlands. [3]Vrije Universiteit, Amsterdam, the Netherlands.

References

1. American Psychiatric Association: *American Psychiatric Association Practice Guidelines for the Treatment of Psychiatric Disorders: Compendium 2006.* Arlington, VA, USA: American Psychiatric Pub; 2006.
2. Hudson JI, Hiripi E, Pope HG Jr, Kessler RC: **The prevalence and correlates of eating disorders in the National Comorbidity Survey Replication.** *Biol Psychiatry* 2007, **61**:348–358.
3. Attia E, Schroeder L: **Pharmacologic treatment of anorexia nervosa: where do we go from here?** *Int J Eat Disord* 2005, **37**(Suppl):S60–S63.
4. Claudino AM, Silvade Lima M, Hay PPJ, Bacalthcuk J, Schmidt UUS, Treasure J: *Antipsychotic Drugs for Anorexia Nervosa (Protocol).* England: The Cochrane Library; 2009.
5. Mondraty N, Birmingham CL, Touyz S, Sundakov V, Chapman L, Beumont P: **Randomized controlled trial of olanzapine in the treatment of cognitions in anorexia nervosa.** *Australas Psychiatry* 2005, **13**:72–75.
6. Bosanac P, Norman T, Burrows G, Beumont P: **Serotonergic and dopaminergic systems in anorexia nervosa: a role for atypical antipsychotics?** *Aust N Z J Psychiatry* 2005, **39**:146–153.
7. Mitchell JE, Steffen K, Cook MT, Roerig J: **Pharmacologic and psychotherapeutic treatment of anorexia nervosa.** *Womens Health (Lond Engl)* 2005, **1**:115–123.
8. Agras WS, Robinson AH: **Forty years of progress in the treatment of the eating disorders.** *Nord J Psychiatry* 2008, **62**(Suppl 47):19–24.
9. Kishi T, Kafantaris V, Sunday S, Sheridan EM, Correll CU: **Are antipsychotics effective for the treatment of anorexia nervosa? Results from a systematic review and meta-analysis.** *J Clin Psychiatry* 2012, **73**:e757–e766.
10. Lebow J, Sim LA, Erwin PJ, Murad MH: **The effect of atypical antipsychotic medications in individuals with anorexia nervosa: a systematic review and meta-analysis.** *Int J Eat Disord* 2012, **46**:332–339.
11. Sim LA, McGovern L, Elamin MB, Swiglo BA, Erwin PJ, Montori VM: **Effect on bone health of estrogen preparations in premenopausal women with anorexia nervosa: a systematic review and meta-analyses.** *Int J Eat Disord* 2010, **43**:218–225.
12. Powers PS, Santana C: **Available pharmacological treatments for anorexia nervosa.** *Expert Opin Pharmacother* 2004, **5**:2287–2292.
13. Lipsey MW, Wilson DB: **The efficacy of psychological, educational, and behavioral treatment. Confirmation from meta-analysis.** *Am Psychol* 1993, **48**:1181–1209.
14. Duval S, Tweedie R: **Trim and fill: a simple funnel-plot-based method of testing and adjusting for publication bias in meta-analysis.** *Biometrics* 2000, **56**:455–463.
15. Higgins JTP, Green SE: *Cochrane Handbook for Systematic Reviews of Interventions Version 5.1.0.* England: The Cochrane Collaboration; 2009.
16. Borenstein M, Hedges LVHJPT, Rothstein HR: *Introduction to Meta-Analysis.* Chichester: Wiley; 2009.
17. Attia E, Haiman C, Walsh BT, Flater SR: **Does fluoxetine augment the inpatient treatment of anorexia nervosa?** *Am J Psychiatry* 1998, **155**:548–551.
18. Attia E, Kaplan AS, Walsh BT, Gershkovich M, Yilmaz Z, Musante D, Wang Y: **Olanzapine versus placebo for out-patients with anorexia nervosa.** *Psychol Med* 2011, **41**:2177–2182.
19. Bissada H, Tasca GA, Barber AM, Bradwejn J: **Olanzapine in the treatment of low body weight and obsessive thinking in women with anorexia nervosa: a randomized, double-blind, placebo-controlled trial.** *Am J Psychiatry* 2008, **165**:1281–1288.
20. Brambilla F, Monteleone P, Maj M: **Olanzapine-induced weight gain in anorexia nervosa: involvement of leptin and ghrelin secretion?** *Psychoneuroendocrinology* 2007, **32**:402–406.
21. Brambilla F, Garcia CS, Fassino S, Daga GA, Favaro A, Santonastaso P, Ramaciotti C, Bondi E, Mellado C, Borriello R, Monteleone P: **Olanzapine therapy in anorexia nervosa: psychobiological effects.** *Int Clin Psychopharmacol* 2007, **22**:197–204.
22. Divasta AD, Feldman HA, Giancaterino C, Rosen CJ, Leboff MS, Gordon CM: **The effect of gonadal and adrenal steroid therapy on skeletal health in adolescents and young women with anorexia nervosa.** *Metabolism* 2012, **61**:1010–1020.
23. Fazeli PK, Lawson EA, Prabhakaran R, Miller KK, Donoho DA, Clemmons DR, Herzog DB, Misra M, Klibanski A: **Effects of recombinant human growth hormone in anorexia nervosa: a randomized, placebo-controlled study.** *J Clin Endocrinol Metab* 2010, **95**:4889–4897.
24. Grinspoon S, Baum H, Lee K, Anderson E, Herzog D, Klibanski A: **Effects of short-term recombinant human insulin-like growth factor I administration on bone turnover in osteopenic women with anorexia nervosa.** *J Clin Endocrinol Metab* 1996, **81**:3864–3870.
25. Grinspoon S, Thomas L, Miller K, Herzog D, Klibanski A: **Effects of recombinant human IGF-I and oral contraceptive administration on bone density in anorexia nervosa.** *J Clin Endocrinol Metab* 2002, **87**:2883–2891.
26. Halmi KA, Eckert E, LaDu TJ, Cohen J: **Anorexia nervosa. Treatment efficacy of cyproheptadine and amitriptyline.** *Arch Gen Psychiatry* 1986, **43**:177–181.
27. Hill K, Bucuvalas J, McClain C, Kryscio R, Martini RT, Alfaro MP, Maloney M: **Pilot study of growth hormone administration during the refeeding of malnourished anorexia nervosa patients.** *J Child Adolesc Psychopharmacol* 2000, **10**:3–8.
28. Kafantaris V, Leigh E, Hertz S, Berest A, Schebendach J, Sterling WM, Saito E, Sunday S, Higdon C, Gollden NH, Malhotra AK: **A placebo-controlled pilot study of adjunctive olanzapine for adolescents with anorexia nervosa.** *J Child Adolesc Psychopharmacol* 2011, **21**:207–212.
29. Lacey JH, Crisp AH: **Hunger, food intake and weight: the impact of clomipramine on a refeeding anorexia nervosa population.** *Postgrad Med J* 1980, **56**(Suppl 1):79–85.
30. Miller KK, Meenaghan E, Lawson EA, Misra M, Gleysteen S, Schoenfeld D, Herzog D, Klibanski A: **Effects of risedronate and low-dose transdermal testosterone on bone mineral density in women with anorexia nervosa: a randomized, placebo-controlled study.** *J Clin Endocrinol Metab* 2011, **96**:2081–2088.
31. Misra M, Katzman D, Miller KK, Mendes N, Snelgrove D, Russell M, Goldstein MA, Ebrahimi S, Clauss L, Weigel T, Mickley D, Schoenfeld DA, Herzog DB, Klibanski A: **Physiologic estrogen replacement increases bone density in adolescent girls with anorexia nervosa.** *J Bone Miner Res* 2011, **26**:2430–2438.
32. Strokosch GR, Friedman AJ, Wu SC, Kamin M: **Effects of an oral contraceptive (norgestimate/ethinyl estradiol) on bone mineral density in adolescent females with anorexia nervosa: a double-blind, placebo-controlled study.** *J Adolesc Health* 2006, **39**:819–827.
33. Vandereycken W: **Neuroleptics in the short-term treatment of anorexia nervosa. A double-blind placebo-controlled study with sulpiride.** *Br J Psychiatry* 1984, **144**:288–292.
34. Walsh BT, Kaplan AS, Attia E, Olmsted M, Parides M, Carter JC, Pike KM, Devlin MJ, Woodside B, Roberto CA, Rockert W: **Fluoxetine after weight restoration in anorexia nervosa: a randomized controlled trial.** *JAMA* 2006, **295**:2605–2612.
35. Walsh BT, Devlin MJ: **Eating disorders: progress and problems.** *Science* 1998, **280**:1387–1390.
36. Brody H: **The placebo response.** *J Fam Pract* 2000, **49**:649–654.

16

Classification of bulimic-type eating disorders: from DSM-IV to DSM-5

Jonathan M Mond

Abstract

Proposed changes to the classification of bulimic-type eating disorders in the lead up to the publication of DSM-5 are reviewed. Several of the proposed changes, including according formal diagnostic status to binge eating disorder (BED), removing the separation of bulimia nervosa (BN) into purging and non-purging subtypes, and reducing the binge frequency threshold from twice per week to once per week for both BN and (BED), have considerable empirical evidence to support them and will likely have the effect of facilitating clinical practice, improving access to care, improving public and professional awareness and understanding of these disorders and stimulating the additional research needed to address at least some problematic issues. However, the omission of any reference to variants of BN characterized by subjective, but not objective, binge eating episodes, and to the undue influence of weight or shape on self-evaluation or similar cognitive criterion in relation to the diagnosis of BED, is regrettable, given their potential to inform clinical and research practice and given that there is considerable evidence to support specific reference to these distinctions. Other aspects of the proposed criteria, such as retention of behavioral indicators of impaired control associated with binge eating and the presence of marked distress regarding binge eating among the diagnostic for BED, appear anomalous in that there is little or no evidence to support their validity or clinical utility. It is hoped that these issues will be addressed in final phase of the DSM-5 development process.

Keywords: DSM-IV, DSM-5, Bulimic-type eating disorders, Bulimia nervosa, Binge eating disorder

Review

Although anorexia nervosa (AN) may be the eating disorder most familiar to the public, and to medical professionals, bulimic-type eating disorders, which occur among individuals of normal or above average body weight, are far more common and affect a much broader section of the population [1-4]. These disorders include bulimia nervosa (BN) and variants of BN that fall short, in one way or another, of the criteria for diagnosis specified in current classification schemes. The most widely recognized scheme for the classification of eating disorders is the American Psychiatric Association (APA) Diagnostic and Statistical Manual of Mental Disorders (DSM), the most recent, fourth revision of which was published in 1994 (DSM-IV) [5]. Minor changes to this volume were made in text revision published in 2000 (DSM-IV-TR) [6]; however, the diagnostic criteria for most disorders, including eating disorders, were unchanged. The purpose of the current article is to review proposed changes to the classification of bulimic-type eating disorders in the upcoming, fifth revision of the DSM (DSM-5) [7].

Correspondence: Jonathan.Mond@anu.edu.au
Research School of Psychology, Australian National University, Canberra ACT 0200, Australia

The status quo: classification of bulimic-type eating disorders in DSM-IV

BN

The current (DSM-IV/DSM-IV-TR) diagnostic criteria for BN are shown in Table 1 (top left). As can be seen, BN is characterized by "recurrent" episodes of binge eating and extreme weight-control behaviors ("inappropriate compensatory behaviors"). Binge eating entails, first, the consumption of an "objectively large" amount food in a discrete period of time and, second, a sense of loss of control over eating during the episode. Extreme weight-control behaviors include self-induced vomiting, misuse of laxatives or diuretics, extreme dietary restriction ("fasting") and excessive exercise. "Recurrent" is defined as at least twice weekly during the past 3 months. That is, episodes of both binge

Table 1 Current (DSM-IV) and proposed (DSM-5) criteria for bulimic-type eating disorders: Bulimia Nervosa, binge eating disorder and eating disorders not otherwise specified (DSM-IV)/feeding or eating disorder not elsewhere classified (DSM-5)

Current (DSM-IV) and proposed (DSM-5) diagnostic criteria for Bulimia Nervosa

Current (DSM-IV)	Proposed (DSM-5)
A. Recurrent episodes of binge eating. An episode of binge eating is characterized by both of the following:	A. Recurrent episodes of binge eating. An episode of binge eating is characterized by both of the following:
(1) Eating, in a discrete period of time (e.g., within any 2-hour period), an amount of food that is definitely larger than most people would eat during a similar period of time and under similar circumstances	(1) Eating, in a discrete period of time (e.g., within any 2-hour period), an amount of food that is definitely larger than most people would eat during a similar period of time under similar circumstances
(2) A sense of lack of control over eating during the episode (e.g., a feeling that one cannot stop eating or control what or how much one is eating)	(2) A sense of lack of control over eating during the episode (e.g., a feeling that one cannot stop eating or control what or how much one is eating)
B. Recurrent inappropriate compensatory behavior in order to prevent weight gain, such as self-induced vomiting; misuse of laxatives, diuretics, enemas, or other medications; fasting; or excessive exercise.	B. Recurrent inappropriate compensatory behaviors in order to prevent weight gain, such as self-induced vomiting; misuse of laxatives, diuretics, or other medications, fasting; or excessive exercise.
C. The binge eating and inappropriate compensatory behaviors both occur, on average, at least twice a week for 3 months.	C. The binge eating and inappropriate compensatory behaviors both occur, on average, at least once per week for 3 months.
D. Self-evaluation is unduly influenced by body shape and weight.	D. Self-evaluation is unduly influenced by body shape and weight.
E. The disturbance does not occur exclusively during episodes of Anorexia Nervosa.	E. The disturbance does not occur exclusively during episodes of Anorexia Nervosa.
Specify type:	
Purging Type: during the current episode of Bulimia Nervosa, the person has regularly engaged in self-induced vomiting or the misuse of laxatives, diuretics, or enemas	
Nonpurging Type: during the current episode of Bulimia Nervosa, the person has used other inappropriate compensatory behaviors, such as fasting or excessive exercise, but has not regularly engaged in self-induced vomiting or the misuse of laxatives, diuretics, or enemas	

Current (DSM-IV) and proposed (DSM-5) diagnostic criteria for binge eating disorder

Current (DSM-IV)	Proposed (DSM-5)
A. Recurrent episodes of binge eating. An episode of binge eating is characterized by both of the following:	A. Recurrent episodes of binge eating. An episode of binge eating is characterized by both of the following:
1. Eating, in a discrete period of time (e.g., within any 2-hour period), an amount of food that is definitely larger than most people would eat in a similar period of time under similar circumstances	1. Eating, in a discrete period of time (e.g., within any 2-hour period), an amount of food that is definitely larger than most people would eat in a similar period of time under similar circumstances
2. A sense of lack of control over eating during the episode (for example, a feeling that one cannot stop eating or control what or how much one is eating)	2. A sense of lack of control over eating during the episode (for example, a feeling that one cannot stop eating or control what or how much one is eating)
B. The binge-eating episodes are associated with three (or more) of the following:	B. The binge-eating episodes are associated with 3 (or more) of the following:
1. Eating much more rapidly than normal	1. Eating much more rapidly than normal
2. Eating until feeling uncomfortably full	2. Eating until feeling uncomfortably full
3. Eating large amounts of food when not feeling physically hungry	3. Eating large amounts of food when not feeling physically hungry
4. Eating alone because of feeling embarrassed by how much one is eating	4. Eating alone because of feeling embarrassed by how much one is eating
5. Feeling disgusted with oneself, depressed, or very guilty after overeating	5. Feeling disgusted with oneself, depressed, or very guilty after overeating
C. Marked distress regarding binge eating is present.	C. Marked distress regarding binge eating is present.
D. The binge eating occurs, on average, at least 2 days a week for 6 months.	D. The binge eating occurs, on average, at least once a week for 3 months.
E. The binge eating is not associated with the regular use of inappropriate compensatory behaviors (e.g., purging, fasting, excessive exercise) and does not occur exclusively during the course of Anorexia Nervosa or Bulimia Nervosa.	E. The binge eating is not associated with the recurrent use of inappropriate compensatory behavior and does not occur exclusively during the course Bulimia Nervosa or Anorexia Nervosa.

Table 1 Current (DSM-IV) and proposed (DSM-5) criteria for bulimic-type eating disorders: Bulimia Nervosa, binge eating disorder and eating disorders not otherwise specified (DSM-IV)/feeding or eating disorder not elsewhere classified (DSM-5) *(Continued)*

Exemplars of the DSM-IV eating disorders not otherwise specified and DSM-5 feeding or eating disorder not elsewhere classified categories[i]	
DSM-IV: Eating Disorders Not Otherwise Specified	**DSM-5: Feeding or Eating Disorder Not Elsewhere Classified**
The Eating Disorder Not Otherwise Specified category is for disorders of eating that do not meet the criteria for any specific Eating Disorder.	**1. Atypical, mixed, or below-threshold presentations:** **Subthreshold Bulimia Nervosa (low frequency or limited duration)**
Examples include:	
3. All of the criteria for Bulimia Nervosa are met except that the binge eating and inappropriate compensatory mechanisms occur at a frequency of less than twice a week or for a duration of less than 3 months.	All of the criteria for Bulimia Nervosa are met, except that the binge eating and inappropriate compensatory behaviors occur, on average, less than once a week and/or for less than for fewer than for 3 months.
4. The regular use of inappropriate compensatory behavior by an individual of normal body weight after eating small amounts of food (e.g., self-induced vomiting after the consumption of two cookies).	**Subthreshold Binge Eating Disorder (low frequency or limited duration)** All of the criteria for Binge Eating Disorder are met, except that the binge eating occurs, on average, less than once a week and/or for fewer than for 3 months.
5. Repeatedly chewing and spitting out, but not swallowing, large amounts of food.	**2. Other specific syndromes not listed in DSM-5:**
6. Binge-eating disorder: recurrent episodes of binge eating in the absence of the regular use of inappropriate compensatory behaviors (see Appendix B in DSM-IV-TR for suggested research criteria).	**Purging Disorder** Recurrent purging behavior to influence weight or shape, such as self-induced vomiting, misuse of laxatives, diuretics, or other medications, in the absence of binge eating.
	Night Eating Syndrome Recurrent episodes of night eating, as manifested by eating after awakening from sleep or excessive food consumption after the evening meal. There is awareness and recall of the eating. The night eating is not better accounted for by external influences such as changes in the individual's sleep/wake cycle or by local social norms. The night eating is associated with significant distress and/or impairment in functioning. The disordered pattern of eating is not better accounted for by Binge Eating Disorder, another psychiatric disorder, substance abuse or dependence, a general medical disorder, or an effect of medication.
	3. Insufficient information: **Other Feeding or Eating Condition Not Elsewhere Classified** This is a residual category for clinically significant problems meeting the definition of a Feeding or Eating Disorder but not satisfying the criteria for any other Disorder or Condition.

[i]Note. Only exemplars of the respective categories relating to bulimic-type eating disorders are shown.

eating and extreme weight control behaviors need to occur at this frequency for the DSM diagnosis of BN to be considered.

A third core feature of BN is the occurrence of extreme concerns about weight or shape or, in the language of the DSM, the "undue influence of weight or shape on self-evaluation". This feature, which is also included among the diagnostic criteria for AN, is considered by many authorities to be a *sine qua non* of eating disorder psychopathology [8,9]. The diagnosis of BN also requires that these symptoms do not occur exclusively during episodes of AN. If individuals who meet diagnostic criteria for AN have regular episodes of binge eating and/or extreme weight-control behaviors, then the diagnosis of BN is "trumped" by that of AN [10].

The final thing to note about the current (DSM-IV) classification of BN is that provision is made for subtyping of individuals with this diagnosis according to the type of extreme weight-control behaviors that they employ in attempting to compensate for their episodes of binge eating. If one or more purging behaviors, namely, self-induced vomiting and/or misuse of laxatives or diuretics, is employed, then the diagnosis of BN purging subtype is given, irrespective of whether extreme dietary restriction and/or excessive exercise is also employed. If only extreme dietary restriction and/or excessive exercise is employed, but not vomiting, laxatives or diuretics, then the diagnosis of BN non-purging subtype is given.

Variants of BN

In DSM-IV, variants of BN (and of AN) that, while "clinically significant", do not meet full diagnostic criteria are designated "Eating Disorders Not Otherwise Specified" (EDNOS). The best-known variant of BN is binge eating disorder (BED), a disorder characterized by regular episodes of binge eating in the absence of the regular extreme weight-control behaviors that are characteristic of BN [9,11]. BED is also the most common variant of BN, in general population samples at least [2,4,12]. As might be expected, individuals with BED tend to be overweight, often very overweight [9,11]. This is contrast to individuals with BN, who tend to be in the normal-weight range. Further, whereas BN is far more common in women than in men, BED may be nearly as common in men as in women [1,4]. This difference reflects the fact that binge eating is common in both men and women, whereas the use of extreme weight-control behaviors, particularly purging behaviors, is uncommon in men [3].

BED was introduced, in DSM-IV, as a provisional diagnosis requiring further research and suggested diagnostic criteria were included in an Appendix [5]. As can be seen in Table 1 (middle left), these criteria include, in addition to the regular occurrence of binge eating and absence of regular extreme weight-control behaviors, the presence of 3 or more of 5 possible behavioral manifestations of binge eating and of "marked distress regarding binge eating". As can also be seen, the operational definition of binge eating suggested for BED is identical to that for BN. For the diagnosis of BED, binge eating must occur, on average, on at least 2 days per week for a period of 6 months or more. This is in contrast to BN, for which the binge eating frequency criterion is couched in terms of the number of episodes, rather than the number of days on which episodes occur, and for which duration of 3 months is sufficient.

Other exemplars of BN-type EDNOS, that is, variants of BN other than BED, mentioned in DSM-IV include disorders that resemble BN except that the binge eating and/or compensatory/extreme weight-control behaviors occur at a frequency of less than twice per week or for a duration of less than 3 months, disorders characterized by "the regular use of inappropriate compensatory behavior by an individual of normal body weight after eating small amounts of food" and disorders characterized by "repeatedly chewing and spitting out, but not swallowing, large amounts of food" (bottom left of Table 1).

The future: classification of bulimic-type eating disorders in DSM-5

BN

The proposed DSM-5 diagnostic criteria for BN are shown in the top right section of Table 1. As can be seen, the major change to the DSM-IV criteria is a revision of the frequency threshold for binge eating and extreme weight-control behaviors, so that an average frequency of once per week - as opposed to twice per week - for these behaviors is sufficient. This change is uncontroversial, since no clinically meaningful differences have been identified between individuals who otherwise meet criteria for BN and who have episodes of binge eating and compensatory behaviors at least once a week and those who otherwise meet criteria for BN and who have episodes of binge eating and compensatory behaviors at least twice per week [13].

A second, key change to the diagnostic criteria for BN, is that the subtyping of this diagnosis into purging and non-purging forms has been replaced by a single diagnosis that includes the use of both purging (self-induced vomiting, misuse of laxatives or diuretics) and non-purging (extreme dietary restriction, excessive exercise) weight-control behaviors. This latter change has been somewhat controversial in that the Eating Disorders Working Group had initially resolved to delete reference not only to the non-purging subtype of BN, but to the use of non-purging weight-control behaviors altogether. In other words, the intention was that BN would be reserved for individuals who employed purging behaviors to compensate for episodes of binge eating, whereas individuals with disorders once classified as BN non-purging subtype would, presumably, be relegated to the "Insufficient Information" section of the DSM-5 "Feeding or Eating Disorder Not Elsewhere Classified" category (bottom right of Table 1). The stated rationale for this recommendation was that:

> ... the non-purging subtype of BN had received relatively little attention and the available data suggested that individuals with this subtype more closely resemble individuals with binge eating disorder. In addition, precisely how to define non-purging inappropriate behaviors (e.g., fasting or excessive exercise) is unclear [7].

Subsequently, however, concerns relating to the elimination of the term "fasting or excessive exercise" from Criterion B prompted the Working Group to change its mind:

> Commentators felt that these forms of inappropriate compensatory behavior, while difficult to define precisely, were observed with sufficient frequency to merit their continued inclusion in the criteria. The Work Group found this persuasive, and those terms are now proposed to be maintained in Criterion B. The text will note the lack of agreement regarding how these terms should be defined and the fact that virtually all research on Bulimia Nervosa, including its treatment, has focused on individuals who actively purge via self-induced vomiting [7].

Hence, while separation of BN into purging and non-purging subtypes will be discontinued, reference to both purging and non-purging compensatory behaviors will be retained.

This change of heart was prudent. For one thing, the fact that disorders characterized by binge eating and the use of non-purging, but not purging, weight-control behaviors, have received relatively little attention is a not a good reason to exclude these disorders from consideration. Rather, reference to these disorders needs to be retained in order to ensure that further research is in fact conducted, in the same way that the inclusion of binge eating disorder as a provisional diagnosis in DSM-IV stimulated new research addressing the prevalence and correlates of this disorder [9,11]. Otherwise the field might end up merely "studying what it defines" (or not studying what it doesn't define) [14]. Further, eliminating reference to non-purging compensatory behaviors altogether would reinforce the impression - that subtyping gave rise to - that bulimic-type eating disorders characterized by purging behaviors are more severe than those involving non-purging behaviors when the reality is that there is little in the way of empirical evidence to support this view [1,12,15-17].

The inference that individuals who compensate for binge eating by means of extreme dietary restriction or excessive exercise, but not purging behaviors, more closely resemble individuals with binge eating disorder (than individuals who binge eat and purge) is also problematic, precisely because "how to define non-purging inappropriate behaviors (e.g., fasting or excessive exercise) is unclear" [12,17-19]. If liberal criteria for these terms (e.g. "restricting dietary intake", "exercising hard") are used, then the distinction between non-purging BN and BED may indeed be blurred e.g. [20]. If, on the other hand, more stringent operational definitions (e.g. "regularly going for a period of 24 hours or more without eating anything", "exercising in a driven or compulsive manner every or nearly every day") are used, then a clear distinction is likely to be observed e.g. [21]. The same issue arises when comparing the severity of purging and non-purging subtypes of BN [12,15,16] and in relation to variants of BN that involve extreme weight-control behaviors in the absence of binge eating (see below).

As long as there are no accepted operational definitions of "extreme dietary restriction" and "excessive exercise", this issue will continue to be a problem for the classification of bulimic-type eating disorders. But it would be better to address this issue, for example, by testing the validity of different possible operational definitions of these terms, than to merely ignore the problem and hope that it will go away [19,22]. Population-based research will be needed to address this issue, since cases of bulimic-type eating disorders that involve non-purging, but not purging, weight-control behaviors are uncommon in clinical samples [23]. The fact that population-based research is more challenging, in terms of requiring greater investment of time and resources, than the use of convenience samples of individuals receiving specialist treatment, might explain why so little research of this kind has been conducted. In addition, the current focus of the DSM on "clinical utility" may provide an incentive for using clinical, rather than epidemiological, samples to inform revisions to classification schemes [24]. Given that the influence of the DSM extends well-beyond mental health care, to primary care practice and the community as a whole, the merits of this focus are debatable [25-27].

Variants of BN

BED

The proposed DSM-5 criteria for BED are shown in the middle-right section of Table 1. As can be seen, the criteria are virtually identical to those suggested in DSM-IV, with one exception. Whereas binge eating on at least two days per week over a period of six months was required for the diagnosis of BED in DSM-IV, binge eating episodes on average at least once per week over a period of three months is required for this diagnosis in DSM-5. All of these changes - assessment of the number of binge eating episodes rather than the number of days on which binge eating occurs, a threshold for binge eating frequency of at least once, rather than at least twice, per week, and binge eating at this frequency for a period of three, rather than six, months - are uncontroversial, in that none of these factors has been found to influence the clinical significance of the disorder [13]. Further, these changes will mean that the criteria for BED are identical to those for BN in each of these respects, thereby eliminating unnecessary confusion.

Of greater consequence is the fact that in DSM-5 BED will no longer be a provisional diagnosis but, rather, a fully-fledged diagnosis, alongside AN & BN. Again this change is uncontroversial, for those in the eating disorders field at least, in that there is more than two decades of research supporting the clinical significance of eating disorders characterized by binge eating but not extreme weight-control behaviors [9,11,28,29]. Inclusion of BED as a formal diagnosis is significant, though, because it will have the effect of reducing the proportion of individuals with eating disorders who would otherwise have fallen into the DSM-5 "Feeding or Eating Disorder Not Elsewhere Classified" category [15,28]. Currently, as many as half of individuals with eating disorders receive the DSM-IV diagnosis of EDNOS and this is the case in both community and clinical samples [30,31]. Not surprisingly, concerns have been expressed about a classification scheme that relegates such a high proportion of cases to a residual category [31,32].

The inclusion of BED as a formal diagnosis also has public policy implications. Eating disorders struggle for recognition within psychiatry, let alone public health, due to the perception that these disorders are either serious but uncommon or common but trivial [1,33]. This perception has been reinforced by the low prevalence of eating disorders meeting (overly restrictive) formal diagnostic criteria. The inclusion of BED as a formal diagnosis will go some way to redressing this misconception, given the comparatively high prevalence of this disorder [2,31,34,35]. The proposed lowering of the threshold for binge eating - from twice per week to once per week - for both BN and BED, which will further reduce the proportion of cases classified as EDNOS, will consolidate change in this regard [2,31,34-36]. To the extent that reimbursement of treatment costs is contingent upon the receipt of a formal diagnosis, reducing the proportion of individuals who are classified as EDNOS should also have the effect of increasing access to specialist treatment [37].

As noted previously, BED is distinguished from other eating disorders in that it is relatively common in both men and women [2,3]. This is significant because it means that eating disorders can, or at least should, no longer be considered to be solely a problem of women [38-40]. However, as is the case with the non-purging form of BN, awareness and understanding of eating-disordered behavior in men may be poor, not only among individuals affected but among health professionals and the community as a whole [38-40]. The inclusion of BED as a formal diagnosis in DSM-5, along with reference to its epidemiology in the accompanying text, will, it is hoped, go some way to redressing this problem. More generally, there is a need to make the DSM classification of eating-disordered behavior less "female-centric" [40,41]. Some reference, in DSM-5, to the fact that this classification has been derived almost entirely from all-female samples may be helpful in promoting greater inclusion of males in future research.

Two aspects of the proposed new diagnostic criteria for BED warrant additional comment, namely, the retention of criteria B (behavioral indicators of impaired control associated with binge eating) and C (presence of marked distress regarding binge eating) and the omission of any reference to the "undue influence of weight or shape on self-evaluation". The decision to retain criteria B and C is notable because there is virtually no empirical evidence to support the validity or clinical utility of either of these criteria [42,43]. Indeed, it has been suggested that the lack of attention given to the behavioral indicators of impaired control may reflect the fact that they are widely seen as being redundant [28]. The same could be said of criterion C [25]. There is also the issue of why these criteria were considered necessary for the diagnosis of BED but not that of BN. It is possible that concerns regarding the proliferation of diagnoses were such that there was a perceived need, on the part of the DSM-IV Eating Disorders Working Group, to take particular care to ensure the "clinical significance" of the new, provisional diagnosis of BED and that these concerns have carried over into the process of including BED as a formal diagnosis in DSM-5 [44]. However, there is considerably more evidence to support the clinical significance of BED now - irrespective of the inclusion of criteria B and C - than there was two decades ago [9,11,28,29].

The omission of any reference to the undue influence of weight or shape on self-evaluation or similar, body-image-related cognitive criterion (such as the "overvaluation of weight or shape") from the proposed DSM-5 criteria for BED also is puzzling, given that evidence from both community and clinical samples suggests, first, that many individuals with BED or variants of BED do not have extreme concerns about weight or shape; and second, that the presence of these concerns distinguishes individuals who have very high levels of distress and disability from those who have minimal distress and disability [25,45-49]. In view of this evidence, there would seem to be a case for the inclusion of "undue influence" as a diagnostic criterion [45] or, perhaps, as a diagnostic specifier [46]. Aside from indicating disorder severity among individuals with BED and sub-threshold variants of BED, a change of this kind would bring the diagnosis of BED into line with those of both AN and BN [8,9,45].

The issue of which of the two options - diagnostic criterion or diagnostic specifier - would be preferable warrants greater consideration. As Grilo and colleagues and others have noted [46,47], inclusion of undue influence as a diagnostic criterion would likely have the effect of excluding from diagnosis some individuals who do in fact experience clinically significant levels of distress and impairment associated with their binge eating. That is, inclusion of undue influence among the diagnostic criteria for BED might result in an unacceptably high rate of "false negative diagnoses". This may be particularly important in specialist treatment settings. On the other hand, reference to undue influence as a diagnostic specifier - but not as a criterion - might lead to the inclusion among diagnosed cases of BED of individuals who are indistinguishable, in terms of levels of eating disorder and comorbid psychopathology, from obese non-binge eaters, that is, an unacceptably high rate of "false positive diagnoses" [45,49]. This may be particularly important in primary care and other non-specialist treatment settings. There are serious adverse consequences potentially associated with both false positive (e.g. unnecessary stigma) and false negative (e.g. ineligibility for reimbursement of treatment costs) diagnoses, hence the relative priority given to minimizing these different errors needs to be carefully considered [24,50,51]. This has been done in relation to mental health problems more generally [24,50,51] but not, to the author's knowledge, in relation to BED or other eating disorders.

In sum, the absence of any reference to undue influence in the proposed DSM-5 criteria for BED, when taken with the decision to retain criteria B and C, is difficult to fathom. However, it is important to note that the (proposed DSM-5) criteria shown in Table 1 are the most recent criteria available, rather than the final, versions of these criteria and that changes may be made before final recommendations are submitted to the APA Board of Trustees [7].

"Purging disorder"

In recent years, there has been considerable interest in a second variant of BN, namely, disorders characterized by the regular use of purging behaviors in the absence of regular episodes of binge eating. The term "purging disorder" has been introduced to refer to disorders of this kind and considerable evidence to support the clinical significance of these disorders has now been amassed [52,53]. Hence, purging disorder is included as an exemplar of the DSM-5 "Feeding or Eating Disorder Not Elsewhere Classified" category (bottom right of Table 1). It is described as being characterized by "Recurrent purging behavior to influence weight or shape, such as self-induced vomiting, misuse of laxatives, diuretics, or other medications, in the absence of binge eating" [53].

As I have argued elsewhere [1,54], there are at least two conceptual problems with the notion of a "purging disorder". First, individuals who report the regular use of purging behaviors in the absence of binge eating often also report regular episodes of subjective binge eating, that is, episodes of perceived over-eating in which a loss of control is experienced but the amount of food consumed is not objectively large, and the available evidence suggests that it is the combination of subjective binge eating and purging behaviors, rather than the occurrence of purging per se, that accounts for the distress and disability associated with these conditions [1,14,54,55]. There is nothing surprising about this latter finding. Evidence from epidemiological studies has consistently shown that, among individuals with bulimic-type eating disorders, the experience of loss of control over eating is a better predictor of distress and disability than the amount of food consumed [1,14,55-60]. This evidence calls into question the validity of the DSM definition of binge eating, which requires not only a loss of control over eating but consumption of an objectively large amount of food.

Whereas "the regular use of inappropriate compensatory behaviors by an individual of normal body weight after eating small amounts of food" is included as an exemplar of EDNOS in DSM-IV, in DSM-5 this terminology is omitted in favor of "purging disorder". The concern with this change is that the focus on purging, rather than the combination of subjective binge eating and purging, may divert attention away from the need for further research addressing the validity of the current DSM definition of binge eating [15,22,55-58]. Since bulimic-type eating disorders characterized by subjective, but not objective, binge eating are relatively uncommon in clinical samples, community-based research will be needed to address this issue and, as also noted above, community-based research may not be a priority for the architects of DSM-5 [24]. On the other hand, the fact that disorders of this kind are uncommon in clinical samples may reflect, in part, the tendency to study - and treat - what we define [14,23].

A concern relating to the inclusion, or at least mention, in the DSM of variants of BN characterized by subjective binge eating is that the assessment of subjective binge eating has been found to be unreliable, far more unreliable than that of objective binge eating [61-63]. This is hardly surprising, given the difficulty of determining whether or not a loss of control over eating is experienced when the amount of food consumed is not unusually large. Further, any change to classification schemes in which eating disorders characterized by SBEs, but not OBEs, are given formal recognition raises vexed conceptual issues, including the very definition of "eating disorder" [64]. As with bulimic-type disorders characterized by non-purging, but not purging, compensatory behaviors, however, simply ignoring the issue is not a good option. Reference to variants of BN characterized by subjective, but not objective, binge eating, in DSM-5 would serve the dual purposes of alerting clinicians - primary care and other non-specialist practitioners in particular - to the occurrence of these disorders while also alerting researchers of the need to address issues of assessment [15,56-58]. It might also be noted that, in adults at least, virtually nothing is known about the prevalence and correlates of variants of BED characterized by SBEs, that is, conditions that involve neither recurrent OBEs nor recurrent extreme weight-control behaviors. Hence, at present, a definition of binge eating solely in terms of loss of control over eating could be considered only in relation to the diagnosis of BN.

A second problem with "purging disorder" is that the use of this term may be taken to infer that variants of BN characterized by subjective, but not objective, binge eating, are worthy of attention if, and only if, they entail the use of purging behaviors. Admittedly, research addressing the clinical significance of disorders characterized by recurrent episodes of subjective binge eating and the recurrent use of non-purging - but not purging - weight-control behaviors is limited. No doubt the lack of any agreed-upon operational definitions of extreme dietary restriction and excessive exercise is a factor in this [12,17,19]. However, findings from at least one population-based study suggested that the combination of binge eating and extreme weight-control behaviors is associated with marked impairment in psycho-social functioning and that this is the case whether for both objective or subjective binge eating and for both purging and non-purging weight-control behaviors [1].

Taken together, the considerations outlined above suggest that the term "compensatory disorder" [1,65] may be preferable to "purging disorder" when referring to disorders characterized by the regular occurrence of extreme weight-control behaviors in the absence of regular (objective) binge eating. A third option that has occasionally appeared in the literature, namely, "subjective bulimia nervosa", may be less desirable because the use of this term may be taken to infer a condition that is less severe or deserving of clinical attention [14,66].

Night eating syndrome

Some comment is warranted concerning so-called "night eating syndrome" (NES), given the intention to include this "disorder", alongside "purging disorder", as an exemplar of the DSM-5 "Feeding or Eating Disorder Not Elsewhere Classified" category. As the name suggests, NES is characterized by recurrent episodes of night eating, as manifested by excessive food consumption at night ("evening hyperphagia") and/or episodes of eating after awakening from sleep ("nocturnal eating") [67]. Negligible food intake at breakfast ("morning anorexia") has also been included as a criterion in some studies [67]. The first scientific study of this behavior, based on a case series study of obese individuals receiving specialist treatment, was published in 1955, i.e. long before the inclusion of either AN or BN in the DSM [68,69]. However, despite this long history, NES has not previously been mentioned in the DSM classification of eating disorders. Hence the proposal to do so in DSM-5 is significant.

The decision to include NES as an exemplar of the DSM-5 Feeding or Eating Disorder Not Elsewhere Classified category is also somewhat surprising, however, given that a recent, comprehensive review of the literature found concluded that there was little evidence to support either the validity or clinical utility of this construct as a potential eating disorder diagnosis [70]. Problems with the existing evidence identified in that review included the lack of agreed upon definitions of and operational criteria for the core features of NES, the reliance on convenience samples of obesity patients in research seeking to elucidate the characteristics and correlates of the behaviors concerned, and, in turn, the lack of any compelling evidence for the delineation of NES from other forms of disordered eating or from normalcy [70]. On the other hand, if specific reference to NES in DSM-5 has the effect of stimulating the additional research needed to address these issues, then the decision to include such reference may be justified.

The decision to include sub-threshold forms of the proposed new BN and BED diagnoses, namely, variants of these disorders characterized by binge eating that occurs less than weekly or for a duration of less than 3 months, as exemplars of the DSM-5 Feeding or Eating Disorder Not Elsewhere Classified category might also be questioned, given that evidence bearing on the clinical significance of these conditions is currently limited [13]. On the other hand, findings from those few studies that have considered bulimic-type eating disorders involving less-than-weekly binge eating suggest that these conditions may be associated with levels of distress and disability comparable to those observed in disorders involving more frequent binge episodes [13]. Hence, it could be argued that further research addressing the optimal diagnostic threshold for binge frequency is warranted and that specific reference to these new sub-threshold variants of BN and BED within the DSM-5 Feeding or Eating Disorder Not Elsewhere Classified category will provide an incentive in this regard. In the meantime, severity of binge eating might be specified as a dimensional rating, so that clinicians and/or researchers would be required to rate the severity of binge eating according to its frequency and, perhaps, an additional, dimensional rating of distress or disability associated with binge eating behaviors [13,56].

Finally, readers may observe that reference to variants of BN characterized by "repeatedly chewing and spitting out, but not swallowing, large amounts of food" as an exemplar of the EDNOS category has been abandoned in DSM-5. This change presumably reflects the perception that these behaviors, which have been observed among individuals with both AN-type and BN-type disorders, are no longer of sufficient importance, in terms of their prevalence and/or clinical significance, to warrant specific mention, although there appears to be little in the way of empirical evidence to support such an assumption [71,72].

Conclusions

Proposed changes to the DSM diagnostic criteria for bulimic-type eating disorders in the lead up to the publication of DSM-5 will go some way to facilitating clinical practice, improving access to care, improving public and professional awareness and understanding of these disorders and stimulating the additional research needed to address at least some problematic issues. However, the omission of any reference to variants of BN characterized by subjective, but not objective, binge eating episodes, and to the undue influence of weight or shape on self-evaluation or similar cognitive criterion in relation to the proposed criteria for BED, is regrettable and other aspects of the proposed criteria, such as retention of behavioral indicators of impaired control associated with binge eating and the presence of marked distress regarding binge eating among the diagnostic criteria for BED, appear anomalous. It is possible that these issues will be addressed in the final phase of the DSM-5 development process.

Postscript

Since this manuscript was reviewed, DSM-5 has been published [73]. There were no changes to the wording of the diagnostic criteria for BN or BED as shown in Table 1. For both diagnoses, these criteria have been supplemented with two sets of specifiers indicating, respectively, the occurrence/state of remission (partial, full) and the current level of severity (mild, moderate, severe, extreme). Also for both diagnoses, operational definitions of each category of remission (in terms of some, or all, of the diagnostic criteria no longer being met for a sustained period of time after full criteria were previously met) and severity (in terms of the weekly frequency of inappropriate compensatory behaviours for BN and weekly frequency of binge eating for BED) are suggested. The inclusion of these specifiers is consistent with the stated intention of the DSM-5 Taskforce to improve clinical utility through the addition of specifiers or dimensions that serve to communicate clinically salient features of a disorder [24].

Concerning the proposed DSM-5 category of "Feeding or Eating Disorder Not Elsewhere Classified", this term has been replaced by a new term, namely, "Other Specified Feeding or Eating Disorder", that subsumes each of the four specific exemplars of this broad category (sub-threshold BN, sub-threshold BED, Purging Disorder and Night Eating Syndrome) shown in Table 1. Accordingly, use of the sub-headings "Atypical, mixed, or below-threshold presentations" and "Other specific syndromes not listed in DSM-5" has been omitted. In addition, the term "Other Feeding or Eating Condition Not Elsewhere Classified" has been replaced by "Unspecified Feeding or Eating Disorder" and the latter is included as a separate, fourth category of disorder, as opposed to being subsumed within the "Other Specified Feeding or Eating Disorder" category. The previously included "Insufficient Information" sub-heading has also been deleted accordingly. These changes presumably reflect a consolidation of efforts to preclude trivialisation of disorders that do not meet formal diagnostic criteria for AN, BN or BED [1,74].

Competing interests

The author declares that he has no competing interests.

References

1. Mond JM, Hay PJ, Rodgers B, Owen C, Crosby R, Mitchell JE: **Use of extreme weight control behaviors with and without binge eating in a community sample of women: Implications for the classification of bulimic-type eating disorders.** *Int J Eat Disord* 2006, **39**:294–302.
2. Hudson JI, Hiripi E, Pope HG, Kessler RC: **The Prevalence and Correlates of Eating Disorders in the National Comorbidity Survey Replication.** *Biol Psychiatry* 2007, **61**:348–358.
3. Hay PJ, Mond JM, Darby A, Buttner P: **Eating disorder behaviours are increasing: Findings from two sequential community surveys in South Australia.** *PLoSONE* 2008, **2**:e1541.
4. Kessler RC, Berglund PA, Chiu WT, Deitz AC, Hudson JI, Shahly V, *et al*: **The prevalence and correlates of binge eating disorder in the World Health Organization World Mental Health Surveys.** *Biol Psychiatry* 2013, **73**:904–91.
5. American Psychiatric Association: *Diagnostic and statistical manual of mental disorders (4th edition) (DSM-IV).* Washington, DC: Author; 1994.
6. American Psychiatric Association: *Diagnostic and statistical manual of mental disorders (4th edition - text revision) (DSM-IV-TR): Washington.* DC: Author; 2000.
7. American Psychiatric Association: *DSM-5 development: Proposed draft revisions to DSM disorders and criteria.* http:www.dsm5.org/ProposedRevision/Pages. Accessed 15/4/12.
8. Fairburn CG, Cooper Z, Shafran R: **Cognitive behaviour therapy for eating disorders: A "transdiagnostic" theory and treatment.** *Behav Res Ther* 2003, **41**:509–528.
9. Devlin MJ, Goldfein JA, Dobrow I: **What is this thing called BED? Current status of binge eating disorder nosology.** *Int J Eat Disord* 2003, **34**:S2–S18.
10. Walsh BT, Garner DM: **Diagnostic issues.** In *Handbook of treatment for eating disorders.* 2nd edition. Edited by Garner DM, Garfinkel PE. New York: Guilford Press; 2002:25–33.
11. Wilfley DE, Wilson GT, Agras WS: **The clinical significance of binge eating disorder.** *Int J Eat Disord* 2003, **34**:S96–S106.
12. Mond JM, Hay PJ, Rodgers B, Owen C, Mitchell JE: **Correlates of the use of purging and non-purging methods of weight control in a community sample of women.** *Aust NZ J Psychiat* 2006, **40**:136–142.
13. Wilson GT, Sysko R: **Frequency of binge eating episodes in bulimia nervosa and binge eating disorder: Diagnostic considerations.** *Int J Eat Disord* 2009, **42**:603–610.
14. Keel PK, Mayer SA, Harnden-Fischer JH: **Importance of size in defining binge eating episodes in bulimia nervosa.** *Int J Eat Disord* 2001, **29**:294–301.
15. Wilfley DE, Bishop ME, Wilson GT, Agras WS: **Classification of eating disorders: Toward DSM-5.** *Int J Eat Disord* 2007, **40**:S123–S129.
16. van Hoeken D, Veling W, Sinke S, Mitchell JE, Hoek HW: **The validity and utility of sub-typing bulimia nervosa.** *Int J Eat Disord* 2009, **42**:595–602.
17. Mond JM, Rodgers B, Hay PJ, Owen C: **Mental health impairment associated with eating-disordered behaviour in a community sample of women.** *J Mental Health* 2011, **20**:456–66.
18. Cooper Z, Fairburn CG: **Refining the definition of binge eating disorder and nonpurging bulimia nervosa.** *Int J Eat Disord* 2003, **34**:S89–S95.
19. Mond JM, Hay PJ, Rodgers B, Owen C: **An update on the definition of "excessive exercise" in eating disorders research.** *Int J Eat Disord* 2006, **39**:147–153.
20. Garfinkel PE, Lin E, Goering P, Spegg C, Goldbloom DS, Kennedy S, *et al*: **Bulimia nervosa in a Canadian community sample: Prevalence and comparison of subgroups.** *Am J Psychiatry* 1995, **152**:1052–1058.
21. Striegel-Moore RH, Cachelin FM, Dohm FA, Pike KM, Wilfley DE, Fairburn CG: **Comparison of binge eating disorder and bulimia nervosa in a community sample.** *Int J Eat Disord* 2001, **29**:157–165.
22. Wade TD: **Epidemiology of eating disorders: Creating opportunities to move the current classification paradigm forward.** *Int J Eat Disord* 2007, **40**:S27–S30.
23. Mond JM, Rodgers B, Hay PJ, Owen C: **Self-recognition of disordered eating among women with bulimic-type eating disorders: A community-based study.** *Int J Eat Disord* 2006, **39**:747–753.
24. First MB: **Clinical utility in the revision of the Diagnostic and Statistical Manual of Mental Disorders.** *Prof Psychol Res Pract* 2010, **41**:465–473.
25. Mond JM, Hay PJ: **Comorbidity and related considerations.** In *Binge eating disorder: A guide for clinicians and advocates.* Edited by Alexander J, Le Grange D, Goldschmidt A. London: Routledge; 2013:66–77.

26. Mond JM, Myers TC, Crosby RD, Hay PJ, Mitchell JE: **Eating disorders in primary care: Hidden morbidity still?** *J Clin Psychol Med Settings* 2010, **17:**56–63.
27. Gurege O: **Research for clinical practice: Focusing on the link.** *Int Rev Psychiatr* 2007, **19:**469–471.
28. Striegel-Moore RH, Franko DL: **Should binge eating disorder be included in the DSM-5? A critical review of the state of the evidence.** *Ann Rev Clin Psychol* 2007, **4:**305–324.
29. Wonderlich SA, Gordon KH, Mitchell JE, Crosby RD, Engel SG: **Validity and clinical utility of binge eating disorder.** *Int J Eat Disord* 2009, **42:**687–705.
30. Mond JM, Hay PJ, Rodgers B, Owen C: **Health service utilization for eating disorders: Findings from a community-based study.** *Int J Eat Disord* 2007, **40:**399–409.
31. Fairburn CG, Cooper Z: **Eating disorders, DSM-5 and clinical reality.** *Br J Psychiatry* 2011, **198:**8–10.
32. Walsh BT, Sysko R: **Broad categories for the diagnosis of eating disorders (BCD-ED): An alternative system for classification.** *Int J Eat Disord* 2009, **42:**754–764.
33. Mond JM, Hay PJ, Rodgers B, Owen C: **Comparing the health burden of overweight and eating-disordered behavior in young adult women.** *J Women's Health* 2009, **18:**1081–1089.
34. Keel PK, Brown TA, Holm-Denoma J, Bodell LP: **Comparison of DSM-IV versus proposed DSM-5 diagnostic criteria for eating disorders: Reduction of eating disorder not otherwise specified and validity.** *Int J Eat Disord* 2011, **44:**553–560.
35. Machado PP, Goncalves S, Hoek HW: **DSM-5 reduces the proportion of EDNOS cases: Evidence from community samples.** *Int J Eat Disord* 2013, **46:**60–65.
36. Trace SE, Thornton LM, Root TL, Mazzeo SE, Lichtenstein P, Pedersen NL, *et al*: **Effects of reducing the frequency and duration criteria for binge eating on lifetime prevalence of bulimia nervosa and binge eating disorder: Implications for DSM-5.** *Int J Eat Disord* 2012, **45:**531–536.
37. Andersen AE, Bowers WA, Watson T: **A slimming program for eating disorders not otherwise specified. Reconceptualizing a confusing, residual diagnostic category.** *Psychiatr Clin N Am* 2001, **24:**271–280.
38. Striegel RH, Bedrosian R, Wang C, Schwartz S: **Why men should be included in research on binge eating: Results from a comparison of psychosocial impairment in men and women.** *Int J Eat Disord* 2012, **45:**233–240.
39. Mitchison D, Mond JM, Slewa-Younan S, Hay P: **Sex differences in health-related quality of life impairment associated with eating disorder features: A general population study.** *Int J Eat Disord* 2013, **46:**375–80.
40. Mond JM, Mitchison D, Hay PJ: **Eating disordered behavior in men: Prevalence, impairment in quality of life, and implications for prevention and health promotion.** In *Current findings on males with eating disorders (pp. 195–208).* Edited by Cohn L, Lemberg R. London: Routledge; 2013.
41. Jones WR, Morgan JF: **Eating disorders in men: A review of the literature.** *J Public Mental Health* 2010, **9:**23–31.
42. White MA, Grilo CM: **Diagnostic efficiency of DSM-IV indicators for binge eating episodes.** *J Consult Clin Psychol* 2011, **79:**75–83.
43. Grilo CM, White MA: **A controlled evaluation of the distress criterion for binge eating disorder.** *J Consult Clin Psychol* 2011, **79:**509–514.
44. Walsh BT: **DSM-5 from the perspective of the DSM-IV experience.** *Int J Eat Disord* 2007, **40:**S3–S7.
45. Mond JM, Hay PJ, Rodgers B, Owen C: **Binge eating with and without the "undue influence of weight or shape on self-evaluation": Implications for the diagnosis of binge eating disorder.** *Behav Res Ther* 2006, **45:**929–938.
46. Grilo CM, Masheb RM, White MA: **Significance of overvaluation of shape/weight in binge eating disorder: Comparative study with overweight and bulimia nervosa.** *Obesity* 2010, **18:**499–504.
47. Goldschmidt AB, Hilbert A, Manwaring JL, Wilfley DE, Pike KM, Fairburn CG, *et al*: **The significance of overvaluation of shape and weight in binge eating disorder.** *Behav Res Ther* 2010, **48:**187–193.
48. Grilo CM: **Why not cognitive body image features such as overvaluation of shape/weight in the binge eating disorder diagnosis?** *Int J Eat Disord* 2013, **46:**208–211.
49. Hill C, Mond JM, Hay PJ: *Binge eating disorder: To include or not to include overvaluation of weight/shape as a diagnostic criterion.* Montreal 2013: Paper presented at the annual meeting of the International Congress of Eating Disorders (ICED); 2013.
50. Spitzer RL, Wakefield JC: **DSM-IV diagnostic criteria for clinical significance: Does it help solve the false positives problem?** *Am J Psychiatry* 1999, **156:**1856–1864.
51. Wakefield JC, Schmitz MF, First MB, Horwitz AV: **Extending the bereavement exclusion for major depression to other losses.** *Arch Gen Psychiatry* 2007, **64:**433–440.
52. Keel PK: **Purging disorder: an ominous variant of bulimia nervosa.** *Int J Eat Disord* 2005, **38:**191.
53. Keel PK, Striegel-Moore RH: **The validity and clinical utility of purging disorder.** *Int J Eat Disord* 2009, **42:**706–719.
54. Mond JM, Hay PJ: **Use of extreme weight control behaviors in the absence of binge eating with and without subjective bulimic episodes: A community-based study.** *Int J Eat Disord* 2010, **43:**35–41.
55. Brownstone LM, Bardone-Cone AN, Fitzsimmons-Craft EE, Printz KS, Le Grange D, Mitchell JE, *et al*: **Subjective and objective binge eating in relation to eating disorder symptomatology, negative affect, and personality dimensions.** *Int J Eat Disord* 2013, **46:**66–76.
56. Mond JM, Latner JE, Hay PJ, Owen C, Rodgers B: **Subjective vs objective bulimic episodes: Another nail in the coffin of a problematic distinction.** *Behav Res Ther* 2010, **48:**661–669.
57. Wolfe BE, Wood Baker C, Smith AT, Kelly-Weeder S: **Validity and utility of the current definition of binge eating.** *Int J Eat Disord* 2009, **42:**674–686.
58. Latner JD, Clyne C: **The diagnostic validity of the criteria for binge eating disorder.** *Int J Eat Disord* 2008, **41:**1–14.
59. Tanofsky-Kraff M: **Binge eating among children and adolescents.** In *Handbook of child and adolescent obesity.* Edited by Jelalian E, Steele R. New York: Springer; 2008:41–57.
60. Bravender T, Bryant-Waugh R, Herzog D, Katzman D, Kriepe RD, Lask B, *et al*: **Classification of eating disturbance in children and adolescents: Proposed changes for the DSM-5.** *Eur Eat Disord Rev* 2010, **18:**79–89.
61. Grilo CM, Masheb RM, Lozano-Blanco C, Barry DT: **Reliability of the Eating Disorder Examination in patients with binge eating disorder.** *Int J Eat Disord* 2004, **35:**80–85.
62. Mond JM, Rodgers B, Hay PJ, Owen C, Beumont PJV: **Temporal stability of the Eating Disorders Examination Questionnaire (EDE-Q).** *Int J Eat Disord* 2004, **36:**195–203.
63. Peterson CB, Miller KB, Johnson-Lind J, Crow SJ, Thuras P: **The accuracy of symptom recall in eating disorders.** *Compr Psychiatry* 2007, **48:**51–56.
64. Hay PJ: **What is an eating disorder? Implications for current and future diagnostic criteria.** *Aust N Z J Psychiatry* 2013, **47:**208–211.
65. Tobin DL, Griffing A, Griffing S: **An examination of subtype criteria for bulimia nervosa.** *Int J Eat Disord* 1997, **22:**179–186.
66. Fairburn CG, Cooper Z: **Thinking afresh about the classification of eating disorders.** *Int J Eat Disord* 2007, **40:**S107–S110.
67. Stunkard AJ, Allison KC, Geliebter A, Lundgren JD, Gluck ME, O'Reardon JP: **Development of criteria for a diagnosis: Lessons from the night eating syndrome.** *Compr Psychiat* 2009, **50:**391–399.
68. Stunkard AJ, Grace WJ, Wolff HG: **The night-eating syndrome: A pattern of food intake among certain obese patients.** *Am J Med* 1955, **19:**78–86.
69. Beumont PJV: **Bulimia: Is is an illness entity?** *Int J Eat Disord* 1988, **7:**167–176.
70. Striegel-Moore RH, Franko DL, Garcia J: **The validity and clinical utility of night eating syndrome.** *Int J Eat Disord* 2009, **42:**720–738.
71. Kovacs D, Mahon J, Palmer RL: **Chewing and spitting out food among eating-disordered patients.** *Int J Eat Disord* 2002, **32:**112–115.
72. Striegel-Moore RH, Franko DL, Thompson D, Barton B, Schreiber GB, Daniels SR: **An empirical study of the typology of bulimia nervosa and its spectrum variants.** *Psychol Med* 2005, **35:**1563–1572.
73. American Psychiatric Association: *Diagnostic and statistical manual of mental disorders (5th edition) (DSM-5).* Washington, DC: Author; 2013.
74. Walsh BT: **Eating Disorders in DSM-5.** *Psychiatr Ann* 2012, **42:**399–400.

17

Impact of female adult eating disorder inpatients' attitudes to compulsive exercise on outcome at discharge and follow-up

Marit Danielsen[1,2*], Øyvind Rø[3,4], Ulla Romild[5] and Sigrid Bjørnelv[1,2]

Abstract

Background: The link between compulsive exercise and eating disorders is well known, but research with clinical samples has been limited. The purpose of the study was to investigate changes in attitudes towards compulsive exercise and its impact on outcome at follow-up in female adult hospitalised patients with eating disorders.

Methods: The sample consisted of 78 patients: Diagnostic distribution: anorexia nervosa 59 % ($n = 46$), approximately 22 % ($n = 16$) in bulimia nervosa, and Eating Disorder not Otherwise Specified respectively. The average follow-up period was 26 months (SD =15 months). Compulsive exercise was measured by the Exercise and Eating Disorder (EED) questionnaire. Other measures were the Eating Disorder Inventory (EDI-2), Body Attitude Test (BAT), Symptom Checklist (SCL-90), Inventory of Interpersonal Problems (IIP 64), Beck Depression Inventory (BDI), and body mass index (BMI). Outcome measures were EDI-2 and BMI (patients with admission BMI ≤ 18.5). Paired sample t-tests and mixed model regression analysis were conducted to investigate changes in compulsive exercise and predictors of outcome respectively.

Results: All measures revealed significant improvements ($p < .01$ – $p < .001$) from admission to follow-up. EED scores significantly predicted changes in EDI-2 scores and BMI ($p < .01$ and $p < .001$ respectively). Other significant predictors were BAT, SCL-90, IIP-64, BMI ($p < .01$–$.001$) (EDI-2 as outcome measure), and BAT and BDI ($p < .001$) (BMI as outcome measure).

Conclusions: The results demonstrated significant improvements in attitudes towards compulsive exercise during treatment and follow-up. The change in compulsive exercise scores predicted the longer-term course of eating disorder symptoms and BMI.

Keywords: Eating disorders, Attitudes, Compulsive exercise, Inpatient, Treatment, Outcome

Background

The DSM-IV and DSM-5 diagnostic criteria highlight excessive or compulsive elements of exercise as recurrent inappropriate behaviour in patients with eating disorders [1, 2]. Such behaviour is characterized as inappropriate when it significantly interferes with a person's life and persists despite injury or medical complications. In cases of anorexia nervosa (AN), the behaviour is described as a cause of weight loss, and in cases of bulimia nervosa (BN) as compensatory behaviour. The only difference between the two editions is that the frequency of compensating behaviour in DSM-5 is reduced from twice a week to weekly [1, 2]. Frequent and intensive physical activity is common in a number of human groups, such as athletes. However, in patients with eating disorders it has been suggested that negative and compulsive attitudes towards exercise are more closely related to symptoms of eating disorders than the excessive amounts of exercise [3, 4].

Numerous definitions and terms have been used in the literature to describe compulsive and/or excessive exercise, yet inconsistency in the definitions renders it difficult for readers to know whether different studies refer

* Correspondence: madaniels@gmail.com
[1]Department of Neuroscience, Faculty of Medicine, Norwegian University of Science and Technology, 7491 Trondheim, Norway
[2]Eating Disorder Unit, Department of Psychiatry, Levanger Hospital, Hospital Trust Nord-Trøndelag, NO-7600 Levanger, Norway
Full list of author information is available at the end of the article

to the same phenomenon [5]. Further, this inconsistency may account for the wide range of prevalence rates reported. Two studies observed an overall prevalence of excessive exercise of 39 and 45 % in transdiagnostic samples, with rates varying according to diagnostic type [6, 7]. In one of the samples, the prevalence was as high as 80 % for patients diagnosed with restrictive anorexia nervosa (AN), 43 % in AN binge-eating/purging subtype, 39. % in bulimia nervosa (BN), and 32 % in eating disorders not otherwise specified (EDNOS) (6). Other studies have shown smaller differences between diagnostic groups [8–10].

There has been an increased interest in the nature of excessive and/or compulsive exercise in eating disorders and the association with symptomatology and treatment outcome [3, 4]. Such attitudes and behaviour have been investigated in treatment programmes with and without exercise interventions. A drive for compulsive exercise present at discharge has been reported as a negative prognostic factor for the long-term course of AN [11]. Carter and colleagues [12] investigated high-level exercise in the first three months after discharge from treatment, and found a significant association with the probability of relapse. Associations between objective measures of amount of exercise (at initiation of treatment) and eating disorder pathology have been investigated. In a review, Gummer and colleagues [13] reported that results were partly conflicting as to whether associations existed. In an inpatient treatment programme (without exercise intervention) the results revealed that a lower amount of pre-treatment exercise was a significant predictor of improvement in eating disorder symptoms [6].

Specific exercise interventions are not commonly incorporated in treatment programmes, and few studies have explored the influence of outcome when such interventions are included [12–14]. In one study with AN, BN, EDNOS, a significant positive correlation was found between reduced exercise dependency and reduced eating disorder symptoms during inpatient treatment [14]. Literature relating to excessive exercise and AN [15, 16] and in transdiagnostic samples [17] has been summarized. A total of 13 studies were evaluated, most of which were characterized by small sample sizes and considerable heterogeneity in definitions, outcome measures, and type of intervention. Despite their methodological heterogeneity, the studies indicate that exercise interventions as a part of treatment have no significant adverse impacts on weight gain for AN patients [15–17]. Four studies found a positive association between exercise interventions and reduced eating disorder symptoms (e.g. body image related symptoms and compensating behaviour) [15, 17]. Moreover, improvements in psychological well-being and quality of life were observed [15]. Of the 13 studies, five investigated adult inpatient samples. None of the studies investigated the course of illness following discharge from inpatient treatment. The authors of the reviews concluded that although initial studies showed promising results, more research is warranted to increase the understanding of compulsive exercise in eating disorders, associations with eating disorder pathology and influence on treatment outcome [15–17]. In order to contribute with increased knowledge to the field, the research focus in this article was directed towards negative and compulsive attitudes to exercise in female adult eating disorder inpatients through a naturalistic follow-up study.

The aims of the study were to:

1. Identify how various dimensions of attitudes towards compulsive exercise change between admission, discharge, and at follow-up in a transdiagnostic sample of hospitalized females with eating disorders.
2. Identify whether changes in attitudes to compulsive exercise predict the course of eating disorder psychopathology and BMI in relation to changes in general mental distress, interpersonal problems, and depression.

Methods

Participants and procedure

The study was conducted as part of a larger follow-up study, and participants in the cohort were recruited from an adult inpatient eating disorder unit in the Central Norway region. Between January 2005 and December 2013, a total of 128 patients were admitted to the unit. Six men were excluded because the EED questionnaire was only validated for women, and 6 female patients were excluded because they decided not to receive treatment after the introductory week. Of the remaining 116 female patients, 78 participated in the follow-up assessment, yielding a response rate of approximately 67 %. A subset of this sample (26 participants) was included in a former study investigating the impact of disturbed body image on treatment outcome [18]. No compensation was given for participation. Written invitations with study information, consent forms, and questionnaires were mailed to former patients for the follow-up assessment.

The data were collected at admission, discharge, and follow-up. The average follow-up period after discharge from treatment was 26 months ($SD = 15$ months, median = 22 months, range = 9.5–92.5 months). The main reason for the variety of the follow-up period is due to the study design. The follow-up study was approved in 2009. All former admitted patients were invited to participate, giving an extended follow-up period for the patients admitted in the earliest years. One of the participants had an extraordinarily long follow-up period of 92 months. The analysis of change during treatment and the analysis of predictors of outcome were performed both with and without the inclusion of the latter participant in the sample. The difference did not have a noteworthy effect on the results and data relating to the participant have been included in all reported results.

The baseline values for participants and non-participants were compared (t-test for independent groups). No differences were found between the groups: age ($t(114) = 0.72$, $p = .472$), body mass index (BMI) ($t(114) = -1.3\ 7$, $p = .173$), EED global score ($t(114) = 0.65$, $p = .520$) and Eating Disorder Inventory (EDI-2) ($t(114) = 1.30$, $p = .197$). Similarly, no differences between participants and non-participants were found in the discharge values: BMI ($t(114) = -0.11$, $p = .910$), EED global score ($t\ (114) = 1.23$, $p = .221$), and EDI-2 sum score ($t(114) = 1.27$, $p = .205$). Among the 78 participants, 78 % ($n = 61$) had completed treatment as planned, 17 % ($n = 13$) had discharged themselves from treatment, and 5 % ($n = 4$) had been discharged in accordance with routine procedures due to breaking the treatment contract.

Diagnostic assessment and clinical interviews at admission were performed by licensed psychologists or psychiatrists, in accordance with DSM-IV diagnostic criteria [1]. The diagnostic distribution in the sample was 59 % ($n = 46$) AN, and approximately 21 % ($n = 16$) in BN and EDNOS respectively. All patients were admitted to inpatient treatment due to having serious symptoms of ED and having received prior treatment without satisfactory effect. The mean duration of illness (self-reported) prior to admission was 5.3 years ($SD = 3.8$, range 1–20 years) and the mean duration of inpatient admission was 134 days ($SD = 56$, range 14–281 days). The mean admission time for AN participants was 149 days ($SD = 61$, range 14–281), BN 115 days ($SD = 36$, range 49–192), and EDNOS 111 days ($SD = 48$, range 15–184). Underweight participants were defined as having a BMI ≤18.5, which has been described by the World Health Organization (WHO) as the threshold for a healthy weight. In this sample, 72 % ($n = 56$) had a BMI below 18.5 at admission ($M = 15.9$, SD 1.6, range 12.4–18.5).

The study received approval from The Regional Committee for Medical and Health Research Ethics and all participants provided written informed consent. The baseline characteristics of the sample are presented in Table 1.

Treatment programme

The treatment programme was multidimensional and has been described in detail elsewhere [18]. In brief, the staff had multidisciplinary backgrounds and the treatment programme was based on psychodynamic theory, with

Table 1 Baseline values for the whole sample and diagnostic groups

	Alle patients	AN	BN	EDNOS			Effect size[3]
	$N = 78$	$n = 46$	$n = 16$	$n = 16$		Bonferroni Post hoc.	Eta squared adjusted for age
	Mean (SD)	Mean (SD)	Mean (SD)	Mean (SD)	F-value[1] p-value[2]	p-value[2]	η^2
Age (years)	21.1 (3.9)	20.4 (3.3)	22.2 (4.5)	22.2 (4.8)	2.00		
Range	16.0 - 36.5	16.0 - 31.7	17.8 - 34.8	16.6 - 36.5			
BMI	17.7 (3.5)	15.5 (1.4)	20.7 (2.5)	20.8 (4.1)	46.10***	AN vs BN and EDNOS***	
Range	13.4 - 34.1	12.4 - 17.6	17.5 - 24.7	18.1 - 34.1			
EED global score	3.0 (0.8)	3.0 (0.7)	3.1 (1.0)	2.9 (0.9)	0.11		.00
EED compulsive	3.4 (1.2)	3.4 (1.2)	3.4 (1.2)	3.5 (1.1)	0.46		.00
EED positive	2.3 (1.4)	2.3 (1.2)	2.6 (0.9)	1.9 (0.9)	1.75		.04
EED bodily signals	2.5 (1.0)	2.6 (1.0)	2.3 (0.9)	2.5 (1.0)	0.32		.00
EED weight & shape	3.6 (1.2)	3.5 (1.2)	4.0 (1.1)	3.5 (1.0)	1.03		.04
EDI-2 sum score	111.2 (40.8)	105.5 (36.0)	138.8 (43.2)	100.1 (41.8)	5.23**	AN vs BN, and BN vs EDNOS*	.13
BAT sum score	66.0 (17.4)	63.8 (16.6)	72.3 (18.1)	66.2 (18.5)	1.44		.04
SCL-90 mean score	1.6 (0.7)	1.6 (0.6)	1.9 (0.7)	1.6 (0.8)	1.60		.04
BDI sum score	30.5 (10.4)	29.9 (8.2)	34.7 (13.1)	27.8 (12.5)	1.95		.05
IIP-64 mean score	1.6 (0.6)	1.6 (0.6)	1.8 (0.6)	1.6 (0.8)	0.79		.02

Note: [1]One way ANOVA between diagnostic groups, df (2, 75). Bonferroni post hoc test, only significant relationships are reported
AN anorexia nervosa, *BN* bulimia nervosa, *EDNOS* eating disorder not otherwise specified
BMI Body mass index, *EED* Exercise and Eating Disorder, EDI-2- Eating Disorder Inventory, *BAT* Body Attitude Test
SCL-90: Symptom Checklist. *BDI* Beck Depression Inventory. IIP-64: Inventory of Interpersonal Problems
[2]*p*-value: * $p < .05$, ** $p < .01$, and *** $p < .001$
[3]Effect size - Eta squared η^2: small effect size =: .02, medium = .13, and large = .26

elements of cognitive behavioural therapy and motivational interviewing. All participants were admitted voluntarily. Following an introductory week, each participant signed a contract formulating their individual goals and formally approving the terms of their treatment.

Physical activity and exercise interventions

Physical activity and exercise interventions were an integrated part of the treatment programme from admission to discharge. According to procedure in the unit, the participants' former exercise experiences were addressed individually at admission, including the reasons why they exercised, how their exercise affected other eating disorder symptoms and vice versa, and the amount of exercise they did. An individualized treatment plan and goals for physical activity as well as an exercise intervention were prepared for each participant.

Each week there was a structured programme with group therapy and individual therapy sessions, which also included body-oriented therapy, adjusted outdoor activity (e.g. walking, horse riding, climbing, kayaking, and skiing in the winter) and regular exercise groups. Underweight participants were required to have a minimum BMI of approximately 17.0 before participation in exercise groups and a planned weight gain had to be met in order to continue participation. Qualified personnel were responsible for planning and supervising the activities. The body-oriented therapy was based upon the theory and principles of Norwegian Psychomotor Physiotherapy (NPMP) [19], which in turn forms part of the Nordic physiotherapy and body-oriented therapy tradition [20]. The initial focus in body image therapy was upon relaxation and body awareness movements. All participants were gradually exposed to diverse approaches that address the relationships between the body, emotions, and interpersonal and social aspects. Regular exercise groups were offered later on in the treatment programme, with one hour of strength training and one hour of aerobic activity. These exercise groups were based on basic training principles such as muscular strength and endurance, cardiovascular endurance, variation, progression, and restitution, and were adjusted to individual needs and capacity. One of the aims was to expose the participants to different levels of intensity, but the exercise was mainly performed at a moderate level. The personnel facilitated a social arena in which participants could enjoy the activities and get new experiences in a non-competitive atmosphere. Individual goals and challenges were addressed before and after exercise sessions to help participants to integrate healthy attitudes and behaviour in accordance with their treatment plan. Participants also received individual supervision, during which a heart rate monitor could be used as an additional tool. Psychoeducation formed part of the intervention and included anatomy, physiology, what constitutes healthy exercise, and what is unhealthy exercise. At discharge, plans were made for the transference of the achieved changes to the participants' daily life at home.

Measures

Compulsive exercise

The Exercise and Eating Disorder (EED) self-report questionnaire [9] is a validated, short questionnaire. It has been developed to cover a broad perspective on attitudes towards compulsive exercise in eating disorders. It is the first clinically-derived questionnaire measuring attitudes towards compulsive exercise in patients with eating disorders and is intended for use in clinical settings [9]. It consists of 18 statements with a four-factor structure and a six-point response scale from zero to five (*never, rarely, sometimes, often, usually, and always*). The global score and subscale scores are based on mean values. Higher scores indicate greater compulsivity and unhealthy exercise. The subscales cover clinically relevant issues:

(1) *Compulsive exercise* (being physically active to avoid dealing with negative emotions; if not active: it feels wrong, I don't eat, I can't relax, I get a bad conscience, my body feels big or nasty; and I listen to my body).
(2) *Positive and healthy exercise* (enjoy being physically active; physically active to be healthy; like to exercise with other people).
(3) *Awareness of bodily signals* (I notice when: I feel fit/am in shape, when I get tired, thirsty, or hungry).
(4) *Exercise for weight and shape reasons* (active in order to: be thin, burn calories, and for appearance reasons).

The EED has been shown to have satisfactory psychometric properties. In the validation study, EED discriminated significantly ($p < .001$) between patients and controls on Global scale, subscales and all single items, showed good internal consistency (Chronbach's alpha .90 in Global scale) and a satisfactory test-retest stability (Pearson's correlation factor = .86 on Global score) [9]. The subscale on compulsive exercise showed the strongest correlation with eating disorder symptomatology (r (441) = 0.70, $p < .01$). In the current study, Cronbach's alpha at admission was .86 for the EED global score, and subscale values were in the range of .65 to .90. At follow-up, the respective values were .94 (global score) and .75 to .94 (subscales). Three versions of the EED were used in the study. Despite some small changes to the wording across the revised versions, the meaning of the content has remained unchanged. Version 2 of the EED included three questions investigating the frequency, intensity, and duration of exercise, all of which have been validated and used elsewhere [21]. Due to differences in the way amount of exercise was reported in Versions 1 and 2 of the EED [9, 22], these quantitative measures are not presented in this article. During the study, the EED global score was used to predict BMI at outcome and follow-up, and the subscale on compulsive exercise was used as a predictor variable in the analyses using EDI-2 as the main outcome measure.

Disturbed body image

The Body Attitude Test (BAT) [23] is a short self-report questionnaire addressing subjective body experience and the attitude that a person with eating disorders has towards their body. It is a self-report measure with 20 items measured on a six-point response scale from *never* to *always.* The items are divided into four subscales: (1) negative appreciation of body size, (2) lack of familiarity with one's own body, (3) general dissatisfaction, and (4) a rest factor with two items which is not considered a separate subscale. The BAT has shown good validity and reliability [23, 24]. Cronbach's alpha values at admission and follow-up for BAT sum score were .92 and .96, while the respective values for the *lack of familiarity with one's own body* subscale were .82 and .92. The BAT has been found to be a significant predictor of changes in EDI-2 from admission to discharge, and most of the predictive value was represented by the BAT subscale on lack of familiarity with one's own body [18]. Therefore, the BAT sum score and *lack of familiarity with one's own body* subscale were respectively selected as covariates for the outcome variables BMI and EDI-2.

Eating disorder symptoms

The Eating Disorder Inventory (EDI-2) [25] is a widely used self-report tool with 91 items and 11 subscales, covering eating disorder symptoms, attitudes, and behaviours. EDI-2 does not cover exercise-related issues. EDI-2 has been validated in Nordic samples [26, 27]. Cronbach's alpha values at admission and follow-up were .95 and .98. The EDI-2 sum scores were one of the outcome measures, and EDI-2 was included as covariate in the analyses with BMI as outcome measure.

General psychopathology

The Symptom Checklist 90 revised version (SCL-90R) [28] was used to measure general psychopathology. The SCL-90R is a validated self-report tool with 90 items divided into 11 subscales [29]. In the study, we only report the mean score of the severity index. Cronbach's alpha values at admission and follow-up were .97 and .99. The mean scores of the SCL-90R were included as a covariate in both models.

Depression

The Beck Depression Inventory (BDI) [30] is a validated self-report inventory with 21 questions measuring the severity of depression. The BDI global score was included as a covariate in both models. Cronbach's alpha value at admission was .89.

Interpersonal problems

The Inventory of Interpersonal Problems (IIP-64) [31] was used as a measure of interpersonal problems. The IIP-64 is a validated self-report inventory consisting of 64 items and eight subscales. Cronbach's alpha values were .96 at admission and follow-up. The mean scores of the IIP-64 were included as covariates.

Body mass index

BMI is calculated using the following formula: kg/m^2. A BMI of 20.0 was the target BMI in the inpatient unit. During treatment, participants were weighed in the morning before breakfast, while wearing only undergarments. At follow-up, body weight was self-reported. When using BMI as the outcome measure, analyses were performed for all underweight patients (admission BMI ≤18.5). The BMI for the whole sample was included as a covariate in the analyses with EDI-2 as an outcome measure. Weight gain during treatment for eating disorders is especially associated with AN. To provide additional information, separate analyses including only AN participants were performed.

Statistical analysis

The Kolmogorov-Smirnov test confirmed normality for the EED global scores at admission, discharge, and follow-up ($D(77) = .066 - .080$, $ps = .200$). The following analyses were performed: descriptive analyses, one-way ANOVA with the Bonferroni post-hoc test, paired sample *t*-test, and Cronbach's alpha. Effect sizes were calculated using Cohen's *d* [32]. Linear mixed model regression analyses were used to investigate the predictive value of the EED. Due to the small size of the diagnostic groups and the lack of significant differences in the EED global scores between groups at admission ($p = .89$), these analyses were performed for the whole sample. In the linear mixed models regression analyses, three models were explored and the results reported: (1) the null model represented the intercept values of the outcome measure and its variances, (2) Model 1 included the covariate of particular interest (i.e. the EED score), and (3) in Model 2 values were adjusted for all significant covariates. R-squared was calculated based on differences of variance between the null model and the other models, and R-squared, the likelihood ratio test (LR test), change in variances, and log-likelihood values were used as measures of model improvement. The intraclass correlation

(ICC), which represents the within-cluster correlation, is reported. Significance levels were set at $p < .05$, and data were analysed and presented for the whole sample and subgroups using SPSS Version 21 and Stata/MP 13 software.

Missing data

In total, the amount of missing data in the returned self-report questionnaires was less than 5 %. Missing data were handled in two ways. Missing single items were replaced by a calculated mean for the specific subscales for each participant. Admission data were completely missing for two participants, while for one participant the discharge data were missing. Data at one or two measure points were missing for eight other participants. Evaluation of the data showed that the missing data were missing at random, and therefore multiple imputations could be performed to replace them.

Results

Study aim 1 – change of measures

The mean values of the EED, global score, and subscales improved significantly (*ps* < .01 to *ps* < .001) from admission to discharge and admission to follow-up. The effect size was large for the global score (.93) and medium to large for the subscales (.49–.84). From discharge to follow-up, the changes were smaller, yet significant for the EED subscales: *compulsive exercise, awareness of bodily signals*, and *exercise for weight and shape reasons* (*ps* < .05). The effect sizes were small (.26–.32).

Significant changes ($p < .001$) were observed for the measures of general psychopathology, body image, and eating pathology across the three time points. Effect sizes from admission to follow-up were large for the BDI (1.00), medium to large for EDI-2, the BAT sum score, the *lack of familiarity with one's own body* subscale, and the SCL-90R (.74, .66, .73, and .63, respectively), and between low to medium for the IIP-64 (0.43). From discharge to follow-up, there were significant changes only in the BAT sum score, with small effect size (.29). No significant changes were observed for the EDI-2, BDI, SCL-90R, and IIP-64 during the follow-up period. The scores at admission, discharge, and follow-up are summarized in Table 2.

Study aim 2

EDI-2 as outcome measure

The initial analyses indicated multicollinearity between the EED global score and BAT sum score. These global scores were therefore replaced with the EED subscale on compulsive exercise and the BAT subscale on lack of familiarity with one's own body as covariates. In the null model, EDI-2 scores from admission to follow-up improved significantly ($p < .001$), but with large values of unexplained variance. Model 1 showed model improvement, R-squared = 47.5 %, and the EED compulsive exercise was a significant predictor ($z = 15.22$, $p < .001$). In Model 2, all covariates except BMI were found to contribute significantly ($p < .001$) and R-squared = 82.3 %. In this model, the EED compulsive exercise score remained significant, but with lower values (z = 2.92, $p < .01$). The reduced z-value indicated shared content between EED with the other covariates, but also accounted for unique explained variance. Significant LR test ($p < .001$) as well as reduced variance and log-likelihood values, and increased R-squared all indicated a further improvement of model fit to the data. The addition of a patient-specific random slope indicated further model improvement (LR test, $p < .01$). The results for the models are presented in Table 3.

BMI as outcome measure (admission BMI (<18.5, n = 56))

No signs of multicollinearity were present in these analyses, and the EED global score and BAT sum score were used as covariates in the models. Model 1 showed improved model fit to the data and R-squared = 24.2 %. The EED global score was a significant predictor of change in BMI ($z = -7.29$, $p < .001$). The negative z-value indicated an association between reduced EED global score and increased BMI. In Model 2, non-significant

Table 2 EED scores (global score and subscales) for the whole sample at admission, discharge and follow-up and differences from admission to follow-up

	Admission $N = 78$		Discharge $N = 78$		Follow-up $N = 78$		Diff[1] A - F	Effect size A - F Cohen's d^3
	Mean (SD)	95 % CI	Mean (SD)	95 % CI	Mean (SD)	95 % CI	*t p*-value[2]	
EED Global score	3.03 (0.81)	2.83; 3.21	2.34 (0.86)	2.15; 2.54	2.13 (1.08)	1.89; 2.37	6.90***	.93
EED Compulsive	3.43 (1.18)	3.16; 3.70	2.68 (1.28)	2.40; 2.98	2.33 (1.43)	2.03; 2.67	6.80***	.84
EED Positive and healthy	2.31 (1.12)	2.05; 2.56	1.55 (0.93)	1.33;1.74	1.77 (1.07)	1.52; 2.00	3.58**	.49
EED Bodily signals	2.50 (0.98)	2.27; 2.71	1.96 (0.89)	1.75; 2.15	1.63 (1.13)	1.35, 1.86	6.17***	.82
EED Weight and shape	3.53 (1.24)	3.30; 3.86	2.94 (1.26)	2.64; 3.21	2.59 (1.47)	2.27; 2.93	5.94***	.69

[1]Paired sample t-test from admission to follow-up A: Admission, F: Follow-up
[2]*P*-values: * $p < .05$, ** $p < .01$, and *** $p < .001$. [3]Cohens *d*: Small effect size = .20, medium = .50, and large = .80

Table 3 Random intercept models with EDI-2 as outcome measure for the whole sample

Fixed part	Null model			Model 1			Model 2		
	Coefficient (SE)	z-value p-value[3]	95 % CI	Coefficient (SE)	z-value p-value[3]	95 % CI	Coefficient (SE)	z-value p-value[3]	95 % CI
Intercept	90.66 (4.25)	21.32***	82.33; 98.99	18.56 (5.69)	3.26**	7.38; 29.72	-3.95 (4.08)	-0.97	11.95; 4.03
EED compulsive				25.55 (1.68)	15.22***	22.25; 28.83	4.58 (1.57)	2.92**	1.50; 7.66
BAT familiarity							1.18 (0.30)	3.93***	0.59; 1.77
BDI sum score							1.09 (0.19)	5.75***	0.72; 1.47
SCL-90R mean score							12.15 (4.05)	3.00**	4.20; 20.10
IIP-64 mean score							13.23 (3.81)	3.48**	5.77; 20.70
Random part									
[1]ψ variance	927.42			548.36			126.65		
[2]θ variance	1447.78			695.34			294.33		
Derived estimates									
R-squared				47.5			82.28		
ICC	0.39						0.30		
Log likelihood	-1225.35			-1145.06			-1029.47		

EED Exercise and Eating Disorders, *BAT* Body Attitude Test, *BDI* Beck depression Inventory, SCL-90R: Symptom checklist revised, IIP-64: Inventory of interpersonal problems
[1]ψ Variance: Variance between patients. [2]θ Variance: Variance within observations in patients
ICC Intraclass correlation. [3]*P* values: * $p < .05$, ** $p < .01$, and *** $p < .001$

covariates (EDI-2, SCL-90, and IIP-64) were removed. Each of these variables was separately included in the model once more, without any change in significance level. Additional significant covariates retained in Model 2 included BAT sum score ($p < .001$) and BDI ($p < .01$), and R-squared = 36.5 %. The EED global score continued to be a significant predictor in Model 2 ($z = -5.78$, $p < .001$). Adjusted for the other covariates, the z-value of the EED was attenuated by 1.51, indicating some shared content of the measures, but also confirmed the importance of the EED as a unique and significant predictor of improvement in BMI. Reduced variance and log-likelihood, increased R-squared, and significant LR test ($p < .001$) all confirmed improvement in the model fit to the data. Inclusion of a patient specific slope did not improve any of the models significantly. Additional analyses of the AN group showed almost similar values to those in the whole underweight group. The results of the models for the whole underweight group and the AN group are presented in Table 4. The values confirmed that Model 2 provides the best fit to the data.

Discussion

Our results showed significant improvement across different dimensions of attitudes towards compulsive exercise in the patient cohort during inpatient treatment and follow-up. Overall, significant changes were either maintained or continued to show additional improvement at follow-up. Further, the results demonstrated that improvements in these compulsive exercise dimensions significantly predicted the course of the illness, as measured by the EDI-2 and BMI. Regarding BMI as outcome measure, additional analyses of the AN group showed almost similar results to those for the whole underweight group.

Although different measures were used, the positive change found in attitudes towards compulsive exercise during treatment is consistent with earlier research [8, 14]. Our follow-up data are the first evidence of show how such attitudes develop in the course following discharge from inpatient treatment. The improvements were significant in three out of four subscales of EED and in the BAT sum score, compared to no changes in other measurements.

Meyer and colleagues [4] propose that weight and shape issues, regulation of negative affect and rigidity, and perceived negative consequences when exercise is restricted or stopped are factors that should be investigated in research directed towards exercise in eating disorders. These factors are in accordance with the view that qualitative measures of excessive exercise are clinically most important [3]. Our research has been conducted in accordance with these recommendations and perspective. The lack of other long-term follow-up studies investigating attitudes towards compulsive exercise limited our ability to compare our findings to existing research directly. However, our results indicate that changes in attitudes towards compulsive exercise during treatment and follow-up may prove to be a beneficial factor that would facilitate treatment progress and outcome. Similar trends have been found in other studies that have reported results during treatment [15–17]. Two studies with comparable treatment settings were

Table 4 Random intercept models, BMI as outcome measure for patients with BMI ≤ 18.5 at admission ($n = 56$) and AN patients ($n = 46$)

Fixed part	Null model			Model 1			Model 2		
	Null model AN[a]			**Model 1 AN**			**Model 2 AN**		
Intercept	Coefficient (SE)	*z*-value *p*-value[3]	95 % CI	Coefficient (SE)	*z*-value *p*-value[3]	95 % CI	Coefficient (SE)	*z*-value *p*-value[3]	95 % CI
BMI	18.53 (0.28)	67.86***	19.04; 20.18	21.80 (0.49)	44.92***	20.86; 22.76	20.66 (0.52)	33.79***	19.64; 21.68
	18.33 (0.25)	**72.63*** **	**17.84; 18.83**	**21.83 (0.59)**	**36.72*** **	**20.67; 23.00**	**20.68 (0.61)**	**33.90*** **	**19.48; 21.87**
EED global score				-1.37 (0.19)	-7.29***	-1.73, -1.00	-1.67 (0.29)	-5.78***	-2.24; -1.10
				-1.45 (0.23)	**-6.34*** **	**-1.90; -1.00**	**-1.82 (0.34)**	**-5.34*** **	**-2.49; -1.15**
BAT sum score							0.07 (0.01)	4.85***	0.04; 0.10
							0.08 (0.02)	**4.85*** **	**0.05; 0.11**
BDI sum score							-0.10 (0.02)	-4.96***	-0.14; -0.06
							-0.11(0.24)	**-4.60*** **	**-0.16; -0.06**
Random part									
[1]ψ variance	0.00				0.00		0.27		
	0.00				**0.00**		**0.31**		
[2]θ variance	7.49				5.68		4.49		
	8.34				**6.39**		**4.88**		
Derived estimates									
R-squared					24.2		36.5		
					23.5		**37.8**		
ICC	0.00				0.00		0.06		
	0.00				**0.00**		**0.06**		
Log likelihood	-405.1				-382.0		-366.9		
	-324.9				**-307.4**		**-293.7**		

[a]All values of AN patients are written in bold
EED, Exercise and Eating Disorders, *BAT* Body Attitude Test, *BDI*: Beck depression Inventory
[1]ψ Variance: Variance between patients. [2]θ Variance: Variance within observations in patients
ICC Intraclass correlation. [3]*p*-values: * $p < .05$, ** $p < .01$, and *** $p < .001$

found [8, 14]. Despite differences in sample sizes and sample characteristics, as well as some inconsistencies in definitions and measurements, these studies found a significant association between reduced exercise dependency and reduced eating disorder symptoms during treatment. The longitudinal design of our study has built upon and extended earlier research, and the main findings emphasize the importance of attitudes towards compulsive exercise for the outcome of eating disorder symptoms following discharge.

To date, researchers have directed more attention towards the relationship between weight gain and exercise interventions in treatment programmes for patients with AN. The results of their research have indicated that the incorporation of exercise interventions in treatment does not have an adverse effect on achieving weight gain [15–17]. Our findings support the existing literature, and the follow-up data strengthen and extend the knowledge in the field.

Relapse after inpatient treatment is common and it has been suggested that it is important to take exercise-related elements into consideration [11, 12]. Moola and colleagues [15] have stated that if patients' exercise beliefs are allowed to remain unchanged during inpatient treatment that might increase their risk of continued unhealthy exercise after discharge. The extent to which improvements in negative attitudes towards compulsive exercise persist following discharge has not been reported previously, nor have earlier studies investigated the predictive significance of attitudes towards compulsive exercise on eating pathology following treatment.

Compulsive exercise is a complex phenomenon. In our study, different domains of attitudes towards exercise were shown to be significant predictors of changes in eating pathology and BMI. In the first model, using the EDI-2, the compulsive exercise subscale of the EED was used as covariate and the results indicated a significant association between compulsive elements of exercise and eating disorder symptoms. In the second model, using BMI as the outcome variable, the EED global score significantly predicted weight gain, thus highlighting the relationship between BMI and various dimensions of attitudes towards exercise. It is important to note that these values were almost similar in the whole underweight group and in additional analyses which included only AN participants. The proportion of explained variance increased in both models when other measures were added as covariates, from 47.5 to 82.3 % (EDI-2 as outcome measure) and 24.2 to 36.5 % (BMI as outcome measure). These findings illustrate the importance of the other covariates, yet exercise remained a significant predictor, indicating that addressing compulsive exercise and attitudes towards exercise in the treatment of eating disorders may be a useful intervention.

Strengths and limitations

The study was a naturalistic cohort study investigating a medium-size sample of female inpatients with eating disorders. All admitted patients were invited to participate. None of the participants were excluded due to symptoms or comorbidity, and this has probably improved the representativeness of our sample and generalizability of our findings to other inpatient settings. The inclusion of follow-up data is a notable strength and adds significantly to existing knowledge of longer term outcomes and compulsive exercise.

However, it is necessary to consider several limitations of the study. The study was a cohort study with no control group and it is uncertain whether the findings related specifically to our treatment programme, which included a physical activity component, or whether they indicate a general pattern of associations between various aspects of eating disorders over time. All participants and only females were recruited from the same inpatient unit, and the findings may not be generalizable to outpatient or other treatment settings. The ability to generalize is also limited by the fact that the EED has only been validated in women. The follow-up of 67.2 % is a weakness, yet no baseline differences were found for age, BMI, EED sum global scores, and EDI-2 scores, or for discharge scores for EED and EDI-2 between participants compared to non-participants. Great variety in lengths of follow-up may also affect the results. Trained and specialized clinicians provided diagnostic quality, yet the diagnostic procedures did not include structured interviews. A transdiagnostic sample was used for the majority of the analyses in the study, due to a lack of diagnostic group differences in EED scores at baseline. Our results might have been influenced by the small sample size of BN and EDNOS participants.

The quantity dimension of exercise was not reported in the study, which may be considered a limitation. Due to differences in how this behaviour has been reported in EED Versions 1 and 2, we decided not to include this information. However, in the validation study an association was found between EED scores and high-level exercise (frequency, intensity, and duration). The majority of patients who were high-level exercisers had high EED scores, whereas among controls the majority of such high-level exercisers had low EED scores. From a clinical perspective, defining the level of exercise as harmful or not should also be evaluated in relation to somatic conditions (e.g. degree of underweight), fitness level (e.g. athletes), and former exercise behaviour [9].

Admission time showed great variation in the study, and prolonged admissions were mainly due to the time necessary to restore weight in severely underweight AN patients, but also related to symptoms of comorbidity. The quiet long admission time may limit the generalizability of the results compared to other shorter inpatient treatment program. There was only one measurement following discharge and the duration of the follow-up interval varied across individual participants. It is important for our results to be replicated in a sample that is large enough to examine different diagnostic groups and different follow-up periods.

So far, there have been no published reports of randomized control trials in which exercise intervention in an inpatient treatment programme has been compared to no exercise intervention, and this makes it difficult to draw conclusions about the impact of exercise interventions. However, the findings in our study show the importance of attitudes towards compulsive exercise for outcome in participants with eating disorders and support the relevance of assessing and addressing attitudes towards compulsive exercise during treatment.

Conclusions

We found a significant reduction in thoughts and attitudes towards compulsive exercise during treatment and that these changes predict outcome, as indicated by reduced eating disorder pathology and increased BMI for underweight participants. The results of the study have implications for future research. In order to evaluate the impact of exercise interventions on outcome, it is important to investigate gender differences, to include a control group and to investigate the relationship to both quality and quantity dimensions.

Abbreviations

AN: anorexia nervosa; BAT: Body Attitude Test; BDI: Beck Depression Inventory; BMI: body mass index; BN: bulimia nervosa; DSM: diagnostic and statistical manual of mental disorders; EDI: Eating Disorder Inventory; EDNOS: eating disorder not otherwise specified; EED: Exercise and Eating Disorder; ICC: intraclass correlation; IIP: Inventory of Interpersonal Problems; LR: likelihood ratio; NPMP: Norwegian Psychomotor Physiotherapy; SCL: Symptom Checklist.

Competing interests

The authors are responsible for the writing this paper and its content. No conflicts of interest are reported.

Authors' contributions

MD was responsible for conducting the study and ØR and SB has contributed through the whole process. The manuscript has been written collaboratively. UR provided statistical support. All authors have read and approved the final manuscript.

Acknowledgements

We wish to thank research staff member Hilde Kristin Vatterholm for her assistance and good work with the data collection. We also extend our gratitude to Catriona Turner for language checking of this manuscript and Deborah L. Reas, PhD, for checking an earlier version of the manuscript.

Funding

The Liaison Committee for Central Norway Regional Health Authority and the Norwegian University of Science and Technology (NTNU).

Author details

[1]Department of Neuroscience, Faculty of Medicine, Norwegian University of Science and Technology, 7491 Trondheim, Norway. [2]Eating Disorder Unit, Department of Psychiatry, Levanger Hospital, Hospital Trust Nord-Trøndelag, NO-7600 Levanger, Norway. [3]Regional Department for Eating Disorders, Division of Mental Health and Addiction, Oslo University Hospital, Oslo, Norway. [4]Division of Mental Health and Addiction, Institute of Clinical Medicine, University of Oslo, Levanger, Norway. [5]Department of Research and Development, Levanger Hospital, Hospital Trust Nord-Trøndelag, NO-7600 Levanger, Norway.

References

1. American Psychiatric Association. Diagnostic and statistical manual of mental disorders. 4th ed. Washington: American Psychiatric Association; 1994.
2. American Psychiatric Association. Diagnostic and statistical manual of mental disorders. 5th ed. Washington: American Psychiatric Association; 2014.
3. Adkins EC, Keel PK. Does "excessive" or "compulsive" best describe exercise as a symptom of bulimia nervosa? Int J Eat Disord. 2005;38:24–9.
4. Meyer C, Taranis L, Goodwin H, Haycraft E. Compulsive exercise and eating disorders. Eur Eat Disord Rev. 2011;19:174–89.
5. Meyer C, Taranis L. Exercise in the eating disorders: terms and definitions. Eur Eat Disord Rev. 2011;19:169–73.
6. Dalle GR, Calugi S, Marchesini G. Compulsive exercise to control shape or weight in eating disorders: prevalence, associated features, and treatment outcome. Compr Psychiatry. 2008;49(4):346–52.
7. Shroff H, Reba L, Thornton LM, Tozzi F, Klump KL, Berrettini WH, et al. Features associated with excessive exercise in women with eating disorders. Int J Eat Disord. 2006;39:454–61.
8. Calogero RM, Pedrotty KN. The practice and process of healthy exercise: an investigation of the treatment of exercise abuse in women with eating disorders. Eat Disord. 2004;12:273–91.
9. Danielsen M, Bjornelv S, Ro O. Validation of the exercise and eating disorders questionnaire. Int J Eat Disord. 2015;48:983–93.
10. Penas-Lledo E, Vaz Leal FJ, Waller G. Excessive exercise in anorexia nervosa and bulimia nervosa: relation to eating characteristics and general psychopathology. Int J Eat Disord. 2002;31:370–5.
11. Strober M, Freeman R, Morrell W. The long-term course of severe anorexia nervosa in adolescents: survival analysis of recovery, relapse, and outcome predictors over 10-15 years in a prospective study. Int J Eat Disord. 1997;22:339–60.
12. Carter JC, Blackmore E, Sutandar-Pinnock K, Woodside DB. Relapse in anorexia nervosa: a survival analysis. Psychol Med. 2004;34:671–9.
13. Gummer R, Giel KE, Schag K, Resmark G, Junne FP, Becker S, et al. High levels of physical activity in anorexia nervosa: a systematic review. Eur Eat Disord Rev. 2015;23:333–44.
14. Bratland-Sanda S, Sundgot-Borgen J, Ro O, Rosenvinge JH, Hoffart A, Martinsen EW. Physical activity and exercise dependence during inpatient treatment of longstanding eating disorders: an exploratory study of excessive and non-excessive exercisers. Int J Eat Disord. 2010;43:266–73.
15. Moola FJ, Gairdner SE, Amara C. Exercise in the care of patients with anorexia nervosa: a systematic review of the literature. Ment Health Phys Act. 2013;6:59–68.
16. Zunker C, Mitchell JE, Wonderlich SA. Exercise interventions for women with anorexia nervosa: a review of the literature. Int J Eat Disord. 2011;44:579–84.
17. Hausenblas HA, Cook BJ, Chittester NI. Can exercise treat eating disorders? Exerc Sport Sci Rev. 2008;36:43–7.
18. Danielsen M, Ro O. Changes in body image during inpatient treatment for eating disorders predict outcome. Eat Disord. 2012;20:261–75.
19. Ekerholt K. Aspects of psychiatric and psychosomatic physiotherapy. Oslo University College, Faculty of Health Sciences, 2010; HiO rapport 3. ISBN 978-82-579-4721-7.
20. Meurle-Hallberg K, Armelius K. Associations between physical and psychological problems in a group of patients with stress-related behavior and somatoform disorders. Physiother Theory Pract. 2006;22:17–31.
21. Kurtze N, Rangul V, Hustvedt BE, Flanders WD. Reliability and validity of self-reported physical activity in the Nord-Trondelag Health Study: HUNT 1. Scand J Public Health. 2008;36:52–61.
22. Danielsen M, Bratberg GH, Ro O. A pilot study of a new assessment of physical activity in eating disorder patients. Eat Weight Disord. 2012;17:e70–7.
23. Probst M, Van Coppenolle H, Vandereycken W. The body attitude test for patients with an eating disorder: psychometric characteristics of a new questionnaire. Eat Disord. 1995;3:133–45.
24. Probst M, Pieters G, Vanderlinden J. Evaluation of body experience questionnaires in eating disorders in female patients (AN/BN) and nonclinical participants. Int J Eat Disord. 2008;41:657–65.
25. Garner DM, Olmsted MP, Polivy J. Development and validation of a multidimensional Eating Disorder Inventory for anorexia and bulimia. Int J Eat Disord. 1983;2:15–34.
26. Clausen L, Rokkedal K, Rosenvinge JH. Validating the eating disorder inventory (EDI-2) in two Danish samples: a comparison between female eating disorder patients and females from the general population. Eur Eat Disord Rev. 2009;17:462–7.
27. Nevonen L, Clinton D, Norring C. Validating the EDI-2 in three Swedish female samples: eating disorders patients, psychiatric outpatients and normal controls. Nord J Psychiatry. 2006;60:44–50.
28. Derogatis LR, Lipman RS, Covi L. SCL-90: an outpatient psychiatric rating scale – preliminary report. Psychopharmacol Bull. 1973;9:13–28.
29. Derogatis LR. The SCL-90-R: Administration, scoring, and procedures. Manual-II. Towson: Clin Psychometric Res; 1983. p. 14–5.
30. Beck AT, Beamesderfer A. Assessment of depression: the depression inventory. Mod Probl Pharmacopsychiatry. 1974;7:151–69.
31. Alden LE, Wiggins JS, Pincus AL. Construction of circumplex scales for the Inventory of Interpersonal Problems. J Pers Assess. 1990;55:521–36.
32. Cohen J. Statistical power analysis for the behavioral sciences. 2nd ed. Hillsdale: Lawrence Erlbaum; 1988.

18

Emotion regulation difficulties in anorexia nervosa: associations with improvements in eating psychopathology

Marsha Rowsell[1], Danielle E. MacDonald[2,3] and Jacqueline C. Carter[1*]

Abstract

Background: Difficulties with emotion regulation have been established as a core deficit in anorexia nervosa (AN). However, limited research has evaluated whether weight gain is associated with improvements in emotion regulation difficulties in AN and whether improvements in emotion regulation are associated with reductions in eating disorder psychopathology. The aims of this study were threefold: 1) to examine the nature and extent of emotion regulation difficulties in AN; 2) to determine whether these difficulties improved during intensive treatment for the eating disorder; and 3) to study whether improvements in emotion regulation were associated with improvements in eating disorder psychopathology.

Method: The participants were 108 patients who met DSM-IV-TR criteria for AN and were admitted to a specialized intensive treatment program. Self-report measures of eating disorder symptoms and difficulties with emotion regulation were administered at admission to and discharge from the program.

Results: Patients with the binge-purge subtype of AN reported greater difficulties with impulse control when upset and more limited access to emotion regulation strategies when experiencing negative emotions than those with the restricting subtype. Among those who completed treatment and became weight restored, improvements in emotion regulation difficulties were observed. Greater pre-to-post treatment improvements in emotional clarity and engagement in goal directed behaviours when upset were associated with greater reductions in eating disorder psychopathology during treatment.

Conclusions: These findings add to growing evidence suggesting that eating disorder symptoms may be related to emotion regulation difficulties in AN and that integrating strategies to address emotion regulation deficits may be important to improving treatment outcome in AN.

Keywords: Anorexia nervosa, Emotion regulation

Background

In her seminal writings, Bruch [1, 2] asserted that problems with emotion regulation, particularly difficulties differentiating and describing emotions, are a core deficit in anorexia nervosa (AN). Recently, a growing body of theoretical and empirical evidence suggests that emotion regulation deficits may play a key role in both the development and maintenance of AN [3–7]. Indeed, several authors have theorized that AN *is* a disorder of emotion regulation and that the symptoms of AN, such as dietary restriction, excessive exercise, and binge/purge behaviors, represent maladaptive attempts to regulate aversive emotional states [8–10].

In a recent review article, Lavender and colleagues [11] examined the research evidence for applying Gratz and Roemer's [12] multidimensional model of emotion dysregulation in conceptualizing emotion regulation difficulties in AN. This review uncovered the following findings: considerable evidence to support the application of this model in AN including evidence of broad deficits in adaptive emotion regulation skills in AN; some evidence of impulse control and distress tolerance

* Correspondence: jacquelinec@mun.ca
[1]Department of Psychology, Memorial University of Newfoundland, St. John's, NL A1B 3X9, Canada
Full list of author information is available at the end of the article

difficulties in AN; substantial evidence of emotion awareness deficits in AN; and some evidence of emotional avoidance in AN.

Indeed, a number of studies have found that difficulties with emotion regulation are associated with eating disorder psychopathology [7, 13]. High levels of negative emotionality have been shown to prospectively increase the risk of eating pathology [14, 15] and, in a recent meta-analysis, lack of adaptive emotion regulation strategies – particularly deficits in problem-solving skills, and greater use of avoidance, rumination and suppression – was associated with greater eating disorder psychopathology [16]. Further, there is evidence that characteristic anxious avoidance, both of emotions and of interpersonal situations that may trigger emotional experiences in AN, often predates the illness and persists after recovery [7, 17, 18].

Several recent studies have found evidence that emotion regulation difficulties may also play a role in the maintenance of AN. It has been consistently found that individuals with AN report greater impairments in emotion regulation compared to controls [19]. Specifically, AN has been shown to be associated with high vulnerability to dysregulated emotions including impaired abilities to experience and differentiate emotions, as well as difficulties with the attenuation and modulation of negative emotional states [19–21]. Individuals with AN have also been found to report higher levels of alexithymia (i.e., difficulty identifying and describing emotions) compared to healthy controls [22, 23]. Further, some research has shown that individuals with AN have greater levels of alexithymia than individuals with other eating disorders such as bulimia nervosa and binge eating disorder [23], suggesting a specific emotion-related deficit in AN rather than a general impairment related to eating disorders more broadly. In addition, several studies have found evidence of distress intolerance, that is, the inability to accept and withstand negative emotional experiences, particularly among those with the restricting subtype of AN [4, 17]. As observed by Lynch and colleagues [24], emotional overcontrol has been linked with social withdrawal, cognitive rigidity, reward insensitivity, strong needs for structure and symmetry, and clinical perfectionism – traits which have been shown to be common among individuals with AN, and which may function to perpetuate the disorder [6, 25, 26].

Studies that have examined differences in emotion regulation deficits between the two subtypes of AN have produced mixed results. In the restricting subtype of AN (AN-R), emotion regulation deficits tend to be characterized by emotional overcontrol, such as emotional inhibition and lack of emotion expression [27]. Certain symptoms of AN-R, such as dietary restriction or excessive exercise, may be conceptualized as maladaptive attempts to avoid emotional arousal and inhibit emotional expression. In support of this theory, Wildes and colleagues [10] found that emotion avoidance partially mediated the relationship between depressive symptoms and eating disorder psychopathology in AN, suggesting that eating disorder symptoms may function to regulate negative mood states. In contrast, the findings of another recent study did not support an emotional avoidance model of AN [28].

In the binge-purge subtype of AN (AN-BP), difficulties with emotion regulation tend to be characterized by impulsivity and difficulties inhibiting maladaptive behavior when experiencing negative emotions [21, 29]. Further, negative emotions have been shown to be a strong proximal trigger for binge eating and purging episodes in AN-BP [10]. Racine and Wildes [30] examined whether specific aspects of the psychopathology of acute AN were uniquely associated with particular types of emotion regulation difficulties. They found that, impulse control difficulties predicted unique variance in both binge eating and purging behaviors, over and above the effects of duration of illness, and depression and anxiety symptoms, respectively. Additionally, limited emotional awareness uniquely predicted the severity of eating disorder cognitions over and above duration of illness, and depression and anxiety symptoms. In another study of inpatients with AN, only one difference was found between patients with AN-R and AN-BP: AN-BP patients had higher impulsivity scores compared to those with AN-R [31]. Further research is needed to clarify differences between the two subtypes of AN with respect to emotion regulation deficits since this may have important potential treatment implications.

The relationship between low body weight in acute AN and emotion regulation difficulties remains unclear. Brockmeyer and colleagues [20] found that lower body mass index was associated with fewer emotion regulation difficulties in a sample of patients with acute AN, suggesting that low weight may function as a persistent but maladaptive means of over-regulating negative affect during the acute illness period. That is, low body weight may lower the frequency or intensity of negative emotions thereby functioning as a form of emotional avoidance. However, given the well-established negative impact of starvation on psychological functioning [32], it is also possible that weight restoration may improve emotion regulation abilities in AN. Only two studies to date have examined whether weight restoration is associated with improvements in emotion regulation in AN. Haynos and colleagues [31] found that difficulties with emotion regulation did not improve with weight restoration through specialized inpatient treatment although significant improvements in both general psychological distress and specific eating disorder psychopathology were found. Conversely, Ben-Porath, Federici, Wisniewski, and

Warren [33] found that problems with emotion regulation improved with weight restoration in AN through a specialized day treatment program that included two hours of dialectical behavioral therapy (DBT) skills training per week. However, because the treatment program in this study included DBT skills training, which is an empirically supported intervention for problems with emotion regulation, it is unknown whether the improvements in emotion regulation were related to skills training or to weight restoration. In addition, while Haynos and colleagues [31] studied a sample of individuals who were all diagnosed with AN, Ben-Porath and colleagues [33] recruited a mixed sample of individuals diagnosed with either AN (~35 %) or BN (~65 %). As such, participants in Ben-Porath study had a greater mean admission BMI than participants in Haynos and colleagues' [31] study, and not all participants in the former study were underweight, making it difficult to compare findings across the studies. Overall, however, it is clear that there is a lack of research with respect to the relationship between weight restoration, improvements eating disorder psychopathology, and changes in emotion regulation difficulties. As such, additional research on this topic is necessary in order to elucidate and clarify the nature of these relationships. In support of this, recently psychological science has shown a renewed interest in the area of study replication [34]. Indeed, researchers have coined replication "the cornerstone of science" [35], highlighting its importance in determining whether any given finding is a false positive or the result of sampling error or non-generalizable sample specific features [34, 35]. Thus, the current study aimed to replicate and extend research on difficulties with emotion regulation in AN.

Study aims and hypotheses

This study had three aims. The first aim was to replicate previous research by comparing patients with AN-R and AN-BP in terms of the nature and extent of difficulties with emotion regulation at the time of admission to intensive treatment using the Difficulties in Emotion Regulation Scale (DERS) which is based on Gratz and Roemer's multidimensional model of emotion regulation and dysregulation [12]. Given previous findings indicating greater impulsivity and more difficulties inhibiting maladaptive behaviors when experiencing negative emotions in AN-BP, it was hypothesized that those with AN-BP would report greater difficulties with emotion regulation overall, as well as greater difficulties with impulse control in particular. Because emotional overcontrol and associated traits have been observed to be common in AN-R, it was hypothesized that patients with the AN-R subtype would have greater difficulties with lack of emotion awareness and non-acceptance of emotions than those with AN-BP.

The second aim of this study was to replicate and extend the work of Haynos and colleagues [31] by examining whether the level of various difficulties with emotion regulation changed during intensive eating disorder treatment among those who successfully completed the program. Given that our program involves extensive psychological treatment including a group focused on enhancing emotion regulation skills, it was hypothesized that, even after controlling for the effects of weight gain across treatment, the overall level of difficulties with emotion regulation would improve from pre-treatment to post-treatment. A secondary exploratory aim was to examine whether there were improvements in the specific facets of emotion regulation difficulties measured by the DERS: awareness and clarity of emotions; emotion acceptance; ability to engage in goal-directed behaviors while experiencing negative emotions; tendency to engage in impulsive behaviors when upset; and access to emotion regulation strategies.

The final aim of this study was to examine whether changes in the various facets of emotion regulation difficulties were associated with changes in eating disorder psychopathology during treatment, after controlling for baseline level of negative affect and amount of weight gain achieved during treatment. Given previous findings suggesting that specific aspects of the psychopathology of AN were uniquely associated with particular types of emotion regulation difficulties, it was hypothesized that greater improvements in the various facets of emotion regulation would be associated with greater improvements in eating disorder psychopathology, even after controlling for the effects of baseline negative affect and weight gain during treatment.

Method

Participants and treatment

The participants were 108 consecutive patients who met *Diagnostic and Statistical Manual of Mental Disorders, Fourth Edition, Text Revision* (DSM-IV-TR) criteria for AN based on assessment using the Eating Disorder Examination (EDE) interview [36, 37]. All participants had a BMI ≤ 17.5 at admission to the program. See Table 1 for demographic and clinical characteristics of the sample. Participants were admitted to the hybrid inpatient/day treatment unit of the Eating Disorders Program at a large general hospital between 2010 and 2014. This program is a specialized hospital-based program operated by an interdisciplinary team consisting of psychiatrists, psychologists, nurses, dieticians, social workers, and occupational therapists. The program goals include medical stabilization, weight restoration, normalized eating through staff-supported meals, as well as eradication of binge eating, purging, and excessive exercise (citation omitted for blind review). Although the underlying orientation of the program is cognitive-

Table 1 Demographic and clinical characteristics of the sample ($N = 108$)

Characteristic	Mean (SD) or %
Female	96.3 %
Age	29.9 (10.9)
Ethnicity	
Caucasian	88.1 %
Asian	3.0 %
Other[a]	10.9 %
Marital Status	
Single	72.6 %
Married/Common-Law	22.6 %
Separated/Divorced	4.7 %
Employment Status	
Student	30.4 %
Employed	48.1 %
Unemployed	21.6 %
AN Subtype	
AN-R	41.5 %
AN-BP	58.5 %
Pre-treatment BMI	14.9 (1.4)
Binge episodes/month Pre-Treatment (AN-BP only)	12.3 (23.1)
Vomit episodes/month Pre-Treatment (AN-BP only)	37.9 (54.9)
Laxative episodes/month Pre-Treatment (AN-BP only)	10.6 (16.5)
Duration of Illness (Years)	10.6 (9.6)
Age of Onset	19.4 (7.7)
Length of Treatment (Weeks)	14.4 (7.1)
Weight Gain During Treatment (kg)	11.5 (6.1)

[a]Other reported ethnicities include Black, West Indian, East Indian, and Hispanic

behavioural, patients attend a variety of groups including interpersonal therapy, and DBT skills training. Once patients reach a BMI of approximately 18, they are transferred from inpatient to day attendance. For the present study, post-treatment BMI and weight were available for the 72 patients who completed the inpatient/day program and achieved a BMI ≥ 19.5. Questionnaire data were available for 53 of the 72 participants who completed treatment and achieved a BMI of at least 19.5. This study was approved by the UHN Research Ethics Board and all participants provided written informed consent to participate.

Assessment measures

Eating disorder psychopathology

The 36-item Eating Disorder Examination–Questionnaire (EDE-Q) was used as a measure of eating disorder psychopathology [38]. This questionnaire is based directly on the EDE interview and is comprised of four subscales (Shape Concern, Weight Concern, Eating Concern, and Dietary Restraint) that can be combined into one Global Score of eating disorder psychopathology ranging from 0 (low) to 6 (high). The EDE-Q has demonstrated good test-retest reliability and strong internal consistency [39]. The Cronbach's alpha for the Global Score in our sample was $\alpha = .91$ and $\alpha = .93$ at pre- and post-treatment, respectively. In addition, the EDE-Q contains items assessing the frequency of eating disorder behaviors including binge eating and compensatory behaviors.

Emotion regulation difficulties

The Difficulties in Emotion Regulation Scale (DERS) is a multidimensional 36-item self-report questionnaire that measures aspects of emotion dysregulation [12]. The DERS provides a total score and six subscale scores including: 1) lack of emotional clarity (Clarity); 2) lack of emotional awareness (Awareness); 3) non-acceptance of emotional responses (Non-acceptance); 4) Impulse control difficulties (Impulse); 5) difficulties engaging in goal directed behavior in the presence of negative emotions (Goals); and 6) limited access to emotion regulation strategies (Strategies). Each item is rated on a 5-point scale ranging from "almost never (0–10 %) to "almost always (91–100 %)". Reliability and validity of this instrument has been established [9]. In the current sample, Cronbach's alpha for the total scale was $\alpha = .96$, and for each of the six subscales it was $\alpha = .86$ (Clarity), $\alpha = .85$ (Awareness), $\alpha = .94$ (Non-Acceptance), $\alpha = .90$ (Impulse), $\alpha = .88$ (Goals), and $\alpha = .92$ (Strategies). At post-treatment, Cronbach's alpha for the total scale was $\alpha = .95$ and for each of the six subscales it was $\alpha = .91$, $\alpha = .89$, $\alpha = .93$, $\alpha = .85$, $\alpha = .91$, and $\alpha = .92$ respectively.

Procedure

Upon being admitted to the program, participants were assessed using the diagnostic items of the EDE interview [35] by a trained interviewer, and objective weight and height were measured. The validity and reliability of the EDE, including interrater reliability, have been well established and were not examined as part of the current study [40].

This information was used by the program psychologist or psychiatrist for diagnosis and subtyping. Prior to beginning the program, all participants completed the EDE-Q and the DERS. The treatment program was delivered as usual, and the EDE-Q and DERS were re-administered at the time of discharge.

Statistical analyses

To determine whether there were any baseline differences between treatment completers and non-completers, these two groups were compared on several pre-treatment variables. Specifically, a series of independent samples *t*-tests were conducted to determine whether treatment completers and non-completers differed on: (a) emotion regulation difficulties at admission; (b) frequency of binge eating episodes, self-induced vomiting episodes, and episodes of laxative misuse at admission; and (c) BMI at admission. To reduce the distributional skewness of behavioral episodes (binge, vomit, and laxative), univariate outliers (i.e., z = +/− 3.29) were identified and replaced with the next highest value in the distribution that was not an outlier [41]. This method corrected distributional problems. Lastly, a chi square test was conducted to examine whether completers and non-completers differed in terms of frequency of AN-subtypes.

In order to address our first aim, an analysis of variance (ANOVA) was conducted to compare the two AN subtypes (AN-R and AN-BP) on the total DERS score. Additionally, a multivariate analysis of variance (MANOVA) was conducted to compare the AN-R and AN-BP subtypes on the six DERS subscales. The overall multivariate effect, as well as the individual univariate effects, were examined.

Secondly, a mixed MANOVA was conducted for the subset of participants who completed treatment ($N = 53$) to evaluate: (a) whether difficulties in emotion regulation would significantly improve from pre-treatment to post-treatment; and (b) potential subtype by time interaction effects. Pre-to-post treatment changes in DERS subscale scores were calculated as change scores. Subsequently, a second mixed MANOVA was conducted to evaluate whether difficulties in emotion regulation would significantly improve from pre-to-post-treatment when controlling for the effect of weight gain during treatment. In this analysis, pre-to-post-treatment weight gain was included as a covariate.

Finally, the hypothesis that change in emotion regulation difficulties would be associated with change in eating disorder psychopathology was investigated using multiple regression analysis. For this analysis, the criterion variable was pre-to-post-treatment change in eating disorder psychopathology as measured by the Global EDE-Q score, and the predictor variables were change in each of the DERS subscales pre-to-post-treatment. Initially we had planned to include baseline anxiety and depression symptoms, as measured by the Brief Symptom Inventory (BSI) [42], and weight gain during treatment, calculated as a change score, as covariates in this regression analysis. However, because we found that change in EDE-Q Global score was not significantly related to the level of anxiety and depression symptoms at pre-treatment ($r = .05$, $p = .72$) or to weight gain during treatment ($r = .11$, $p = .43$), the analyses were conducted without controlling for these variables. First, a series of univariate regression analyses were conducted to determine whether improvement in each facet of emotion regulation was associated with improvement in eating disorder psychopathology across treatment. Based on the results of these separate univariate regressions, a stepwise multiple regression analysis was then conducted with all six DERS subscales included as potential predictors. Based on the results of this model, a second multiple regression analysis was performed, including only the predictors that provided a significant contribution to the initial stepwise model, entered together at the same step.

Results

Comparisons between completers and Non-completers

With respect to potential differences between program completers and non-completers, there were no statistically significant differences between these two groups on baseline DERS Goals, $t(106) = .07$, $p = .94$; Impulse, $t(106) = 1.38$, $p = .17$; Awareness, $t(106) = .07$, $p = .94$; Strategies, $t(106) = 1.61$, $p = .11$; Clarity, $t(106) = 1.35$, $p = .18$; Non-acceptance, $t(106) = .62$, $p = .54$; and total, $t(106) = 1.20$, $p = .23$ scores. Mean subscale and total DERS scores were comparable, though somewhat higher, than previous reports of AN samples [e.g., 30, 31]. Furthermore, completers and non-completers did not significantly differ in terms of baseline frequency of binge eating, $t(59) = .29$, $p = .78$, or self-induced vomiting, $t(59) = 1.15$, $p = .26$. However, non-completers reported significantly more episodes of laxative misuse at baseline than completers, $t(59) = 2.59$, $p = .01$. Moreover, completers and non-completers did not differ significantly in terms of AN subtype, $\chi 2$ (1) = 3.60, $p = .06$. Finally, completers and non-completers did not significantly differ in term of baseline BMI, $t(106) = -1.87$, $p = .07$. Overall, these findings suggest that there were few meaningful pre-existing differences between completers and non-completers. See Table 2 for means and standard deviations of pre-treatment variables for completers versus noncompleters.

Subtype comparisons

In accordance with our first hypothesis, there was a significant difference with respect to baseline emotion regulation difficulties, as measured by the DERS total subscale, between AN-R and AN-BP subtypes, $F(1, 104) = 9.28$, $p = .003$, $R^2 = .08$. Additionally, significant differences in baseline emotion regulation difficulties, as measured by DERS subscales, were yielded between the AN-R and AN-BP subtypes, Wilks's $\lambda = .83$, $F(6, 99) = 3.38$, $p = .004$. Examination of the univariate effects indicated that the AN-BP subtype exhibited significantly greater impairments with respect to the Impulse subscale, $F(1,104) = 16.63$, $p < .001$, $R^2 = .14$, and Strategies subscale, $F(1,104) = 10.48$, $p = .002$, $R^2 = .09$. This indicates that, when experiencing negative emotions, patients with the AN-BP subtype reported greater difficulties with impulse control and more limited access to emotion regulation strategies than those with the AN-R subtype. There were no significant group differences with

Table 2 Means and standard deviations of pre-treatment variables for completers ($N = 72$) and non-completers ($N = 36$)

Variable	Mean (SD) Completers	Non-Completers
DERS-Goals	18.99 (4.75)	19.06 (5.08)
DERS-Impulse	16.60 (6.64)	18.52 (7.20)
DERS-Awareness	20.97 (5.23)	21.06 (6.20)
DERS-Strategies	25.53 (8.63)	28.44 (9.31)
DERS-Clarity	16.40 (4.51)	17.72 (5.29)
DERS Non-Acceptance	20.01 (7.06)	20.94 (7.98)
DERS-Total	118.50 (26.42)	125.75 (34.91)
Binge episodes/month (AN-BP)	13.86 (30.35)	25.46 (63.79)
Vomit episodes/month (AN-BP)	33.58 (55.86)	54.58 (82.82)
Laxative episodes/month (AN-BP)	7.11 (16.00)	24.80 (50.61)
BMI	15.11 (1.33)	14.56 (1.54)

Note. DERS = difficulties in emotion regulation scale

respect to the remaining DERS subscales, $ps > .05$. See Table 3 for these DERS subscale scores by subtype, as well as DERS total scores (which were not included in the model but are provided in the table for descriptive purposes).

Pre-to-post treatment analyses

In accordance with our second hypothesis, the results from our first mixed MANOVA showed an overall multivariate effect of time on participants' emotion regulation difficulties from pre-treatment to post-treatment, Wilks's $\lambda = .52$, $F(6, 46) = 7.01$, $p < .001$. Given that the multivariate effect of time on emotion regulation difficulties was statistically significant, univariate effects were examined. The univariate effects for time indicated significant differences for each of the DERS subscale change scores from pre-treatment to post-treatment, indicating that across subtypes, participants made significant changes over time on all six of the DERS subscales: (1) Goals, $F(1, 51) = 4.94$, $p = .03$; (2) Impulse, $F(1, 51) = 26.50$, $p < .001$; (3) Awareness, $F(1, 51) = 16.18$, $p < .001$; (4) Strategies, $F(1, 51) = 10.06$, $p < .01$; (5) Clarity, $F(1, 51) = 15.51$, $p < .001$; and (6) Non-Acceptance, $F(1, 51) = 5.51$, $p = .02$. Additionally, the multivariate interaction effect of subtype and time was statistically significant, Wilks's $\lambda = .75$, $F(6,46) = 2.52$, $p = .03$, indicating that there were significant differences between AN-R and AN-BP in terms of degree of improvement in emotion regulation during treatment. The univariate effects indicated a significant group by time interaction on the Impulse subscale, $F(1, 51) = 13.71$, $p = .001$. Examination of the means indicated that AN-BP improved more during treatment than AN-R, with respect to the ability to inhibit impulsive behaviors when experiencing negative emotions. See Table 4 for these DERS subscale change scores by subtype, as well as DERS total change scores (which were not included in the model but are provided in the table for descriptive purposes).

When pre-to-post treatment weight gain was included as a covariate in our second mixed MANOVA, there was no longer a multivariate effect of time on emotion regulation difficulties from pre-treatment to post-treatment, Wilks's $\lambda = .85$, $F(6, 45) = 1.32$, $p = .27$, indicating that across subtypes, patients did not exhibit overall improvements in emotion regulation after controlling for the effects of weight gain. However, the multivariate interaction effect of subtype by time remained statistically significant after controlling for the effects of weight gain, Wilks's $\lambda = .75$, $F(6, 45) = 2.54$, $p = .03$. This indicates that even after controlling for the effects of weight gain, a significant difference was observed between AN-R and AN-BP in terms of improvement on the Impulse subscale, $F(1,50) = 14.14$, $p < .001$. Examination of the means indicated that AN-BP improved more during treatment than AN-R, with respect to inhibiting impulsive behaviors when experiencing negative emotions.

Table 3 Means and standard deviations for the DERS subscales at pre-treatment for AN-BP and AN-R subtypes

Measure	Mean (SD) AN-BP ($n = 62$)	AN-R ($n = 44$)	p
DERS-Goals	19.52 (4.26)	18.02 (5.43)	.12
DERS-Impulse	19.32 (6.42)	14.18 (6.35)	< .001
DERS-Awareness	21.42 (5.19)	20.18 (6.01)	.25
DERS-Strategies	28.63 (7.46)	23.18 (9.87)	.002
DERS-Clarity	17.23 (4.18)	16.02 (5.45)	.24
DERS-Non-acceptance	21.31 (7.23)	18.55 (7.24)	.06
DERS-Total	127.42 (25.53)	110.29 (31.66)	.003

Note. DERS = difficulties in emotion regulation scale
Note. DERS total scores were not included in the multivariate model but are provided in the table for descriptive purposes. The p value for the total score comes from an independent samples t test run for descriptive purposes only

Table 4 Overall means and standard deviations of DERS subscales from Pre- to post-treatment ($n = 53$)

Measure	Mean (SD) Pre-Treatment	Post-Treatment	p
DERS-Goals	18.26 (4.78)	16.87 (5.31)	.03
DERS-Impulse	16.23 (6.64)	12.26 (4.95)	< .001
DERS-Awareness	20.51 (5.49)	17.43 (5.15)	< .001
DERS-Strategies	24.74 (8.80)	21.04 (8.00)	.003
DERS-Clarity	16.26 (4.24)	13.19 (4.72)	< .001
DERS-Non-acceptance	19.57 (6.99)	17.53 (6.79)	.02
DERS-Total	115.57 (25.76)	98.32 (25.75)	< .001

Note. DERS = difficulties in emotion regulation scale
Note. DERS total scores were not included in the multivariate model but are provided in the table for descriptive purposes. The p value for the total score comes from an independent samples t test run for descriptive purposes only

Emotion regulation difficulties and eating psychopathology

To address the third aim of this study, a series of univariate regression models were conducted to assess whether change in each of the DERS subscales were predictors of change in eating disorder psychopathology (i.e., Global EDE-Q). Findings from these analyses indicated that for each DERS subscale, changes during treatment significantly predicted changes in eating disorder psychopathology across time, *ps* $< .05$, above and beyond the impact of weight gain. Next, a stepwise multiple regression analysis was conducted with all six DERS subscales included as potential predictors. As mentioned, since depression and anxiety scores were not associated with changes in EDE-Q Global score, they were not included as covariates in the following models. Results indicated that only changes in the Goals and Clarity subscales during treatment provided significant predictive contributions to the model, *ps* $< .05$. Accordingly, only these two subscales were included in a subsequent multiple linear regression model with the DERS Goals and Clarity subscales entered together. Overall, this model significantly predicted changes in eating disorder psychopathology during treatment, F (2, 51) =14.29, $p < .001$, R^2 = .36 (See Table 5 for beta weights and other statistics for the individual predictors). This indicates that greater improvements during treatment with respect to emotional clarity and engagement in goal directed behaviours when upset accounted for approximately 36 % of corresponding improvements in eating disorder psychopathology.

Discussion

This study examined difficulties with emotion regulation in a sample of patients with AN who were admitted to a specialized intensive hospital-based treatment program. Our first objective was to compare the two AN subtypes in terms of emotion regulation deficits at baseline. As predicted, it was found that patients with AN-BP reported greater difficulties with emotion regulation overall, and in particular with refraining from impulsive behaviors when experiencing negative emotions and accessing adaptive emotion regulation strategies. This is consistent with the findings of Fischer and colleagues [29] who also found that the binge-purge subtype of AN was associated with greater impulse control difficulties but different from those of Haynos and colleagues [31] who found no differences in emotion regulation between subtypes. Contrary to our predictions, we did not find that patients with the AN-R subtype had greater difficulties with emotion awareness or non-acceptance of emotions compared to those with the AN-BP subtype. Instead, these emotion regulation difficulties appear to be equally common in both subtypes. This indicates individuals with both subtypes of AN struggle with a broad range of emotion regulation deficits with respect to understanding, accepting, and effectively managing their emotions. Greater difficulties with impulse control in AN-BP patients may reflect the fact that by definition they are more likely to engage in impulsive and uncontrolled behaviors while under distress (i.e., binge eating, purging) as part of their disorder, whereas individuals with AN-R typically do not. Thus, although both groups experience significant difficulties, these effects were particularly pronounced for patients with AN-BP, suggesting that this group may in fact be particularly impaired.

Our second objective was to examine whether emotion regulation difficulties improved during treatment among those who successfully completed the program. In contrast to the findings of Haynos and colleagues [31], but in line with the findings of Ben-Porath and colleagues [33], and consistent with our own predictions, patients with both AN subtypes made improvements with respect to all facets of emotion regulation from pre-treatment to post-treatment in this study. Although both groups made significant improvements during treatment, AN-BP patients made more pronounced improvements during treatment on impulse control, compared to AN-R patients. This may reflect the fact that AN-BP patients had higher baseline difficulties with impulse control, therefore leaving them with greater room for improvement during treatment. Nevertheless, patients who completed treatment experienced improvements overall in their ability to use strategies to regulate their emotions, to more effectively inhibit impulsive behaviours, and to remain goal directed while under distress, and improved in their awareness of emotions, acceptance of emotions, and ability to differentiate between emotions.

After controlling for the effects of weight gain on pre-to-post treatment changes in emotion regulation difficulties, improvements in emotion regulation skills overall were no longer statistically significant. However, the multivariate interaction remained significant, indicating that even after controlling for the effects of weight regain, the AN-BP group continued to experience greater improvements in impulse control compared to AN-R patients. The fact that pre-to-post treatment improvements in emotion regulation overall were no longer

Table 5 Multiple regression model predicting improvements in EDE-Q global score from improvements in DERS subscales during treatment ($n = 53$)

Model	Predictor	*B*	*SE*	β	*t*	*p*	*r*
1	DERS-Goals	.08	.03	.34	2.87	.006	.48
	DERS-Clarity	.08	.03	.39	3.25	.002	.51

Note. DERS = difficulties in emotion regulation scale

observed after controlling for the effect of weight gain may suggest that weight restoration improves emotion regulation difficulties independent of the effects of psychological therapy. However, this conceptualization is inconsistent with the results of Haynos and colleagues [31] who found no improvement in emotion regulation skills following weight restoration. One possibility for these seemingly inconsistent findings is that weight restoration and emotion regulation skills training may work together to improve emotion regulation skills in individuals with AN. Treatment programs in both our study and Ben-Porath and colleagues' [33] study involved a substantial focus on psychological interventions including group dialectic behavior therapy (DBT) skills training. This approach is unique from the treatment program in Haynos and colleagues' [31] study, which did not have an emotion regulation focus. These between-study differences in treatment programs may explain why Haynos and colleagues [31] did not observe emotion regulation improvements following weight restoration, whereas our study and Ben-Porath and colleagues' study [33] did show that emotion regulation improved following weight restoration. Unfortunately, a limitation of the current study is that we did not have a comparison treatment condition and therefore there is no way of knowing for certain whether the observed changes were due to differences in treatment programs or to other factors such as improved nutrition and weight status. Of note, since EDE-Q and DERS data were not available for patients who dropped out of treatment or were discharged prematurely, these finding only apply to treatment completers.

Our final objective was to examine whether changes in difficulties with emotion regulation predicted changes in eating disorder psychopathology during treatment. Weight gain during treatment was not a significant predictor of improvements in eating disorder psychopathology, so we did not control for the effects of weight gain. It was found that improvements in the ability to differentiate emotions, and the ability to remain goal-directed when experiencing negative emotions predicted improvements in eating disorder psychopathology from pre-treatment to post-treatment. These findings are consistent with recent research by Racine and Wildes [5] who found that emotion regulation deficits predicted AN symptom severity over the year following intensive treatment [30]. It is possible that eating disorder symptoms reduce emotional clarity, and with improvement to eating disorder psychopathology this emotional clarity also improves. Alternatively, it is possible that as individuals learn to identify and differentiate their emotions, they are better able to cope with them rather than engaging in eating disorder behaviours. Additionally, it is likely that during treatment, individuals learn strategies to inhibit urges and remain goal directed even while under distress, which may result in improvements both to emotion regulation and to eating disorder psychopathology. Although it cannot be determined from this study whether improvements in emotion regulation result in improved eating disorder psychopathology or vice versa, or whether in fact the treatment exerts separate but concurrent effects on both sets of problems, this finding demonstrates that changes in both variables are certainly associated.

Taken together, the findings of this study suggest that while weight restoration may play an important role in the treatment of AN, individuals who make more substantial improvements in a range of emotion regulation skills during treatment are also more likely to make improvements to their eating disorder psychopathology, and that this latter relationship appears to occur independently from weight regain. While causal conclusions cannot be drawn about the observed correlational relationships, the findings suggest that recovery from AN may be associated with: 1) an initial focus on weight restoration; and 2) a subsequent emphasis on emotion regulation skills training.

The present findings have a number of potential clinical implications. Some authors have argued that existing treatments for AN have paid insufficient attention to the issue of emotion dysregulation, particularly the ability to tolerate and effectively regulate emotions, and that this may partially explain the lack of effective treatments for adult AN [13, 24]. To date, treatments designed to improve emotion regulation skills, such as DBT, have been tested almost exclusively in eating disorder patients with bulimia nervosa and binge eating disorder [43–45] . Interventions to target emotional over-control typical in AN has received almost no research attention [24]. Our findings suggest that increasing emotion awareness and improving the ability to tolerate distress and engage in adaptive behaviors when distressed is an important part of overcoming AN. Racine and Wildes [30] have found evidence that improvements in emotion regulation are likely to have a positive impact on the longitudinal course of AN. Our results support this hypothesis and suggest that both weight restoration and improvements in emotion regulation are important targets of treatment in AN. In future research, it will be important to examine in randomized controlled studies whether integrating emotion regulation skills training into existing treatments for AN improves treatment outcome.

The current study had a number of limitations. First, we utilized self-report questionnaire measures to assess eating disorder behaviors. Previous research has shown that self-report questionnaires are somewhat less reliable than interview measures of these symptoms [46], suggesting that future research may benefit from a replication of this study employing interview measures of eating disorder behaviors. Second, post-treatment DERS and EDE-Q data were available for treatment completers only. Although there were no baseline differences between completers and non-completers, it is possible that the results might have been different if we had been able to include non-completers in our analyses. Third, this was a correlational study and it is therefore important to be cautious about interpreting the results. Specifically, we cannot conclude that improvements in emotion regulation played a causal role in determining the level of improvement in eating disorder psychopathology. Fourth, there were no follow-up assessments of patients beyond the discharge assessment and we therefore do not know whether the relationships that we observed persisted after treatment. Finally, this study was conducted using a sample of patients with AN attending an inpatient treatment program who are likely to represent more severe cases. It will be important to investigate in future studies whether the observed relationships hold true in a less severely ill sample, such as individuals receiving outpatient treatment in the community.

Conclusion

In conclusion, findings from the present study add to growing evidence that eating disorder symptoms may serve an emotion regulation function in AN. Specifically, the findings suggest that improvements in emotion regulation skills during treatment are associated with improvements in eating disorder psychopathology, above and beyond the effect of weight restoration on eating disorder psychopathology. Thus, developing interventions to address emotion regulation deficits may be an important component to improving treatment outcome in AN.

Competing interests

The authors declare that they have no competing interests.

Authors' contributions

MR took primary responsibility for all aspects of this study and manuscript including: reviewing relevant literature to developing the study rationale and the specific research questions; developing the study methodology; developing the analytic approach; conducting the analyses and interpreting the results; as well as writing up the paper for publication. DM contributed to developing the study methodology and analytic approach; conducting the analyses and interpreting the results; and writing up the paper for publication. JC contributed to reviewing the relevant literature and developing the study rationale; developing the analytic approach; developing the study methodology; interpreting study results; and writing up the paper for publication. All authors read and approved the final manuscript.

Author details

[1]Department of Psychology, Memorial University of Newfoundland, St. John's, NL A1B 3X9, Canada. [2]Department of Psychology, Ryerson University, Toronto, Ontario M5G 2C4, Canada. [3]Department of Psychiatry, University Health Network, Toronto, Ontario M5G 2C4, Canada.

References

1. Bruch H. Eating disorders: obesity, anorexia nervosa and the person within. New York: Basic Books; 1973.
2. Bruch H. Psychotherapy in anorexia nervosa. Int J Eat Disord. 1982;1(4):3–14.
3. Engel S, Wonderlich S, Crosby R, Mitchell J, Crow S, Gordon K, et al. The role of affect in the maintenance of anorexia nervosa: evidence from a naturalistic assessment of momentary behaviors and emotion. J Abnorm Psychol. 2013;122(3):709–19.
4. Harrison A, Sullivan S, Tchanturia K, Treasure J. Emotional functioning in eating disorders: attentional bias, emotion recognition and emotion regulation. Psychol Med. 2010;40(11):1887–97.
5. Racine S, Wildes J. Dynamic longitudinal relations between emotion regulation difficulties and anorexia nervosa symptoms over the year following intensive treatment. J Consult Clin Psychol. 2015;83(4):785–95.
6. Schmidt U, Treasure J. Anorexia nervosa: valued and visible. A cognitive-interpersonal maintenance model and its implications for research and practice. Br J Clin Psychol. 2006;45(3):343–66.
7. Treasure J, Schmidt U. DBS for treatment-refractory anorexia nervosa. Lancet. 2013;381(9875):1338–9.
8. Corstorphine E. Cognitive-emotional-behavioural therapy for the eating disorders: working with beliefs about emotions. Eur Eat Disord Rev. 2006;14:448–61.
9. Fox J. A qualitative exploration of the perception of emotions in anorexia nervosa: a basic emotion and developmental perspective. Clin Psychol Psychother. 2009;16(4):276–302.
10. Wildes J, Ringham R, Marcus M. Emotion avoidance in patients with anorexia nervosa: initial test of a functional model. Int J Eat Disord. 2010; 43(5):398–404.
11. Lavender J, Wonderlich S, Engel S, Gordon K, Kaye W, Mitchell J. Dimensions of emotion dysregulation in anorexia nervosa and bulimia nervosa: A conceptual review of the empirical literature. Clin Psychol Rev. 2015;40: 111–122.
12. Gratz K, Roemer L. Multidimensional assessment of emotion regulation and dysregulation: development, factor structure, and initial validation of the difficulties in emotion regulation scale. J Psychopathol Behav Assess. 2004;26(1):41–54.
13. Haynos AF, Fruzzetti AE. Anorexia nervosa as a disorder of emotion dysregulation: evidence and treatment implications. Clin Psychol Sci Pract. 2011;18:183–202.
14. Leon GR, Fulkerson JA, Perry CL, Keel PK, Klump KL. Three to four year prospective evaluation of personality and behavioral risk factors for later disordered eating in adolescent girls and boys. J Youth Adolesc. 1999;28:181–96.
15. Stice E. Risk and maintenance factors for eating pathology: a meta-analytic review. Psychol Bull. 2002;128(5):825–48.
16. Aldao A, Nolen-Hoeksema S, Schweizer S. Emotion-regulation strategies across psychopathology: a meta-analytic review. Clin Psychol Rev. 2010;30(2):217–37.
17. Corstorphine E, Mountford V, Tomlinson S, Waller G, Meyer C. Distress tolerance in the eating disorders. Eat Behav. 2007;8:91–7.
18. Troop N, Holbrey A, Trowler R, Treasure J. Ways of coping in women with eating disorders. J Nerv Ment Dis. 1994;182(10):535–40.
19. Harrison A, Sullivan S, Tchanturia K, Treasure J. Emotion recognition and regulation in anorexia nervosa. Clin Psychol Psychother. 2009;16(4):348–56.
20. Brockmeyer T, Holtforth M, Bents H, Kämmerer A, Herzog W, Friederich H. Starvation and emotion regulation in anorexia nervosa. Compr Psychiatry. 2012;53(5):496–501.
21. Brockmeyer T, Skunde M, Wu M, Bresslein E, Rudofsky G, Friederich H, et al. Difficulties in emotion regulation across the spectrum of eating disorders. Compr Psychiatry. 2014;55(3):565–71.
22. Gilboa-Schechtman E, Avnon L, Zubery E, Jeczmien P. Emotional processing in eating disorders: specific impairment or general distress related deficiency? Depress Anxiety. 2006;23(6):331–9.
23. Nowakowski ME, McFarlane T, Cassin S. Alexithymia and eating disorders: a critical review of the literature. J Eat Disord. 2013;1:21.
24. Lynch TR, Gray KL, Hempel RJ, Titley M, Chen EY, O'Mahen HA. Radically open-dialectical behavior therapy for adult anorexia nervosa: feasibility and outcomes from an inpatient program. BMC Psychiatry. 2013;13:293.
25. Cassin S, von Ranson K. Personality and eating disorders: a decade in review. Clin Psychol Rev. 2005;25(7):895–916.
26. Shafran R, Cooper Z, Fairburn C. Clinical perfectionism: a cognitive-behavioural analysis. Behav Res Ther. 2002;40(7):773–91.
27. Geller J, Cockell SJ, Hewitt PL, Goldner EM, Flett GL. Inhibited expression of negative emotions and interpersonal orientation in anorexia nervosa. Int J Eat Disord. 2000;28(1):8–19.

28. Haynos A, Crosby R, Engel S, Lavender J, Wonderlich S, Le Grange D, et al. Initial test of an emotional avoidance model of restriction in anorexia nervosa using ecological momentary assessment. J Psychiatr Res. 2015;68:134–9.
29. Fischer S, Smith G, Cyders M. Another look at impulsivity: a meta-analytic review comparing specific dispositions to rash action in their relationship to bulimic symptoms. Clin Psychol Rev. 2008;28(8):1413–25.
30. Racine SE, Wildes JE. Emotion dysregulation and symptoms of anorexia nervosa: the unique roles of lack of emotional awareness and impulse control difficulties when upset. Int J Eat Disord. 2013;46(7):713–20.
31. Haynos AF, Roberto CA, Martinez MA, Attia E, Fruzzetti AE. Emotion regulation difficulties in anorexia nervosa before and after inpatient weight restoration. Int J Eat Disord. 2014;47(8):888–91.
32. Keys A, Brožek J, Henschel A, Mickelsen O, Taylor H. The biology of human starvation. (2 vols). Oxford: Univ. of Minnesota Press; 1950.
33. Ben-Porath D, Federici A, Wisniewski L, Warren M. Dialectical behavior therapy: does it bring about improvements in affect regulation in individuals with eating disorders? J Contemp Psychother. 2014;44(4):245–51.
34. Maxwell S, Lau M, Howard G. Is psychology suffering from a replication crisis? what does 'failure to replicate' really mean? Am Psychol. 2015;70(6):487–98.
35. Moonsinghe R, Khoury MJ, Janssens ACJW. Most published research findings are false-But a little replication goes a long way. PLoS Med. 2007;4(2):e28.
36. Association AP. Diagnostic and statistical manual of mental disorders. 4th ed. Washington, DC: American Psychiatric Association; 2000.
37. Fairburn CG, Cooper Z. The Eating Disorder Examination. C. G. Fairburn GTW, C. G. Fairburn, G. T. Wilson (Eds). New York: Guilford Press; 1993.
38. Fairburn CG, Bèglin SJ. Assessment of eating disorders: interview or self-report questionnaire. Int J Eat Disord. 1994;16:363–70.
39. Luce KH, Crowther JH. The reliability of the eating disorder examination-self-report questionnaire version (EDE-Q). Int J Eat Disord. 1999;25(3):349–51.
40. Rizvi S, Peterson C, Crow S, Stewart AW. Test-retest reliability of the eating disorder examination. Int J Eat Disord. 2000;28(3):311–6.
41. Tabachnick BG, Fidell LS. Using multivariate statistics. 5th ed. Needham Heights: Pearson; 2001.
42. Derogatis LR, Melisaratos N. The brief symptom inventory: an introductory report. Psychol Med. 1983;13(3):595–605.
43. Safer D, Robinson A, Jo B. Outcome from a randomized controlled trial of group therapy for binge eating disorder: comparing dialectical behavior therapy adapted for binge eating to an active comparison group therapy. Behav Ther. 2010;41(1):106–20.
44. Safer D, Telch C, Agras W. Dialectical behavior therapy for bulimia nervosa. Am J Psychiatry. 2001;158(4):632–4.
45. Telch C, Agras W, Linehan M. Dialectical behavior therapy for binge eating disorder. J Consult Clin Psychol. 2001;69(6):1061–5.
46. Carter JC, Aime AA, Mills JS. Assessment of bulimia nervosa: a comparison of interview and self-report questionnaire methods. Int J Eat Disord. 2001; 30(2):187–92.

Predictors of therapeutic alliance in two treatments for adults with severe and enduring anorexia nervosa

Colleen Stiles-Shields[1*], Bryony H. Bamford[2], Stephen Touyz[3], Daniel Le Grange[4,5], Phillipa Hay[6] and Hubert Lacey[7]

Abstract

Background: Therapeutic alliance (TA) has been found to be a significant predictor of outcome for patients with severe and enduring anorexia nervosa (SE-AN), accounting for more variance than treatment type. To better understand how to promote TA for this population, the aim of the current study was to investigate predictors of TA in adults with SE-AN.

Methods: Participants were 63 adult females with SE-AN presenting to an outpatient, multi-site randomized controlled trial conducted at two clinical sites. Participants' perception of the quality of their therapeutic relationship, demographic information, and eating disorder symptomatology were assessed via interview and questionnaire measures.

Results: Baseline ratings of how successful participants believed treatment would be for them was the only variable to significantly predict early ($p = .01$), mid ($p = .009$), and late treatment alliance ($p = .03$). No other variables investigated predicted the quality of patient rated TA at any point in treatment ($ps > .57$).

Conclusions: Results suggest instilling hope in treatment outcome may enhance TA, and in turn, outcomes for patients with SE-AN in outpatient therapy.

Keywords: Therapeutic alliance, Anorexia nervosa, Cognitive behavioral therapy, Specialist supportive clinical management, Predictors

Background

Therapeutic alliance (TA) is a relational bond that develops between a patient and clinician via collaborative work and trust, as both endeavor to establish and accomplish treatment goals [1]. Cited as a critical non-specific factor in the treatment of depression [2], TA has been shown to predict outcomes across a variety of treatments and disorders, including in chronic presentations [3–10]. In the treatment of eating disorders, TA is often considered an important element of interventions, but with mixed effect on treatment success [11–16].

TA has been shown to play a central role in preventing premature treatment drop-out in an inpatient population with anorexia nervosa (AN) [17, 18], with even initial impressions promoting treatment compliance [17]. Further, in a sample of adults with severe and enduring anorexia nervosa (SE-AN), TA was found to be a significant predictor of eating disorder symptoms at end of treatment (EOT) and at follow-up [19]. Indeed, TA actually accounted for more of the variance in outcome than treatment type. As such, correlates of TA are a critical domain to explore for patients with SE-AN.

While TA is recognized as an important predictor of treatment engagement, less is known about the factors that may contribute to the development of a strong alliance in patients with AN, particularly those with a severe and enduring course of illness. Research within the field of anxiety and depression indicates that patients with more severe symptoms report poorer TA [20]; however, these associations between symptom severity and TA have not been replicated in adults with bulimia nervosa (BN) [21]. The quality of the therapeutic relationship has been noted as worse in individuals with chronic eating disorders [22], suggesting that duration of illness, or number of previous treatment episodes may adversely affect treatment engagement and TA. Additionally, when

* Correspondence: ColleenSS@u.northwestern.edu
[1]Department of Preventive Medicine, Northwestern University Feinberg School of Medicine, Chicago, IL, USA
Full list of author information is available at the end of the article

exploring psychotherapy processes, patient preconceptions and expectations regarding improvement have been found to be associated with stronger alliance and better overall treatment outcomes [23, 24]. This finding has been supported within a treatment trial for BN [21]. Further, there is recent evidence to suggest that positive early symptom change may be responsible for enhancing TA in patients with BN [11, 14]. Despite these findings, there is still a dearth of research investigating whether, and which, patient characteristics influence TA in SE-AN. Greater understanding of patient characteristics that may influence therapeutic alliance and treatment engagement is needed to help clinicians identify specific treatment adaptations that may be needed to better tailor treatment to individual need.

The aim of this paper is to explore possible correlates of TA that may be present, irrespective of treatment or therapist variation. In line with previous research highlighted above, we hypothesized that characteristics associated with SE-AN (i.e., longer treatment duration, increased severity, higher previous treatment episodes, lower motivation and expectation of treatment success, and lower body mass index) would predict poorer participant-rated TA for adults with SE-AN.

Methods

This study is a secondary analysis of data from a randomized clinical trial (RCT) conducted at two clinical sites (The University of Sydney and St. George's Hospital, University of London), with a Data and Coordinating Center (The University of Chicago Medicine). The RCT compared the efficacy of Cognitive Behavioral Therapy for anorexia nervosa (CBT-AN) and Specialist Supportive Clinical Management (SSCM) for a sample of adults with SE-AN. Specific treatment effects have been analysed and are reported in the main outcome paper [25]. Participants received 30 individual, outpatient treatment sessions provided over eight months.

Participants

Recruitment of participants occurred from July 2007 to November 2010 through advertising to eating disorder clinics, clinicians, and generic websites.

Participants were eligible for randomization if they met the *Diagnostic and Statistical Manual for Mental Disorders*, 4th Edition, Text Revision (DSM-IV-TR) [26] criteria for AN, excluding criterion D (amenorrhea); had an illness duration of at least 7 years; were at least 18 years of age; and were female. Exclusion criteria included presenting with a current manic episode or psychosis; current alcohol or substance abuse or dependence; significant current medical or neurological illness (including seizure disorder), with the exception of nutrition-related alterations that are impacted by weight; current engagement in psychotherapy and being unwilling to suspend such treatment for the duration of their participation in the study; and plans to move beyond commuting distance for the study site in the following 12 months or not living within commuting distance to the study site.

In compliance with the Institutional Review Boards (IRB) of the two intervention sites and the data and coordinating center, participants completed written informed consent prior to assessment. In addition to IRB approval, the trial was approved by the Human Research Ethics Committee (approval number 02-2007/9669) and was registered with the Australian New Zealand Clinical Trials Registry (ACTRN12607000440426).

Treatments and therapists

Participants were randomized to either CBT-AN or SSCM by a biostatistician independent from both intervention sites. Randomization was conducted using Ephron's biased coin approach, stratified within sites by: 1) subtype of illness (Restrictive and Binge-Purge) and 2) psychopharmacological medication status. Treatment occurred in outpatient settings at The University of Sydney and St. George's Hospital, University of London. Treatments and therapist characteristics are described in detail in previous papers [25, 27].

Measures

Physical assessment

Participants were weighed in light, indoor clothing with their shoes removed. Weight and height were measured by a trained research assistant using a calibrated digital or balance-beam scale and stadiometer, respectively, to calculate body mass index (BMI = kg/m^2).

Helping Relationships Questionnaire (HRQ)

The HRQ measures the patient's perspective of the therapist-patient relationship via an 11 self-report items [28]. Items for the HRQ are rated on a 6-point likert scale, ranging from -3 ("Strongly feel it is not true") to +3 ("Strongly feel it is true"). Total scores, computed by summing all items, range from -33 to 33, with higher total scores reflecting greater TA. The HRQ was administered at week two, mid-treatment, and EOT. Participant responses with missing items on the HRQ were excluded from analyses involving HRQ total scores. The HRQ has strong psychometrics and has been shown to correlate with treatment outcome [29, 30].

The Eating Disorder Examination (EDE)

The EDE is a semi-structured investigator-based interview measuring cognitive and behavioral symptoms related to eating disorders [31]. The EDE was used to generate DSM-IV-TR diagnoses for an ED and to assess the severity of symptomatology. Subscales include:

Weight Concern, Shape Concern, Eating Concern, and Restraint; global scores reflect the overall severity of ED symptoms.

The Anorexia Nervosa Stages of Change Questionnaire (ANSOCQ)

The ANSOCQ is a 20-item self-report questionnaire assessing a patient's readiness for recovery from AN, with higher total scores reflecting greater readiness for recovery [32].

The Treatment Suitability and Patient Expectations (TSPE)

The TSPE is a 2-item self-report questionnaire designed to assess a patient's belief regarding her expectation of improvement in her treatment assignment ("How successful do you think your treatment here will be?") and suitability of her assigned treatment. The TSPE items are answered using an 11-point scale ranging from 0 (not at all) to 10 (completely acceptable or extremely suitable). The TSPE is given following the first therapy session, once the patient has met with her therapist and is aware of which treatment to which she has been randomized. The patient is asked to comment on "overall" improvement, rather than improvement on any specific domains (e.g., weight gain, quality of life). The TSPE has been utilized in multiple trials with patients with eating disorders [25, 33–35]. Cronbach's alphas for the TSPE ranged from .75 to .92 over the assessment time points in this trial.

Assessment time points

The physical assessment, EDE and ANSOCQ were administered at baseline (pre randomization), session 15, and EOT. The HRQ and the TSPE were given following the first therapy session, session 15, and EOT.

Data analysis

Stepwise multiple regressions were conducted to investigate the predictive utility of patient motivation, believed suitability of treatment, symptom severity, duration of illness, number of previous specialist ED treatment experiences, and BMI on early treatment alliance. Stepwise multiple regressions were also conducted to investigate the predictive power of the variables detailed above, as well as early treatment alliance, on participant ratings of mid and end of treatment alliance. An alpha level of .05 was used to provide maximum power to identify potential predictors of therapeutic alliance.

Post hoc analyses were conducted to better understand the role of significant predictor(s) of TA. An independent *t*-Test was used to examine any differences occurring based on treatment assignment and a pearson correlation was run to understand the predictor(s) relationship to outcome. To determine if a significant meditational effect was present among the significant predictor(s) of TA, TA, and eating disorder symptom outcomes (defined by EDE global score), the methodology outlined by Baron and Kenny was utilized to evaluate if mediation was supported [36].

Results

A total of 63 participants were randomized to CBT-AN ($n = 31$) or SSCM ($n = 32$). The range of age for study participants was 20-62 ($M = 33.4 \pm 9.6$), with duration of illness ranging from 7 to 49 years ($M = 16.6 \pm 8.5$). The mean BMI for the sample was 16.2 (SD = 1.3, range = 11.8-18.5). The majority of participants met criteria for AN restricting subtype ($n = 47$, 74.6 %). No significant differences on any baseline characteristics were found between treatment groups, sites, or group-by-site interactions [25]. Table 1 shows baseline demographics for all predictor variables.

Baseline ratings of how successful participants believed treatment would be was the only variable to significantly predict early ($\beta = 0.67$, SE = 0.94, $p = .01$), mid ($\beta = 0.80$, SE = 0.80, $p = .009$), and late treatment alliance ($\beta = 0.66$, SE = 1.98, $p = .03$; see Table 2). Motivation, symptom severity, duration of illness, age, number of previous specialist ED treatment experiences, early therapeutic alliance, and BMI did not significantly predict alliance at any point in treatment ($ps > .57$; see Table 3).

Patient expectations of treatment success

Participant ratings of anticipated treatment success did not significantly differ based on treatment assignment (CBT-AN $M = 7.04 \pm 1.97$, SSCM $M = 7.17 \pm 1.56$, $p = .78$). The TSPE item was significantly correlated with EOT ($r(47) = -.40$, $p = .005$) and follow-up ($r(44) = -.48$, $p = .001$) EDE global scores.

Mediation analyses

Given the present findings that anticipated treatment success significantly predicted TA, and past findings from this sample indicating TA as a significant predictor of outcome [19], additional analyses were conducted to determine the possibility of a mediating relationship, such that expectations for therapy impacts overall TA, which impacts treatment outcomes (see Fig. 1). Utilizing Baron and Kenny's (1986) four step approach, a full mediation effect is suggested for early TA, such that: step 1) expectations of treatment success (TSPE item 2) significantly predicts EOT symptomology (EDE global score; $p = .005$); step 2) expectations of treatment success (TSPE item 2) significantly predicts early TA ($p < .001$); step 3) early TA significantly predicts EOT symptomology ($p = .02$); and step 4) expectations of treatment success no longer significantly predicts EOT symptomology after controlling for early TA ($p = .07$) [36]. A partial mediation effect is suggested for late TA, such that: step 1) expectations of treatment success significantly predicts EOT symptomology ($p = .005$); step 2) expectations of

Table 1 Baseline characteristics of predictor variables for therapeutic alliance

Variable	Mean	Standard Deviation	Range (Minimum, Maximum)
Age	33.41	9.57	42 (20, 62)
Duration of Illness	16.57	8.45	42 (7, 49)
ANSOCQ	16.57	17.89	77 (0, 77)
BMI	16.20	1.34	6.67 (11.80, 18.47)
EDE Global Score	3.10	1.31	5.26 (.41, 5.67)
Frequency of Specialist ED Interventions	6.80	4.16	16 (2, 18)
TSPE: Suitability of Treatment	7.41	1.78	9 (1, 10)
TSPE: Success of Treatment	7.08	1.75	9 (1, 10)

Note. ANSOCQ = The Anorexia Nervosa Stages of Change Questionnaire; BMI = Body Mass Index; EDE = Eating Disorders Examination; ED = Eating Disorders; TSPE = Treatment Suitability and Patient Expectations

treatment success significantly predicts late TA ($p < .02$); step 3) late TA significantly predicts EOT symptomology ($p = .002$); and step 4) expectations of treatment success significantly predicts EOT symptomology after controlling for early TA ($ps = .03$).

Discussion

This study examined predictors of TA in a treatment trial offering two psychological therapies for SE-AN. Contrary to our hypotheses, nearly all of the variables examined were not found to be significant predictors of TA at the start of treatment, mid treatment, or EOT. Indeed, patient expectations for treatment, an item in the TSPE which was given following the first therapy session, was found to be the only significant predictor of TA throughout treatment. Mediation analyses suggested that this early treatment factor impacts outcomes such that patient treatment expectations drive the development of TA, which impacts treatment outcomes.

These findings are in contrast to previous research suggesting that increased duration of illness, severity of illness, and decreased motivation may have a negative impact on TA [3, 20–22]. A number of recent studies confirm the difficulties in engaging individuals with SE-AN in psychological treatments [37–39]. This has likely contributed to a prejudice that may be held by many treating clinicians, both in their own expectations for outcome as well as their belief that patients with SE-AN are not interested in positive treatment outcomes. However, it appears that within this sample, illness duration, illness severity, previous failed treatment experiences, and baseline BMI had no significant predictive capacity on patients' therapeutic relationships. While this study did not include patients with a short duration of AN, reported levels of TA in the current study were consistent with the use of the HRQ with other samples with eating disorders [33]. As such, clinicians should remain highly cautious when assuming that illness characteristics can impact the likelihood of forming an engagement. Additionally, this study found that early TA had little predictive validity on later TA ratings. This suggests that when initial impressions are made, other factors may override them and have a greater influence on the strength of the therapeutic relationship as treatment progresses.

Patients' belief in the ability of the treatment to contribute to overall improvement of symptoms was the only significant contributor to their experience of TA at all stages of treatment. This finding is consistent with the literature on adults with BN [21], and longstanding work noting the importance of hope and alliance in treatments [40]. Further, it suggests that clinicians attempting to engage patients with SE-AN in meaningful psychological work should focus early in treatment on

Table 2 Significant predictors of therapeutic alliance determined through stepwise regression

Stepwise regression variable	ΔR^2	ΔF	B	SE	*B*	*p*
Early Treatment Alliance Model						
Baseline Rating of Anticipated Treatment Success	.45	8.97	2.83	0.94	.67	.01
Mid Treatment Alliance Model						
Baseline Rating of Anticipated Treatment Success	.64	12.68	2.86	0.80	.80	.009
Late Treatment Alliance Model						
Baseline Rating of Anticipated Treatment Success	.44	7.09	5.27	1.98	.66	.03

Note. Variables excluded for early treatment alliance model: number of previous specialist eating disorder interventions, baseline motivation score, duration of illness, age, baseline Body Mass Index (BMI), rating of treatment suitability, and baseline eating disorder severity ($ps > .68$); variables excluded for mid and end of treatment alliance models: early treatment rating of therapeutic alliance, number of previous specialist eating disorder interventions, baseline motivation score, duration of illness, age, baseline BMI, rating of treatment suitability, and baseline eating disorder severity ($ps > .57$)

Table 3 Variables excluded as significant predictors of therapeutic alliance determined through stepwise regression

Stepwise regression variable	Beta In	*t*	*p*
Early Treatment Alliance Model			
Previous specialist ED intervention	.362	1.73	.12
Baseline ANSOQC Total	.142	.57	.58
Duration of illness	-.052	-.22	.83
Age	-.026	-.11	.92
Baseline BMI	-.173	-.72	.49
Baseline rating of treatment suitability	.278	1.03	.33
Baseline EDE Global score	-.039	-.17	.87
Mid Treatment Alliance Model			
Previous specialist ED intervention	.119	.49	.64
Baseline ANSOQC Total	.366	1.64	.15
Duration of illness	-.353	-1.70	.14
Age	-.435	-1.81	.12
Baseline BMI	-.403	-1.63	.16
Baseline rating of treatment suitability	-.225	-.74	.49
Baseline EDE Global score	-.281	-1.26	.25
Early Treatment HRQ Total	.087	.27	.80
Late Treatment Alliance Model			
Previous specialist ED intervention	-.091	-.34	.74
Baseline ANSOQC Total	-.176	-.61	.56
Duration of illness	-.229	-.86	.41
Age	-.021	-.07	.95
Baseline BMI	.300	.98	.36
Baseline rating of treatment suitability	-.147	-.44	.67
Baseline EDE Global score	-.049	-.18	.86
Early Treatment HRQ Total	.205	.66	.53

Note. ED = Eating Disorder; ANSOQC = The Anorexia Nervosa Stages of Change Questionnaire; BMI = Body Mass Index; EDE = Eating Disorders Examination; HRQ = Helping Relationships Questionnaire

bolstering patient expectations about the intervention they are undertaking. This may include providing psychoeducation regarding the efficacy of CBT-AN and SSCM for SE-AN [25], or the benefits of symptom change even when remission is not possible [27]. Where available, these early treatment actions may aid the process of building a positive TA throughout treatment, which in turn supports better outcomes [19, 41]. Indeed, as more research is conducted to identify the most effective means to treat adults with SE-AN, bolstering TA is a likely channel to improve outcomes for currently available treatments [42].

To our knowledge, this is the first study to examine predictors of TA in a sample of SE-AN. Engagement in treatments for SE-AN remains a struggle for clinicians. Therefore, examining predictors of TA as a means to enhance the likelihood of forming a positive TA is crucial. There were several strengths to this study, including assessments with well-validated measures. Despite these strengths, limitations should be considered in the interpretation of these findings. While the sample sizes were sufficient to show differences in outcomes, they were also moderate in size. Further, despite its use across a number of RCTs [25, 33–35], the two-item TSPE remains unvalidated. The TSPE was also administered following the first session, which means it is possible that patient expectations were also influenced by the rapport experienced with the therapist during the first session. For this reason, we are cautious to over interpret these findings until they can be confirmed in future research examining treatment expectation prior to meeting the therapist. Additionally, this sample includes only individuals with SE-AN. While it remains unclear how these results generalize to individuals with a shorter duration or less severe presentations, the authors see this as a future research question, rather than a limitation of the study. It is also of note that the number of analyses conducted increases the risk for Type I error. Future studies should

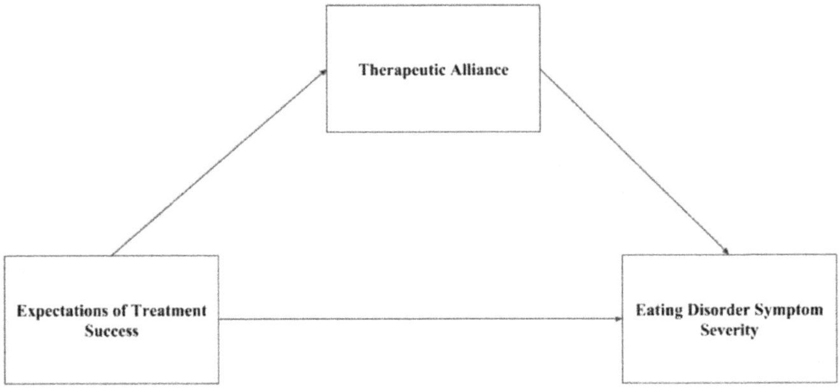

Fig. 1 Therapeutic alliance mediates the relationship between treatment expectations and outcome

explore predictors of TA in larger samples, including both individuals with BN and with patients with a shorter duration of AN. This would also exclude the possibility of any floor effects influencing the non-significant finding for duration of illness arising from the chronic nature of this group. It may also be beneficial to explore patient characteristics in conjunction with therapist characteristics.

Conclusions

Results of this study suggest that an initial patient expectation for successful outcome significantly predicts patient-reported TA throughout treatment. Further, a mediational relationship between early patient treatment expectations, TA, and outcomes appears to exist for this sample of adults with SE-AN. Most cases of SE-AN are defined for clinicians by patients' egosyntonic wish to preserve maladaptive behaviors that they identify as having a "functional" purpose [37]. Through this lens, therapeutic relationships can at times be sacrificed, regardless of chronicity. However, recent findings show that positive and strong TA can be established in individuals with SE-AN [19]. The present study expands insight into TA for individuals with SE-AN, demonstrating that TA can be bolstered with early treatment expectations for successful treatment.

Abbreviations

AN: anorexia nervosa; ANSOCQ: anorexia nervosa stages of change questionnaire; BMI: body mass index; BN: bulimia nervosa; CBT-AN: cognitive behavioral therapy for anorexia nervosa; DSM-IV-TR: Diagnostic and Statistical Manual for Mental Disorders, 4th Edition, Text Revision; EDE: eating disorder examination; EOT: end of treatment; HRQ: helping relationships questionnaire; IRB: Institutional review board; RCT: randomized controlled trial; SE-AN: severe and enduring anorexia nervosa; SSCM: specialist supportive clinical management; TA: therapeutic alliance; TSPE: treatment suitability and patient expectations.

Competing interests

Daniel Le Grange receives consultant fees from the Training Institute for Child and Adolescent Eating Disorders, LLC. Dr. Le Grange also receives royalties from Guilford Press and Routledge. Stephen Touyz has received fees for serving as consultant to Shire Pharmaceuticals advisory board member. Phillipa Hay receives Honoraria from PLOSMedicine. Stephen Touyz and Phillipa Hay receive royalties from Hogrefe Publications, McGraw Hill Pubs and honoraria from Biomed Central.

Authors' contributions

CSS and BHB conceived of the study and helped draft the manuscript. ST, PH, HL, and DLG served as primary investigators of the RCT and helped draft the manuscript. All authors read and approved the final manuscript.

Funding

Funding for this work was supported by: National Health and Medical Research Council (Australia) PG 457419 (Drs. Touyz, Le Grange, Lacey and Hay), South-west London and St. George's NHS Trust (Dr. Lacey), the Butterfly Foundation (Dr. Touyz), University of Western Sydney (Dr. Hay), and F31 MH106321 (Ms. Stiles-Shields).

Author details

[1]Department of Preventive Medicine, Northwestern University Feinberg School of Medicine, Chicago, IL, USA. [2]The London Centre for Eating Disorders and Body Image, London, UK. [3]University of Sydney, School of Psychology, Sydney, Australia. [4]Department of Psychiatry, University of California, San Francisco, San Francisco, CA, USA. [5]Department of Pediatrics, University of California, San Francisco, San Francisco, CA, USA. [6]Centre for Health Research, School of Medicine, Western Sydney University, Sydney, Australia. [7]St. George's, University of London, Eating Disorders Research Group, London, UK.

References

1. Bordin E. The generalizability of the psychoanalytic concept of the working alliance. Psychother Theory Res Pract. 1979;16:252–60.
2. Ilardi SS, Craighead WE. The role of nonspecific factors in cognitive-behavior therapy for depression. Clin Psychol Sci Pract. 1994;1:138–55.
3. Macneil C, Hasty M, Evans M, Redlich C, Berk M. The therapeutic alliance: is it necessary or sufficient to engender positive outcomes? Acta Neuropsychiatrica. 2009;2:95–8.
4. Martin D, Garske J, Davis M. Relation of the therapeutic alliance with outcome and other variables: A meta-analytic review. J Consult Clin Psychol. 2000;68:216–20.
5. Tasca GA, Lampard AM. Reciprocal influence of alliance to the group and outcome in day treatment for eating disorders. J Counseling Psychol. 2012;59:507.
6. Arnow BA, Steidtmann D, Blasey C, Manber R, Constantino MJ, Klein DN, Markowitz JC, Rothbaum BO, Thase ME, Fisher AJ, Kocsis JH. The relationship between the therapeutic alliance and treatment outcome in two distinct psychotherapies for chronic depression. J Consult Clin Psychol. 2013;81:627.
7. Horvath AO, Del Re AC, Fluckiger C, Symonds D. Alliance in individual psychotherapy. Psychother. 2011;48:9–16.
8. Horvath AO, Luborsky L. The role of the therapeutic alliance in psychotherapy. J Consult Clin Psychol. 1993;61:561–73.
9. Del Re AC, Flückiger C, Horvath AO, Symonds D, Wampold BE. Therapist effects in the therapeutic alliance–outcome relationship: A restricted-maximum likelihood meta-analysis. Clin Psychol Rev. 2012;32:642–9.
10. Ardito RB, Rabellino D. Therapeutic alliance and outcome of psychotherapy: Historical excursus, measurements, and prospects for research. Front Psychol. 2011;2:270.
11. Brown A, Mountford V, Waller G. Therapeutic alliance and weight gain during cognitive behavioural therapy for anorexia nervosa. Behav Res Ther. 2013;51:216–20.
12. Loeb K, Wilson G, Labouvie E, Pratt E, Hayaki J, Walsh B, et al. Therapeutic alliance and treatment adherence in two interventions for bulimia nervosa: A study of process and outcome. J Consult Clin Psychol. 2005;73:1097–107.
13. Bourion-Bedes S, Baumann C, Kermarrec S, Ligier F, Feillet F, Bonnemains C, Guillemin F, Kabuth B. Prognostic value of early therapeutic alliance in weight recovery: A prospective cohort of 108 adolescents with anorexia nervosa. J Adolesc Health. 2013;52:344–50.
14. Graves TA, N. T, Thompson-Brenner H, Franko DL, Eddy KT, Bourion-Bedes S, Brown A, Constantino MJ, Flückiger C, Forsberg S, et al. A Meta-Analysis of the Relation between Therapeutic Alliance and Treatment Outcome in Eating Disorders. Clin Psychol Rev. Under Review.
15. Forsberg S, LoTempio E, Bryson S, Fitzpatrick KK, Le Grange D, Lock J. Therapeutic alliance in two treatments for adolescent anorexia nervosa. Int J Eat Disord. 2013; 46:34–8.
16. Waller G, Evans J, Stringer H. The therapeutic alliance in the early part of cognitive-behavioral therapy for the eating disorders. Int J Eat Disord. 2012; 45:63–9.
17. Sly R, Morgan JF, Mountford VA, Lacey JH. Predicting premature termination of hospitalised treatment for anorexia nervosa: The roles of therapeutic alliance, motivation, and behaviour change. Eat Behav. 2013;14:119–23.
18. Gallop R, Kennedy SH, Stern D. Therapeutic alliance on an inpatient unit for eating disorders. Int J Eat Disord. 1994;16:405–10.
19. Stiles-Shields C, Touyz S, Hay P, Lacey JH, Crosby RD, Rieger E, Bamford BH, Le Grange D. Therapeutic alliance in two treatments for adults with severe and enduring anorexia nervosa. Int J Eat Disord. 2013;46:783–9.
20. Raue P, Castonguay L, Goldfried M. The working alliance: A comparison of two therapies. Psychother Res. 1993;3:197–207.
21. Constantino M, Arnow B, Blasey C, Agras W. The association between patient characteristics and the therapeutic alliance in cognitive-behavioral

and interpersonal therapy for bulimia nervosa. J Consult Clin Psychol. 2005; 73:203–11.
22. de la Rie S, Noordenbos G, Donker M, van Furth E. The quality of treatment of eating disorders: a comparison of the therapists' and the patients' perspective. Int J Eat Disord. 2008;41:307–17.
23. Messer S, Wolitzky D, Muran J, Barber J. The therapeutic alliance: An evidence based guide to practice. New York: Guilford Press New York; 2010.
24. Watson JC, Kalogerakos F. The therapeutic alliance in humanistic psychotherapy. In Muran CJ, Barber JP, editors. The therapeutic alliance: An evidence-based guide to practice. New York: Guilford Press; 2010. p. 191-209.
25. Touyz S, Le Grange D, Lacey H, Hay P, Smith R, Maguire S, Bamford B, Pike KM, Crosby RD. Treating severe and enduring anorexia nervosa: a randomized controlled trial. Psychol Med. 2013;43:2501–11.
26. American Psychiatric Association. Diagnostic and statistical manual of mental disorders (DSM-IV-TR). Washington, DC: APA; 2000.
27. Hay PJ, Touyz S, Sud R. Treatment for severe and enduring anorexia nervosa: A review. Aust N Z J Psych. 2012;46:1136–44.
28. Luborsky L. Principles of Psychoanalytic Psychotherapy. New York: Basic Books; 1984.
29. Alexander L, Luborsky L. The penn helping alliance scales. In: Breenberg LS, Pinsoff WM, editors. The Psychotherapeutic Process: A Research Handbook. New York: Guilford Press; 1986. p. 325–66.
30. Luborsky L, McLellan AT, Woody GE, O'Brien CP, Auerbach A. Therapist success and its determinants. Arch Gen Psych. 1985;42:602.
31. Cooper Z, Fairburn CG. The eating disorder examination: a semi-structured interview for the assessment of the specific psychopathology of eating disorders. Int J Eat Disorder. 1987;6:1–8.
32. Rieger E, Touyz S, Beumont P. The Anorexia Nervosa Stages of Change Questionnaire (ANSOCQ): information regarding its psychometric properties. Int J Eat Disord. 2002;32:24–38.
33. Zaitsoff SL, Celio Doyle A, Rienecke Hoste R, Le Grange D. How do adolescents with bulimia nervosa rate the acceptability and therapeutic relationship in family-based treatment? Int J Eat Disord. 2008;41:390–8.
34. Le Grange D, Crosby RD, Rathouz PJ, Leventhal BL. A randomized controlled comparison of family-based treatment and supportive psychotherapy for adolescent bulimia nervosa. Arch Gen Psych. 2007;64:1049–56.
35. Lock J, Le Grange D, Agras S, Moye A, Bryson S, Jo B. Randomized clinical trial comparing family-based treatment to adolescent focused therapy for adolescents with anorexia nervosa. Arch Gen Psych. 2010;67:1025–32.
36. Baron RM, Kenny DA. The moderator-mediator variable distinction in social psychological research: Conceptual, strategic, and statistical considerations. J Pers Soc Psychol. 1986;51:1173–82.
37. Strober M. The chronically ill patient with anorexia nervosa: Development, phenomenology and theraputic considerations. In: Grilo CM, Mitchell JM, editors. The Treatment of Eating Disorders. London: The Guildford Press; 2010. p. 225–38.
38. Wonderlich S, Mitchell JE, Crosby RD, Myers TC, Kadlec K, LaHaise K, Swan-Kremeier L, Dokken J, Lange M, Dinkel J. Minimizing and treating chronicity in the eating disorders: a clinical overview. Int J Eat Disord. 2012;45:467–75.
39. Strober M, Johnson C. The need for complex ideas in anorexia nervosa: Why biology, environment, and psyche all matter, why therapists make mistakes, and why clinical benchmarks are needed for managing weight correction. Int J Eat Disord. 2012;45:155–78.
40. Frank JD. Common features of psychotherapy. Aust N Z J Psychiatry. 1972;6:34–40.
41. Ackerman SJ, Hilsenroth MJ. A review of therapist characteristics and techniques positively impacting the therapeutic alliance. Clin Psychol Rev. 2003;23:1–33.
42. Crits-Christoph P, Baranackie K, Kurcias J, Beck AT, Carroll K, Perry K, Luborsky L, McLellan A, Woody G, Thompson L. Meta-analysis of therapist effects in psychotherapy outcome studies. Psychother Res. 1991;1:81–91.

Do female dieters have an "eating disorder" self-schema?

Sarah Greer[2] and Myra Cooper[1*]

Abstract

Background: The processing of schema-related information is important in the maintenance of specific eating disorder (ED)-related belief systems and psychopathology. To date, most research on differences in the processing of ED schematic information has used interview or self-report questionnaire measures. Dieting is a known risk factor for EDs and dieters have been included in some studies. However, they have not been compared with non-dieters on a novel, objective measure of ED related schema processing.

Methods: The current study recruited healthy female volunteers from the community and divided them into dieting ($n = 25$) and non-dieting ($n = 24$) groups using rigorous criteria. ED self-schemas with content unrelated to eating, weight and shape were measured using a self-schema processing task.

Results: Dieters endorsed significantly more ED relevant words compared to non-dieters, whereas non-dieters rejected significantly more ED relevant words compared to dieters. Reaction times to endorsements and rejections were non-significant when the two groups were compared. In a surprise recall task, dieters recalled significantly more ED relevant words.

Conclusion: The results of this study support the presence of ED self-schemas with negative content unrelated to eating, weight and shape in otherwise healthy dieters. Implications for future research and the early identification of individuals vulnerable to EDs are discussed.

Keywords: Eating disorders, Dieting, schema, self-schema, Core beliefs, Information processing

Background

Self-schemata are "cognitive generalisations about the self, derived from past experience that organise and guide the processing of self-related information contained in the individual's social experiences" ([1], p64). Identifying and modifying maladaptive self-schemata (also termed core or negative self-beliefs), is now often considered to be a key focus of eating disorder (ED) treatment [2–4]. As described by Young [5, 6] these schemata typically develop early in life, and although commonly associated with personality disorders, also have a strong association with EDs (for example, as measured by the Young Schema Questionnaire (YSQ, [7]) [8]. Although it has proved difficult to identify schema patterns typical of eating or other psychiatric disorders using the YSQ, self-schemata or negative self-beliefs that may be uniquely associated with EDs, compared to depressive and anxious patients and symptoms have been found using exploratory, data driven work [9, 10]. This is important as people with EDs often have high levels of anxiety and depression, and it is theoretically and clinically useful to identify core beliefs particularly characteristic of the ED. In terms of measurement, with the exception of Benas and Gibb [11], who used computer-based tasks to measure reaction times to specific content, most studies have assessed self-schema in EDs using self-report questionnaires or semi-structured interviews (e.g., [10, 12, 13]). Experimental designs, for example, Markus's [1] "Me/Not" paradigm, have not generally been used but may provide a more objective assessment of any biased self-processing relevant to EDs.

Dieting is a risk factor for EDs, and a strong predictor of ED symptoms [14, 15]. Dieters may be best defined as those *attempting* to restrict food intake rather than only those succeeding; as attempt rather than success is important in

* Correspondence: myra.cooper@hmc.ox.ac.uk
[1]Isis Education Centre, University of Oxford, Warneford Hospital, Oxford OX3 7JX, UK
Full list of author information is available at the end of the article

cognitive behaviour models of EDs [16]. Dieting measured using the Eating Disorder Examination Questionnaire (EDE-Q; [17]) predicted the development of an ED [16]; thus the EDE-Q may be a particularly useful measure of dieting in EDs. Given the role of dieting in EDs, one group who may have accessible ED related self-schemata are dieters.

The notion dieters have an active ED self-schema was tested by Pringle, Harmer and Cooper [18]. They used a self-schema processing task (SSPT) based on Markus's [1] "Me/Not Me" paradigm. The task measured endorsement and reaction times to ED relevant, depression relevant, generic negative and generic positive/neutral words, drawn from Cooper and Cowen's [9] work on self-schema. An ED-relevant schema was associated with higher levels of ED-related symptoms [18]. As described by Cooper and Cowen, an ED-relevant self schema contains extreme negative content, that is unrelated to eating, weight and shape, and is at least partly distinct from the negative self schema associated with depression [9]. A follow-up study indicated that an ED self-schema was related to risk of developing an ED twelve months later [19]. An ED self-schema may thus represent one mechanism through which dieting increases vulnerability to developing an ED.

The study by Pringle and colleagues [18] used a cross sectional design. To date no study has investigated whether dieters have an ED self-schema, compared to non-dieters. In the current study it was hypothesised that dieters will endorse more ED self-schema-relevant words and show faster reaction times for "Me" endorsements to ED words compared to depression, generic negative words and generic positive/neutral words, than non-dieters. It was also hypothesised that dieters would have higher levels of recall of words related to ED self-schema compared to all three other groups. Dieter and non-dieter groups were rigorously defined to ensure they did not contain participants with EDs or other psychiatric disorders; thus an 'at risk' rather than symptomatic group enabled potential vulnerability to be tested.

Method

Recruitment

Following Oxford University ethical approval, women aged 18 to 35 were recruited through advertisements that sought healthy volunteers. Advertisements were placed in online newspapers, student newsletters, social networking sites, and notice boards at colleges and gyms. Presentations were made at undergraduate lectures at local universities, gym classes and meetings of dieting organisations (e.g., "Weight Watchers"). Advertisements sought women who were actively dieting, attempting to diet or trying to eat healthily as well as those who were not (i.e., non-dieters). Potential participants responded by completing an online survey, which was used to screen to ensure basic study criteria were met.

Screening

Inclusion criteria were: Female, between and including the ages of 18 – 35 years.

Exclusion criteria were: Psychiatric history, including an ED; self-declared proficiency in English less than comfortably fluent.

Participants

Of the 181 women who began the online survey, 138 met screening criteria, completed the survey, and indicated willingness to be contacted for further testing. Of these, 72 agreed to meet and completed the Structured Clinical Interview for DSM-IV Axis I disorders (SCID; [20]). Ten met Axis I criteria, or were taking medication that might affect task performance [21]. These people were excluded, leaving 62 potential participants. All participants gave informed consent at each stage of the study. Figure 1 depicts the screening and participant selection process.

Creating dieting and non-dieting groups

Technical difficulties were experienced with one participant's data. Another participant's data was removed after she disclosed difficulties understanding the SSPT words. The sample then included 60 females. A ranking was established using scores on the Restraint subscale to identify participants with the highest and lowest dieting behaviours. Two groups were thus identified for the final analyses: "dieters" ($n = 25$), and "non-dieters" ($n = 24$); numbers were in line with previous research in this area and adequate for the analyses planned [22]. Dieters had a Restraint subscore of 2.4 and above and non-dieters had a score of 1.4 and below.

Power

An exact calculation of number of participants needed and power could not be made due to a lack of previously relevant studies. However, Cohen's (1988) rule of thumb suggested 26 participants in each cell for 80 % power using analysis of variance, assuming a large effect size, and with alpha set at 0.05.

Measures

The Self-Schema Processing Task (SSPT) [18]. The SSPT task involves four sets of 30 "self words" matched for length and word frequency: ED relevant (e.g., evil, repulsive), depression relevant (e.g., numb, excluded), generic negative (e.g., hostile, bossy) and generic positive/neutral (e.g., honest, pleasant). The ED and depression relevant words were taken from Cooper and Cowen [9], and negative and positive words from Anderson [23]. The groups of words were matched for number of letter in each word and word frequency using the MRC Psycholinguistic database [18].

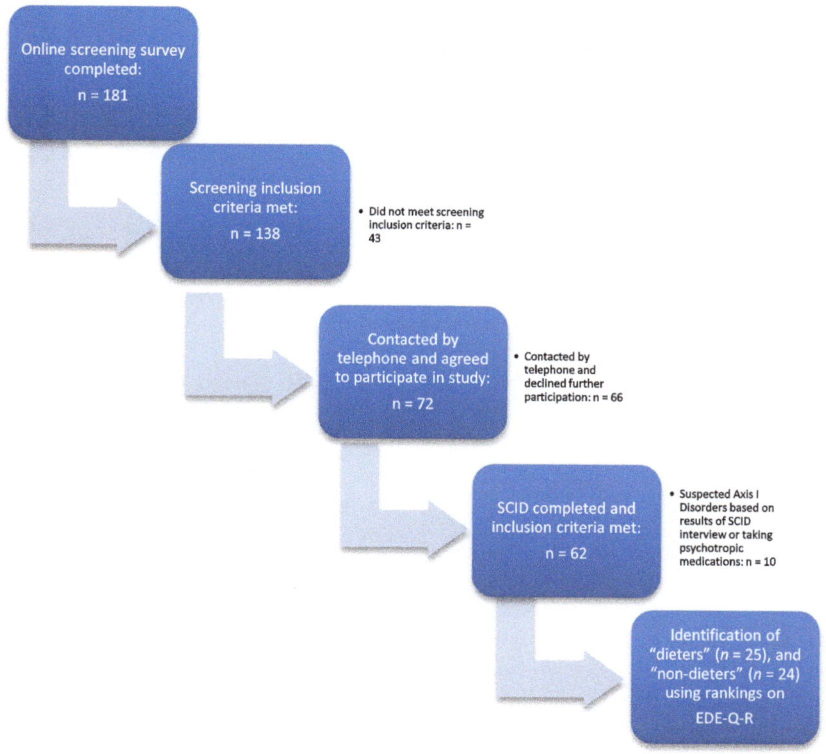

Fig. 1 Flow chart showing recruitment pathway and selection of participants

Participants were shown a word on a laptop screen and asked to indicate whether they felt the word described or applied to them, i.e., was "me" or "not me", by pressing labelled keys on the keyboard. A "fixation cross" appeared on the screen for 1 s and disappeared to reveal the target word [24]. Words were presented for 500 milliseconds, with participants asked to respond as quickly and as accurately as possible. Two scores were used here, reaction time in milliseconds and number of words endorsed (and subsequently, recalled).

Eating Disorder Examination-Questionnaire-Restraint Subscale (EDE-Q-R). The EDE-Q is a 36 item self-report questionnaire derived from the Eating Disorder Examination (EDE) interview [25]. It has good reliability and acceptable criterion validity, including in women in community samples [26]. A measure of dieting behaviour was obtained here using the "Restraint" subscale.

Eating Attitudes Test (EAT-26) [27]. This is a widely used self-report measure of ED symptoms. High internal consistency (alpha = .90) and acceptable criterion-related validity have been reported [28].

Hospital Anxiety and Depression Scale (HADS). The HADS [29] is a self-assessment scale of anxious and depressive symptoms with well-established psychometric properties, and detects depression and anxiety in individuals in a variety of settings [30].

Rosenberg Self Esteem Scale (RSE). The RSE is a widely used self-report measure of global self-esteem. It is composed of 10 statements related to self-worth and self-acceptance [31]. It has high reliability and validity and has been called, "the standard by which new self-esteem measures are evaluated" ([32], p.123).

National Adult Reading Test (NART; [33]). This is a widely used estimate of general intelligence or IQ, with good psychometric properties. It was included because of potential confounds with the complexity of the words used in the SSPT and with level of education and dieting behaviour.

Visual Analogue Scales (VAS). These measured emotions on the day of testing. The emotions measured were: happy, sad, angry, frightened, anxious, disgusted and surprised. These were included because of potential confounds between mood at time of testing and SSPT responses.

Procedure

Testing (individually based) began with administering the SSPT, followed by "filler" tasks to provide a 5–10 min delay before the surprise free recall task. The session also included the NART; 32), and a measure of emotions using the VAS.

Data analysis

Mixed design ANOVAs were planned for endorsements, reaction time and recall on the SSPT (group × "Me/Not Me" × word category), provided data met the relevant assumptions.

Results

Participant characteristics

Of the final sample ($n = 49$), most were White/Caucasian (90 %), followed by Mixed (6 %), Asian or British Asian (2 %) and Other (2 %). Information on participants' age, Body Mass Index (BMI), EAT-26 scores, and NART scores is provided in Table 1. BMI data was missing for one participant in the dieting group. Mean EAT-26 scores for both dieting and non-dieting groups were in the normal range, i.e., below the clinical cut-off of 20 points [27], supporting the non-clinical definition of these groups.

Also important for a healthy, non-clinical sample, mean scores for anxiety and depression symptoms on the HADS were in the normal range (below cut-off of 7 points) [29]. No other variables differed significantly between the dieters and non-dieters. This included years in education ($X^2 = 1.25$, p = .52) and English as a mother tongue ($p = .66$),

EDE-Q Restraint scores

These can be seen in Table 1. As expected, the dieting group had a significantly higher score on the EDE-Q-R than the non-dieting group (t (1, 47) = −12.82, $p < .001$).

SSPT: endorsements

Endorsement data can be seen in Table 2.

Table 2 Mean number of words endorsed as "Me" and "Not me" on the SSPT

	Dieters		Non-dieters	
	($n = 25$)		($n = 24$)	
	"Me"	"Not Me"	"Me"	"Not Me"
	Mean (SD)	Mean (SD)	Mean (SD)	Mean (SD)
Eating disorder relevant	2.4 (2.8)	27.6 (2.8)	0.5 (.72)	29.5 (0.7)
Depression relevant	3.5 (5.7)	26.4 (5.9)	1.46 (2.0)	28.5 (2.0)
Generic negative	4.8 (4.4)	25.1 (4.4)	3.7 (2.8)	26.21 (3.0)
Generic positive/neutral	22.8 (5.0)	7.0 (4.8)	24.2 (3.8)	5.8 (3.8)

SD standard deviation, *SSPT* self-schema processing task

Assumptions of normality were not met and there was a significant amount of variance between groups. This prevented meaningful interpretation of a mixed design ANOVA (group x "Me"/"Not Me" endorsements x word category). Separate ANOVAS[1] were therefore conducted for "Me"/"Not Me" endorsements in each of the four categories of words (i.e., ED relevant, depression relevant, generic negative, and generic positive/neutral), with a between-group factor of dieting/non-dieting. There was a significant group effect for number of ED relevant words endorsed as "Me", (F (1, 47) = 10.71, $p = .002$). No other significant group effects were found. All statistics can be seen in Table 3.

Post hoc tests indicated that dieters endorsed significantly more ED-relevant words as "Me", than non-dieters ($U = 156.0$, $z = -3.05$, $p = .002$, $r = -.44$). No other comparisons were significant.

SSPT: reaction times

A mixed design (group x "Me"/"Not Me" reaction times x word category) ANOVA was performed. However, owing to the forced-choice design (i.e., "Me" or "Not Me") of the SSPT, participants could potentially respond identically to

Table 1 Demographic and between-group statistics for the dieting and non-dieting groups

	Dieters	Non-dieters		
	($n = 25$)	($n = 24$)		
	Mean (SD)	Mean (SD)	t value	Significance level
Age (years)	23.48 (4.8)	25.67 (3.5)	1.81	.08
Current BMI	22.85 (2.5)	24.28 (4.8)	1.29	.20
EDE-Q-R scores	3.57 (1.0)	0.77 (0.5)	12.82	.0001***
EAT-26 scores	14.72 (13.8)	11.42 (9.9)	.97	.34
Anxiety (HADS)	5.12 (3.5)	5.21 (3.2)	.09	.93
Depression (HADS)	2.36 (2.3)	2.38 (2.2)	.02	.98
Estimated IQ (NART)	108.44 (8.2)	105.7 (5.6)	1.38	.18
Self-Esteem (RSE)[a]	17.96 (6.6)	20.17 (4.6)	1.36	.18

BMI body mass index, *EAT-26* eating attitudes test, *EDE-Q-R* eating disorders examination questionnaire (Restraint subscale), *HADS* hospital anxiety and depression scale, *IQ* intelligence quotient, *NART* National Adult Reading Test, *RSE* (rosenberg self-esteem scale), *SD* standard deviation

[a]Higher scores indicate higher levels of self-esteem

***$p < .0001$

Table 3 F-Scores for group effects on endorsements of word categories and reaction times (SSPT)

	Endorsements				Reaction Times			
	"Me"	P	"Not Me"	P	"Me"	P	"Not Me"	P
ED relevant	10.71	.002**	10.25	.002**	1.19	.28	2.21	.14
Depression relevant	2.94	.09	2.89	.09	.44	.51	.98	.33
Generic negative	1.14	.29	1.62	.21	.69	.41	1.99	.17
Generic positive/ neutral	1.17	.28	1.02	.32	1.00	.32	1.10	.30

ED eating disorder, *SSPT* self-schema processing task
$^{**}p < .01$

all words within the same category. Unfortunately, this led to a large amount of missing data as a number of participants responded "Not Me" to all words in some categories. This meant that nearly half ($n = 23$) the sample could not be included, resulting in an underpowered analysis ($n = 26$) that could not be meaningfully interpreted.

In an exploratory analysis, the mean reaction times for categories of words and dieting groups were analysed using ANOVAs to look at between group differences, as for endorsements (see data in Table 4). Dieters and non-dieters' mean reaction times to words from all four categories were not significantly different (all p values > .1).

Recall task

A repeated measures ANOVA indicated that the pattern of dieters' recall of words from each of the four categories did not differ significantly from that of non-dieters' (F (3, 141) = 1.344, $p = .26$), and these are represented in Fig. 2.

Mean number of words recalled by participants in the SSPT surprise recall task can be seen in Table 5. Post hoc tests indicated that recall of ED relevant, but no other, words differed significantly between groups (t (1, 47) = −2.31), $p = .025$), with dieters recalling more ED relevant words than non-dieters.

Table 4 Mean reaction times in milliseconds on the SSPT

	Dieters		Non-dieters	
	($n = 14$)		($n = 12$)	
	"Me"	"Not Me"	"Me"	"Not Me"
	Mean (SD)	Mean (SD)	Mean (SD)	Mean (SD)
Eating disorder relevant	703.6 (546.9)	414.2 (193.9)	536.7 (525.1)	338.5 (160.3)
Depression relevant	602.7 (648.7)	511.6 (375.6)	487.2 (565.9)	422.9 (230.7)
Generic negative	663.6 (375.5)	482.6 (243.5)	573.3 (385.5)	394.6 (187.9)
Generic positive/ neutral	517.6 (241.7)	778.3 (415.9)	448.5 (242.3)	665.0 (333.2)

SD standard deviation, *SSPT* self-schema processing task

VAS emotions

Of the VAS emotions only "sad" scores differed significantly, $U = 192.50$, $z = -2.15$, $p = .031$, $r = -.31$. Dieters reported greater feelings of sadness on the day of testing than non-dieters.

Covariates

Owing to the significant difference between dieting and non-dieting groups on the "sad" emotion VAS, this variable was included in the significant analyses as a covariate to determine its potential impact. "Sad" scores were associated with endorsements of ED relevant words (F (1, 46) = 16.71, $p < .001$); however, the main between-group effect of ED relevant words on endorsements remained significant (F (1, 46) = 5.06, $p = .03$) with "sad" as a covariate.

Discussion

As expected, the dieting group differed significantly from the non-dieting in greater endorsement of ED relevant words, but not depression relevant, generic negative and generic positive/neutral words, on the SSPT. This finding adds to that of Pringle et al. [18], who found that longer reaction times to reject ED relevant words as "Not Me" were predictive of sub-clinical ED symptoms in dieters. The current findings indicate that dieters with no significant ED symptoms also endorse significantly more ED relevant words as "Me" when compared to non-dieters.

Unlike Pringle's study [18] there were no significant differences between groups on reaction times measures, for either endorsements or rejections of ED relevant words. However, this data included missing values for several participants. These analyses were therefore most likely underpowered. Imputing missing data was considered but thought inadvisable as the data imputation method that seemed most appropriate is normally used in repeated measures designs [34], and this was not the method used here. To improve power, future studies might consider using pre-designated and equally occurring categories (e.g., identifying the colour of a word). However, using a method without "Me" and "Not Me" endorsements/rejections might be seen as differing significantly from the original theory underlying the schema paradigm [1]. More radically, it could be asked whether both reaction times and endorsements are always necessary to identify the presence of a schema, or even whether endorsements are more valid (and easier to measure) demonstrations of schematic functioning.

While ratings were relatively low, dieters scored significantly higher on a VAS measure of sadness than non-dieters. The mean difference in "sad" ratings between groups was significantly associated with number of endorsements of ED relevant words. Nevertheless, the

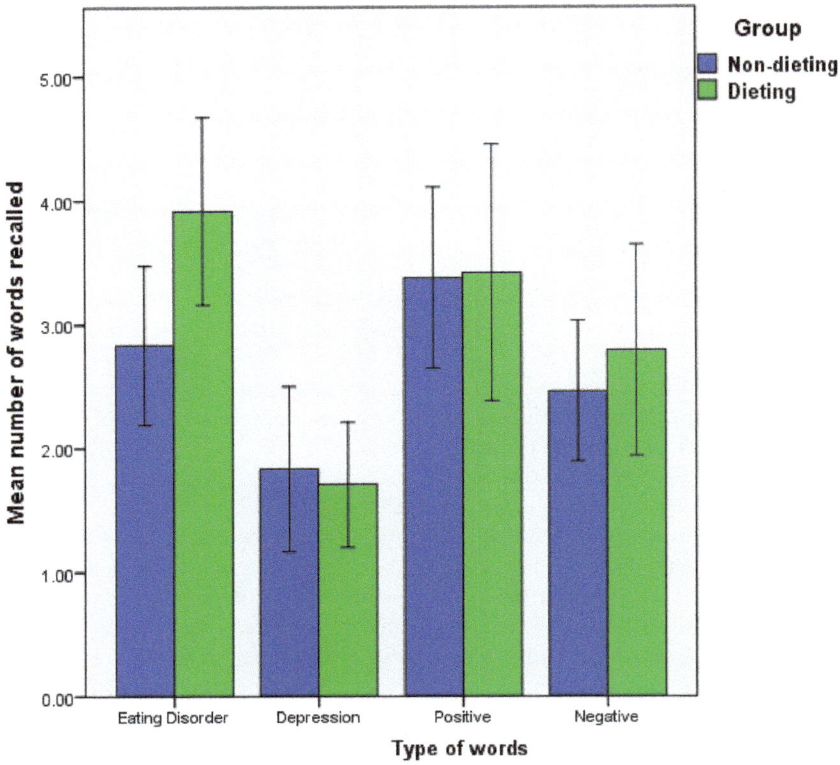

Fig. 2 Mean number of words of each type recalled by non-dieters and dieters

main effect of endorsement and dieting group remained significant after controlling for sadness, suggesting that sadness did not provide a complete explanation for the difference between the groups on endorsements. There was no significant relationship between "sad" ratings and the number of ED words recalled by dieters or non-dieters. Greater recall by the dieters could not therefore be attributed to any differences between the two groups in VAS sad ratings.

Given the high comorbidity of EDs with mood and anxiety disorders [35], higher "sadness" ratings are not wholly unexpected. However, it is also possible that this emotion is linked to the experience of dieting, as dieters are thought to hold a negative view of the self [36]. Theoretical models of EDs postulate an association between core belief activation and distress [3], providing some support for this assertion in an "at risk" group.

One possibility is that these "unrelated content" tasks might be behavioural biomarkers of, for example, risk for EDs (as suggested by the data in Pringle et al., 18). More generally, these data add to the research suggesting an important role for ED-relevant self-schemas, in both ED groups and as a dimensional construct [9, 12, 18, 19]. Future research in dieters and other groups "at risk" of an ED might usefully include measures investigating content not only related to eating, weight and shape, but also to generic or ED-related self-schemas.

The study had some limitations. The sample size was relatively small, and this was particularly true for investigating self-schema reaction times. Nevertheless, schema processing differences were found between the two groups on number of endorsements and in the surprise recall test, thus two out of the three main hypotheses were confirmed, with only differences in reaction time between the dieters and non-dieters not proving significant. A measure of self-reported hunger was not administered on the day of testing given dieters who do not demonstrate ED

Table 5 Mean number of words recalled by participants from the SSPT

	Dieters ($n = 25$) Mean (SD)	Non-dieters ($n = 24$) Mean (SD)
Eating disorder relevant*	3.92 (1.8)	2.83 (1.5)
Depression relevant	1.80 (1.3)	1.83 (1.6)
Generic negative	2.68 (2.1)	2.46 (1.4)
Generic positive/neutral	3.40 (2.4)	3.38 (1.7)

SD standard deviation
Difference between groups, *$p < .05$

symptoms are not suffering from the effects of semi-starvation [37]. Nevertheless, more subtle differences in hunger may have been present and future studies might usefully measure this. Self-report data were used to calculate BMI; ideally height and weight should have been measured on the day of testing.

The planned data analytic strategy was altered as data on the SSPT did not meet the assumptions for parametric analyses. While it may subsequently have been desirable to adjust significance levels for the increased number of analyses conducted, the study was an exploratory one and, as such, no adjustments were made in order to minimise the risk of error arising from this procedure [36]. Post hoc comparisons were conducted in the absence of a significant omnibus effect; again, while this can be inadvisable, it can also be a useful analysis to minimise the risk of a Type 1 error, which it is important to guard against in an exploratory study such as this [38]. Finally, the nature of the data did not allow analysis of 'me' and 'not me' data together, but inspection of the means indicates that dieters and non-dieters both appeared to endorse many more negative words as 'not me', than 'me'. This is perhaps not surprising in a relatively healthy population.

The study had several strengths. Participants were rigorously screened and had higher dietary restraint scores than some previous studies of dieters [16, 17]. Screening ensured that they did not have a psychiatric disorder, including an ED. Findings of interest, therefore, can be attributed to the "at risk" status rather than the presence of any significant ED symptoms.

Conclusion

Future research may benefit from investigating self and ED schema processing in those with EDs. A depressed group might be a useful comparison in any such study. It may be possible to establish some criteria by which schematics and aschematics in those "at risk," might be identified. Given that not all dieters will develop an ED, investigating the profile of each (schematic or aschematic) might refine our notion of who is most at risk [18], and could benefit clinical outcomes through the early identification of vulnerable individuals [37].

Endnotes

[1]This is considered equivalent to an independent sample *t*-test of between-group means.

Competing interests

The authors declare that they have no competing interests.

Authors' contributions

SG designed the study, collected and analysed the data under the supervision of MJC for the award of Doctor of Clinical Psychology at the University of Oxford. SG prepared a first draft of the paper. MJC completed remaining drafts and the final version. Both authors read and approved the final manuscript.

Author details

[1]Isis Education Centre, University of Oxford, Warneford Hospital, Oxford OX3 7JX, UK. [2]Richmond Hospital, 7000 Westminster Hwy, Richmond, BC V6X 1A2, Canada.

References

1. Markus H. Self-schemata and processing information about the self. J Pers Soc Psychol. 1977;35:63–78. doi:10.1037/0022-3514.35.2.63.
2. Cooper MJ. Cognitive behavioural models in eating disorders. In: Fox J, Goss K, editors. Eating and its disorders. Chichester, UK: John Wiley & Sons; 2012.
3. Cooper MJ, Todd G, Wells A. Treating bulimia nervosa and binge eating: An integrated metacognitive and cognitive therapy manual. London: Taylor & Francis; 2009.
4. Waller G, Cordery H, Corstorphine E, Hinrichsen H, Lawson R, Mountford V, et al. Cognitive-behavioral therapy for the eating disorders: A comprehensive treatment guide. Cambridge: Cambridge University Press; 2007.
5. Young JE. Cognitive therapy for personality disorders: A schema-focused approach. Sarasota, FL: Professional Resource Press; 1990.
6. Young JE. Cognitive therapy for personality disorders: A schema-focused approach. Revth ed. Sarasota, FL: Professional Resource Press; 1994.
7. Young JE, Brown G. Young Schema-Questionnaire (2nd. edition). In: Young JE, editor. Cognitive therapy for personality disorders: A schema-focused approach (Rev. edition). Sarasota, FL: Professional Resource Press; 1994.
8. Leung N, Waller G, Thomas G. Core beliefs in anorexic and bulimic women. J Nerv Ment Dis. 1999;187:736–41.
9. Cooper MJ, Cowen P. Negative self-beliefs in relation to eating disorder and depressive symptoms: different themes are characteristic of the two sets of symptoms in those with eating disorders and/or depression. J Cogn Psychother: an Int Q. 2009;23:147–60. doi:10.1891/0889-8391.23.2.147.
10. Fairchild H, Cooper M. A multidimensional measure of core beliefs relevant to eating disorders: preliminary development and validations. Eating Behaviours. 2010;1:239–46. doi:10.1016/j.eatbeh.2010.05.004.
11. Benas JS, Gibb BE. Cognitive biases in depression and eating disorders. Cogn Ther Res. 2009;35:68–78. doi:10.1007/s10608-009-9279-1.
12. Cooper M, Todd G, Wells A. Content, origins and consequences of dysfunctional beliefs in anorexia nervosa and bulimia nervosa. J Cogn Psychother. 1998;12:213–30.
13. Cooper MJ, Turner H. Underlying assumptions and core beliefs in anorexia nervosa and dieting. Br J Clin Psychol. 2000;39:215–8.
14. Stice E, Agras WS. Predicting onset and cessation of bulimic behaviours during adolescence: a longitudinal grouping analysis. Behav Ther. 1998; 29:257–76. doi:10.1016/S0005-7894(98)80006-3.
15. Stice E. A prospective test of the dual-pathway model of bulimic pathology: mediating effects of dieting and negative affect. J Abnorm Psychol. 2001;110:124–35. doi:10.1037/0021-843X.110.1.124.
16. Fairburn CG, Cooper Z, Doll HA, Davies BA. Identifying dieters who will develop an eating disorder: a prospective, population-based study. Am J Psychiatr. 2005;162:2249–55. doi:10.1176/appi.ajp.162.12.2249.
17. Fairburn CG, Beglin SJ. Assessment of eating disorders: interview or self-report questionnaire? Int J Eat Disord. 1994;16:363–70.
18. Pringle A, Harmer CJ, Cooper MJ. Investigating vulnerability to eating disorders: biases in emotional processing. Psychol Med. 2009;40:645–55. doi:10.1017/S0033291709990778.
19. Pringle A, Harmer CJ, Cooper MJ. Biases in emotional processing are associated with vulnerability to eating disorders over time. Eat Behav. 2010; 12:56–9. doi:10.1016/j.eatbeh.2010.08.003.
20. First MB, Spitzer RI, Gibbon M, Williams JBW. Structured clinical interview for axis I and II DSM-IV disorders: Patient edition (SCID-IV/P). New York: New York State Psychiatric Institute, Biometrics Research Department; 1996.
21. Harmer CJ, Shelley NC, Cowen PJ, Goodwin GM. Increased positive versus negative affective perception and memory in healthy volunteers following selective serotonin and norepinephrine reuptake inhibition. Am J Psychiatr. 2004;161:1256–63. doi:10.1176/appi.ajp.161.7.1256.
22. Cohen J. A power primer. Psychol Bull. 1992;112:155–9.
23. Anderson NH. Likeableness ratings of 555 personality-trait words. J Pers Soc Psychol. 1968;9:272–9.
24. MacDonald MR, Kuiper NA. Efficiency and automaticity of self-schema processing in clinical depressives. Motiv Emot. 1985;9:171–84. doi:10.1007/BF00991574.

25. Fairburn CG, Cooper Z. The eating disorder examination. In: Fairburn CG, Wilson GT, editors. Binge eating: Nature, assessment and treatment. 12th ed. New York: Guilford Press; 1993. p. 317–60.
26. Rø Ø, Reas DL, Lask B. Norms for the eating disorder examination questionnaire among female university students in Norway. Nord J Psychiatry. 2010;64:428–32.
27. Garner DM, Garfinkel PE. The eating attitudes test: an index of the symptoms of anorexia nervosa. Psychol Med. 1979;9:273–9. doi:10.1017/S0033291700030762.
28. Garner DM, Olmsted MP, Bohr Y, Garfinkel PE. The eating attitudes test: psychometric features and clinical correlates. Psychol Med. 1982;12:871–8.
29. Zigmond AS, Snaith RP. The hospital anxiety and depression scale. Acta Psychiatr Scand. 1983;67:361–70. doi:10.1111/j.1600-0447.1983.tb09716.x.
30. Bjelland I, Dahl AA, Haug TT, Neckelmann D. The validity of the hospital anxiety and depression scale: an updated literature review. J Psychosom Res. 2002;52:69–78.
31. Rosenberg M. Society and the adolescent self-image. Princeton, NJ: Princeton University Press; 1965.
32. Blascovich J, Tomaka J. Measures of self-esteem. Measures of Personality and Social Psychological Attitudes. 1991;1:115–60.
33. Nelson HE, Willison J. National adult reading test (NART) manual. 2nd ed. Windsor, UK: NFER-Nelson; 1991.
34. Elliott P, Hawthorne G. Imputing missing repeated measures data: How should we proceed? Aust N Z J Psychiatry. 2005;39:575–82. doi:10.1111/j.1440-1614.2005.01629.x.
35. Russell S, Fuscaldo G, Ealey W. Eating disorders with comorbid depression and anxiety: literature review. Melbourne: Beyond Blue Limited; 2008.
36. Bender R, Lenge S. Adjusting for multiple testing – when and how? J Clin Epidemiol. 2001;54:343–9.
37. Heatherton TF, Baumeister RF. Binge eating as escape from self-awareness. Psychol Bull. 1991;110:86–108. doi:10.1037/0033-2909.110.1.86.
38. Hancock GR, Klockars AJ. The quest for α: developments in multiple comparison procedures in the quarter century since games (1971). Rev Educ Res. 1996;66:269–306.

Neurobiological model of the persistence of anorexia nervosa

Joanna E. Steinglass* and B. Timothy Walsh

Abstract

Anorexia Nervosa (AN) is characterized by the maintenance of an undernourished, or starved, state. Persistent restrictive eating, or the recurrent intake of a diet that is inadequate to sustain a healthy weight, is the central behavior maintaining AN. To understand this disturbance, we need to understand the neural mechanisms that allow or promote the persistent choice of inadequate caloric intake. While a range of neural disturbances have been reported in AN, abnormalities in systems relevant to reward processing and the development of habit systems have been consistently described in both structural and functional neuroimaging studies. Most recently, brain and behavior have been directly examined by investigating the neural underpinnings of restrictive food choice. These recent data suggest that, among individuals with AN, dorsal frontostriatal circuits play a greater role in guiding decisions regarding what to eat than among healthy individuals. This line of research attempts to leverage advances in the field of cognitive neuroscience to further our understanding of persistent maladaptive choices of individuals with AN, in the hope that such advances will help in the development of novel treatments for this potentially fatal disorder.

Keywords: Anorexia nervosa, Cognitive neuroscience, Habit systems, Reward systems, Eating behavior

Background

Anorexia Nervosa (AN) is characterized by the maintenance of an undernourished, or starved, state. Affecting approximately 1 % of women [1] across all socioeconomic classes [2], AN is characterized by severe restriction of food intake resulting in an inappropriately low body weight, fear and anxiety about weight gain, and preoccupation with body shape and weight [3]. The recurrent intake of a diet that is inadequate to sustain a healthy weight is the central behavior maintaining this condition. To understand this disturbance, it is useful to consider the neural mechanisms that promote the persistent choice of inadequate caloric intake, a behavior that clearly becomes maladaptive and self-destructive. Here, we review a cognitive neuroscience model of AN that focuses on the persistence of maladaptive behavior.

AN commonly begins during adolescence, with a peak age at first presentation between 14 and 18 years [4, 5]. Unlike many psychiatric illnesses, in which early onset signifies a more severe course of illness, adolescents with AN have a better prognosis than adults: studies of adolescents receiving treatment for AN show that, at 1 year of follow-up, approximately 75 % are in partial or full remission [6–8]. However, when the disease progresses into adulthood, the treatment outlook is disheartening [8, 9]. No pharmacotherapies have proven effective, psychosocial interventions are often inadequate, and relapse rates are high – up to 50 % of adult patients require rehospitalization within a year of discharge [10, 11]. Mortality among young women with AN is at least six times that expected for their age [12], the highest of any psychiatric disorder, and the likelihood of death increases with duration of illness [13]. A better understanding of the neural underpinnings of AN may help to develop novel treatments and improve outcomes for these severely ill individuals.

* Correspondence: js1124@cumc.columbia.edu
1051 Riverside Drive, Unit 98, New York, NY 10032, USA

Review

The importance of eating behavior in AN

Eating is a multifaceted behavior, affected by multiple social, psychological and biological factors. The neurobiological value of food as a primary reward has been long noted [14–16], and much is understood regarding appetitive and inhibitory control around normal eating

[17–19]. Yet, models of the neural mechanisms of normal eating have not contributed greatly to the understanding of eating disorders – perhaps because these models, largely based on studies of rodents, do not clarify the influences that promote maladaptive eating behavior among humans with eating disorders [19].

The aberrations in eating behavior that occur among individuals with eating disorders have been usefully examined via objective assessment in eating laboratories. Most such studies have compared the eating of individuals without eating disorders to that of individuals with binge eating, such as occurs in bulimia nervosa (BN) and binge eating disorder (BED). Laboratory studies have documented that individuals with BN and with BED consume significantly more calories than controls when asked to binge, and that some satiety cues are abnormal. These studies have also documented that, when not binge eating, individuals with BN tend to consume fewer calories than healthy volunteers [20, 21]. These studies laid a foundation for using the laboratory setting to examine abnormally reduced food intake such as occurs in AN.

Restrictive caloric intake in AN has been objectively assessed [22, 23]. One of the first observational studies of intake among individuals with AN demonstrated lower caloric intake compared with healthy controls (HC) (1289 ± 150 vs 2220 ± 108 kcal, $p < 0.05$) as well as restricted fat intake (17.6 ± 2.3 % vs 28.4 ± 1.3 % of total calories consumed, $p < 0.05$) [24]. Additional studies of eating behavior have demonstrated significantly restricted dietary intake among individuals with AN, not only when acutely ill but also immediately after weight restoration. In a single item meal study using an unfamiliar food, patients with AN ate significantly less than HC (104 ± 102 vs 490 ± 188 g, $p < 0.01$) and showed no significant improvement in intake even after they had gained to a normal weight (178 ± 203 g, $p = 0.85$) [25]. In another study, hospitalized patients with AN participated in a Multi-item Meal (www.phenxtoolkit.org [26]) in the laboratory before and after weight restoration treatment, and were compared with HC. Participants were brought to the eating laboratory where they were presented with an array of foods. Individuals with AN ate significantly fewer calories compared with HC, both at admission, when they were severely underweight (364 ± 208 vs. 775 ± 228 kcal, $p = 0.001$), and after full weight restoration (516 ± 273 vs. 758 ± 346 kcal, $p = 0.03$). Furthermore, individuals with AN were particularly avoidant of calories from fat at admission (18 ± 10%vs. 38 ± 7 % of total calories consumed, $p = 0.001$) and after weight restoration (23 ± 9 % vs. 38 ± 18 %, $p = 0.004$) [27]. Assessment of dietary histories of outpatients has also documented restricted intake [28] and specifically avoidance of fat among individuals with AN (15.7 ± 1.7 % vs. 24.8 ± 1.3 % of total calories consumed, $p < 0.05$) [24]. Critically, restrictive eating patterns including reduced caloric intake, limited diet variety and the consumption of foods with low energy density are related to poor outcome over time [29, 30].

"Dieting" is the colloquial term for restricting caloric intake, or, attempting to restrict caloric intake below the amount required to maintain weight. Self-reported dieting is almost universal among adolescent girls, and occurs in up to 75 % of healthy adult populations as well [31]. In the majority of individuals, dieting is ineffective in altering long term weight [32, 33]. For as many as 38 % of dieters, the behavior becomes frankly pathological, termed "disordered eating" [34, 35], and 25 % of those individuals develop eating disorders [36]. Dieting is a signature behavior across eating disorders [37], where persistent efforts to restrict intake are accompanied by disturbed psychological functioning. AN is persistent dieting at its most extreme. Consideration of the importance of dieting in eating disorders is not new – some approaches to probing the neurobiology of AN have usefully incorporated hypotheses about the relationship between neurobiology and dieting, possibly as a "self-medication" for anxiety [38, 39]. Yet, the neural mechanisms of persistent, maladaptive caloric restriction – a signature behavior of several eating disorders - have not been rigorously examined.

Eating is complex and multi-determined [40, 41]. However, the findings described above demonstrate that the salient behavioral disturbance of individuals with AN is the selection of low-calorie foods in a remarkably stereotyped fashion that promotes persistence of illness. A logical and important next step is to ask what drives this behavior neurobiologically.

Cognitive neuroscience of anorexia nervosa

Cognitive neuroscience aims to illuminate the neural basis of human behavior, and to link advances in psychology with biological science. This approach has great potential as we aim to understand the neural mechanisms of the salient maladaptive behaviors in AN. Some proposed models have used a "bottom-up" approach, in which basic processes are studied in order to evaluate aberrancies in brain functioning. For example, study of cognitive domains (e.g., set shifting [42–44]), showed neuropsychological abnormalities; individuals with AN have more difficulty shifting between cognitive tasks, perhaps related to a tendency toward psychological rigidity. However, cognitive findings are not entirely consistent across studies, and these broad executive functioning deficits do not identify specific underlying neural targets [45, 46]. A similar "bottom-up" approach examined basic processes such as taste and yielded evidence of differences in neural activation related to probes of images and actual sensory processing [38, 47]. But, these behavioral and neural abnormalities have not been directly linked to eating disorder behavior. Nonetheless, these studies, and others reviewed below, have consistently shown abnormalities in reward systems and in frontostriatal systems and have paved the way for our current, "top-down," approach that probes the neural activity directly related to disturbances in eating behavior.

The neurobiology of reward in AN

Mesolimbic neural systems of reward processing encompass the midbrain/ventral tegmental area, ventral striatum (including nucleus accumbens, NAcc), and orbitofrontal cortex (OFC). Several studies have examined neural correlates of reward processing among individuals with AN using structural and functional MRI, as well as PET. Structural MRI studies have shown volumetric abnormalities among individuals with AN within reward-sensitive regions, including the OFC, though the directionality of these abnormalities (increased vs decreased volumes) has been inconsistent [48, 49]. Task-based fMRI studies have examined responses to monetary and taste rewards in AN. When asked to respond to monetary stimuli, individuals with AN showed abnormalities in striatal and prefrontal cortex activity [50, 51]. Abnormal task-related responses to images of food and receipt of sweet vs. non-sweet liquids have also been shown with abnormally increased activity within the OFC and the NAcc [52–54]. One PET study indicated increased dopamine receptor density in the NAcc of 10 women recovered from AN [55]. However, Broft et al. found no differences in striatal dopamine receptor binding potential in AN nor any impact of weight gain [56]. Broadly, across a range of imaging techniques and study designs, studies suggest abnormalities within reward circuitry in AN. Early data also indicate abnormalities in the organization of this neural circuit, with heightened connectivity based on resting fMRI and diffusion tractography MRI between the NAcc and the OFC among adolescents and young adults with AN [57].

The functioning of reward systems in AN is likely impacted by both food restriction and adolescence itself. Studies in rodents suggest that food restriction sensitizes reward circuits [58]. For example, following 1-week of food restriction, rats showed increases in dopamine release in response to cocaine and amphetamines [59]. Food restriction in rodents and non-human primates resulted in subsequent increases in drug self-administration [58, 60]. Studies of reward systems in adolescence have also shown increased salience of rewards. For example, an fMRI study compared activation of the NAcc and OFC in children, adolescents, and adults during a task that paired stimulus selection with varying amounts of monetary reward. Relative to the adults and children, the teens showed the strongest blood-oxygenation level dependent (BOLD) signal response within the NAcc to the monetary rewards [61]. Similarly, in a Go/No-Go Task that induces a decrease in impulse control with rewarding relative to neutral stimuli, adolescents showed the largest decrement in impulse control and this behavior was associated with increased NAcc activity [62]. Since AN is defined by food restriction and usually begins during adolescence, these studies underscore the potential relevance of the organization and function of reward systems in AN. Indeed, several reward-centered models of the pathophysiology of AN have emerged [63–67]. While these models differ somewhat in their focus, they overlap in suggesting that AN is associated with abnormalities in the mesolimbic reward systems.

The neurobiology of frontostriatal systems in AN

Habit formation is the process by which a behavior associated with receipt of a reward, if repeated frequently ("practiced"), becomes almost automatic and far less dependent on the receipt of the reward [68]. As behavior shifts from goal-directed to habitual, there is an accompanying shift in the neural systems supporting behavior [69–71]. Human and animal research indicate that once the behavior achieves the characteristics of habit (i.e., becomes outcome independent), it is under the control of neural systems that include the dorsal striatum (basal ganglia, caudate and putamen) and associated dorsolateral frontal cortex. These circuits are thought to be of particular interest in persistent, maladaptive behaviors seen across psychiatric illnesses [72].

A range of disturbances in dorsal frontostriatal systems has been described in AN. PET studies have shown hypermetabolic abnormalities in the caudate among patients with AN, as compared with healthy controls (HC) and with individuals with BN [73–76]. A PET dopamine binding study also reported that dopamine binding potential in the dorsal caudate correlated with harm avoidance, a trait commonly found in individuals with AN [55]. Structural studies, including a meta-analysis, have shown decreased volume in the caudate among individuals with AN [48]. One fMRI study of a monetary guessing game found increased neural activity in the caudate among recovered AN [50]. A study using food pictures for symptom provocation found greater caudate activation among individuals who had recovered from AN as compared with HC [77]. These data have yielded several models proposing frontostriatal dysfunction in AN [65, 78–82].

A habit centered model

We have recently suggested that persistent dieting in AN has the behavioral characteristics of "habit" [68]: restrictive intake in AN is learned, not innate, occurs repeatedly, and, once learned, is elicited by specific stimuli for the individual [78]. As these behaviors are learned through reinforcement, the mesolimbic reward system is highly relevant for understanding the development and persistence of AN. Habitual behaviors are defined as being relatively insensitive to the receipt of a desirable outcome –a person continues the behavior even if their desire for the outcome has changed [69]. Most importantly, once the behavior is established, it takes great effort from the individual to change the behavior. Individuals with AN develop – i.e., learn - dieting behavior, typically during adolescence. The dieting behavior is reinforced for a number of reasons, many specific to the affected individual (e.g., the pleasure of achieving weight loss; the receipt of compliments; a sense of satisfaction for having achieved a challenging goal, a heightened sense of self-control). As noted above, adolescence is a stage of life when reward salience is unusually high, which may also contribute to the development and perpetuation of behaviors in young people [61, 62]. Among individuals with AN, the effects of starvation on the brain likely also contribute to altered decision-making. The dieting behavior is repeated, and with repetition becomes more automatic, such that ultimately the behavioral routines are elicited by cues (e.g., the onset of a meal leads to initiation of a series of ritualized behaviors that collectively serve to minimize intake).

A key prediction of the habit model of AN is that restrictive intake in AN is associated with activity in the dorsal striatum. We recently tested this hypothesis in a group of older adolescents and adults with AN, using a Food Choice Task performed during fMRI scanning [83]. In this task [84], participants are asked to make a series of choices between a food that they themselves have rated as "Neutral" on both healthiness and tastiness, and a series of 75 other food items. Participants are aware that after the task they will receive one of their selections to eat as a snack, so their choices have real implications. As expected (and as previously shown [84]), the participants with AN were substantially less likely to choose the high fat food items ($F_{1,40} = 32.2$, $p < 0.0001$).We also found that caloric intake in the laboratory meal the following day was significantly associated with proportion of high fat items selected in the task ($r = 0.61$, $p < 0.01$), indicating that this assessment captures the restrictive intake so characteristic of AN.

In order to examine the neural correlates of the behavior, we measured the correlation between BOLD signal and each participant's choices by entering individual choice ratings in a parametric analysis to determine the link between behavior and BOLD activity. Whole brain analyses in controls and individuals with AN during food choice showed no significant differences between groups in the mesolimbic reward regions (even at a lenient threshold), but significantly different patterns of activation in the dorsal striatum. Region of interest (ROI) analyses focused on the dorsal striatum, as per the *a priori* hypothesis, and, as hypothesized, in AN, food choices were strongly associated with dorsal striatum activity, a pattern that was not found in the control group ($p < 0.05$).

This study also yielded intriguing behavioral findings that demonstrate the complex relationship between "self-control" and "habit" in maladaptive eating behavior. Individual ratings of healthiness and tastiness of each food item were used to identify trials in which "self-control" would need to be engaged to make the "correct" (i.e., healthy) choice; that is, to choose foods that were Healthy even when they were rated by the participant as Not Tasty, or, conversely, to *not* choose foods rated Not Healthy but Tasty [85]. Compared to controls, individuals with AN tended to rate Not Healthy foods as Not Tasty, leading to their having fewer choices in which "self-control" was needed ($t_{40} = 3.10$, $p = 0.004$). Even so, individuals with AN made the self-controlled choice significantly more often when the opportunity arose ($t_{40} = -4.89$, $p = 0.00002$).

Conclusions

The origins of AN are complex. Our current understanding is that innate factors, including genetic ones, contribute significant risk but are not determinative. Acting on such underlying vulnerabilities, psychosocial and environmental factors, typically combined with the stresses of adolescence, trigger a commitment to calorie restriction and weight loss that initially appears no different from that experienced by a majority of adolescent girls in developed countries. In those who develop AN, however, food restriction becomes all-consuming, relentless, and remarkably stereotyped. Among the substantial number who develop chronic illness, dietary practices are deeply entrenched and difficult to alter, underlying the persistence of the disorder.

The stereotyped nature of the behaviors characteristic of AN and their persistence suggest that affected individuals share similar disturbances in neural circuits related to restrictive food intake. The field of cognitive neuroscience aims to understand how the brain governs mental processes and ultimately behavior. We have adopted a "top-down" approach based in cognitive neuroscience to attempt to elucidate the core behavioral disturbances of AN. In this model, we propose that some aspect of dieting behavior is initially rewarding, but that this behavior persists in individuals with AN as maladaptive behavior because it is ultimately mediated by neural circuits linked to habit formation.

We and others have found that the characteristic patterns of food restriction can be readily assessed by objective measurement of eating behavior. By adapting techniques utilized by cognitive neuroscientists to examine the neural basis for self-control in avoiding "junk food," we have developed a Food Choice Task using images of foods that accurately captures the restriction of caloric intake of AN and that is predictive of actual food intake. Conducting this task during fMRI, we have found that the neural circuits engaged by individuals with AN during food choice differ significantly from those engaged by healthy controls, and are circuits associated with habit formation.

We emphasize that this line of work has only just begun, and that many questions are unanswered. The recently acquired fMRI data addressed the hypothesis that persistent maladaptive behavior in AN is mediated by dorsal frontostriatal circuits that underlie habit behavior. Yet, this was not a definitive test of whether restrictive intake is a "habit." Additionally, it is not known if the neural circuits engaged by successful dieters who do not develop AN differ from those of individuals with the disorder. It is not known how the neural circuits related to food choice change as AN becomes chronic nor how they change with treatment. There is compelling evidence that psychological and emotional factors impact food restriction in AN, and it is not clear how such factors affect the neural circuits associated with food choice. However, it is our hope that the integration of the perspective of cognitive neuroscience into the study of AN will be a source of new lines of thinking and of probing this enigmatic disorder.

Competing interests
The authors declare that they have no competing interests.

Authors' contributions
JES and BTW participated equally in the project development, interpretation, and writing of this manuscript. All authors read and approved the final manuscript.

Acknowledgments
We wish to gratefully acknowledge Karin Foerde, PhD and Daphna Shohamy, PhD who have guided our understanding of cognitive neuroscience and are partners in our research efforts. This work was supported, in part, by New York State Psychiatric Institute, the Irving Institute for Clinical and Translational Research at Columbia University Medical Center, the Hilda and Preston Davis Foundation, the National Eating Disorders Association, the Global Foundation for Eating Disorders, and the National Institute of Mental Health.

References
1. Hudson JI, Hiripi E, Pope Jr HG, Kessler RC. The prevalence and correlates of eating disorders in the National Comorbidity Survey Replication. Biol Psychiatry. 2007;61(3):348–58.
2. Gard MC, Freeman CP. The dismantling of a myth: a review of eating disorders and socioeconomic status. Int J Eat Disord. 1996;20(1):1–12.
3. APA. Diagnostic and Statistical Manual of Mental Disorders. 4th ed. Washington: American Psychiatric Association Press; 2000.
4. Herpertz-Dahlmann B. Adolescent eating disorders: update on definitions, symptomatology, epidemiology, and comorbidity. Child Adolesc Psychiatr Clin N Am. 2015;24(1):177–96.
5. Swanson SA, Crow SJ, Le Grange D, Swendsen J, Merikangas KR. Prevalence and correlates of eating disorders in adolescents. Results from the national comorbidity survey replication adolescent supplement. Arch Gen Psychiatry. 2011;68(7):714–23.
6. Lock J, Le Grange D, Agras WS, Moye A, Bryson SW, Jo B. Randomized clinical trial comparing family-based treatment with adolescent-focused individual therapy for adolescents with anorexia nervosa. Arch Gen Psychiatry. 2010;67(10):1025–32.
7. Agras WS, Lock J, Brandt H, Bryson SW, Dodge E, Halmi KA, et al. Comparison of 2 family therapies for adolescent anorexia nervosa: a randomized parallel trial. JAMA Psychiatry. 2014;71(11):1279–86.
8. Watson HJ, Bulik CM. Update on the treatment of anorexia nervosa: review of clinical trials, practice guidelines and emerging interventions. Psychol Med. 2013;43(12):2477–500.
9. Hay P. A systematic review of evidence for psychological treatments in eating disorders: 2005–2012. Int J Eat Disord. 2013;46(5):462–9.
10. Eckert ED, Halmi KA, Marchi P, Grove W, Crosby R. Ten-year follow-up of anorexia nervosa: clinical course and outcome. Psychol Med. 1995;25(1):143–56.
11. Pike KM. Long-term course of anorexia nervosa: response, relapse, remission, and recovery. Clin Psychol Rev. 1998;18(4):447–75.
12. Arcelus J, Mitchell AJ, Wales J, Nielsen S. Mortality Rates in Patients With Anorexia Nervosa and Other Eating Disorders: A Meta-analysis of 36 Studies. Arch Gen Psychiatry. 2011;68(7):724–31.
13. Sullivan PF. Mortality in anorexia nervosa. Am J Psychiatry. 1995;152(7):1073–5.
14. Schultz W. Predictive reward signal of dopamine neurons. J Neurophysiol. 1998;80(1):1–27.
15. Hassani OK, Cromwell HC, Schultz W. Influence of expectation of different rewards on behavior-related neuronal activity in the striatum. J Neurophysiol. 2001;85(6):2477–89.
16. Dagher A. Functional brain imaging of appetite. Trends Endocrinol Metab. 2012;23(5):250–60.
17. LaBar KS, Gitelman DR, Parrish TB, Kim YH, Nobre AC, Mesulam MM. Hunger selectively modulates corticolimbic activation to food stimuli in humans. Behav Neurosci. 2001;115(2):493–500.
18. Smeets PA, Charbonnier L, van Meer F, van der Laan LN, Spetter MS. Food-induced brain responses and eating behaviour. Proc Nutr Soc. 2012;1–10.
19. Saper CB, Chou TC, Elmquist JK. The need to feed: homeostatic and hedonic control of eating. Neuron. 2002;36(2):199–211.
20. Kissileff HR, Walsh BT, Kral JG, Cassidy SM. Laboratory studies of eating behavior in women with bulimia. Physiol Behav. 1986;38(4):563–70.
21. Walsh BT, Hadigan CM, Kissileff HR, LaChaussee JL. Bulimia nervosa. A syndrome of feast and famine. In: Anderson GH, Kennedy SH, editors. The biology of feast and famine. Relevance to eating disorders. San Diego: Academic; 1992. p. 1–20.
22. Heaner MK, Walsh BT. A history of the identification of the characteristic eating disturbances of Bulimia Nervosa, Binge Eating Disorder and Anorexia Nervosa. Appetite. 2013;65:185–8.
23. Hetherington MM, Rolls BJ. Eating behavior in eating disorders: response to preloads. Physiol Behav. 1991;50(1):101–8.
24. Hadigan CM, Anderson EJ, Miller KK, Hubbard JL, Herzog DB, Klibanski A, et al. Assessment of macronutrient and micronutrient intake in women with anorexia nervosa. Int J Eat Disord. 2000;28(3):284–92.
25. Sysko R, Walsh BT, Schebendach J, Wilson GT. Eating behavior among women with anorexia nervosa. Am J Clin Nutr. 2005;82(2):296–301.
26. Hamilton CM, Strader LC, Pratt JG, Maiese D, Hendershot T, Kwok RK, et al. The PhenX Toolkit: get the most from your measures. Am J Epidemiol. 2011;174(3):253–60.
27. Mayer LE, Schebendach J, Bodell LP, Shingleton RM, Walsh BT. Eating behavior in anorexia nervosa: Before and after treatment. Int J Eat Disord. 2012; 45(2):290–293.
28. Huse DM, Lucas AR. Dietary patterns in anorexia nervosa. Am J Clin Nutr. 1984;40(2):251–4.
29. Schebendach JE, Mayer LE, Devlin MJ, Attia E, Contento IR, Wolf RL, et al. Dietary energy density and diet variety as predictors of outcome in anorexia nervosa. Am J Clin Nutr. 2008;87(4):810–6.
30. Schebendach J, Mayer LE, Devlin MJ, Attia E, Walsh BT. Dietary energy density and diet variety as risk factors for relapse in anorexia nervosa: A replication. Int J Eat Disord. 2012;45(1):79–84.
31. Jeffery RW, Adlis SA, Forster JL. Prevalence of dieting among working men and women: the healthy worker project. Health Psychol. 1991;10(4):274–81.

32. Lowe MR, Annunziato RA, Markowitz JT, Didie E, Bellace DL, Riddell L, et al. Multiple types of dieting prospectively predict weight gain during the freshman year of college. Appetite. 2006;47(1):83–90.
33. French SA, Jeffery RW, Folsom AR, McGovern P, Williamson DF. Weight loss maintenance in young adulthood: prevalence and correlations with health behavior and disease in a population-based sample of women aged 55–69 years. Int J Obes Relat Metab Disord. 1996;20(4):303–10.
34. Reba-Harrelson L, Von Holle A, Hamer RM, Swann R, Reyes ML, Bulik CM. Patterns and prevalence of disordered eating and weight control behaviors in women ages 25–45. Eat Weight Disord. 2009;14(4):e190–8.
35. Liebman M, Cameron BA, Carson DK, Brown DM, Meyer SS. Dietary fat reduction behaviors in college students: relationship to dieting status, gender and key psychosocial variables. Appetite. 2001;36(1):51–6.
36. Shisslak CM, Crago M, Estes LS. The spectrum of eating disturbances. Int J Eat Disord. 1995;18(3):209–19.
37. Fairburn CG. Cognitive Behavior Therapy and Eating Disorders. New York: Guilford Press; 2008.
38. Kaye WH, Wierenga CE, Bailer UF, Simmons AN, Bischoff-Grethe A. Nothing tastes as good as skinny feels: the neurobiology of anorexia nervosa. Trends Neurosci. 2013;36(2):110–20.
39. Kaye W. Neurobiology of anorexia and bulimia nervosa. Physiol Behav. 2008;94(1):121–35.
40. Steinglass JE, Sysko R, Mayer L, Berner LA, Schebendach J, Wang Y, et al. Pre-meal anxiety and food intake in anorexia nervosa. Appetite. 2010;55(2):214–8.
41. Lavender JM, De Young KP, Wonderlich SA, Crosby RD, Engel SG, Mitchell JE, et al. Daily Patterns of Anxiety in Anorexia Nervosa: Associations With Eating Disorder Behaviors in the Natural Environment. J Abnorm Psychol. 2013;122(3):672–83.
42. Steinglass JE, Walsh BT, Stern Y. Set shifting deficit in anorexia nervosa. J Int Neuropsychol Soc. 2006;12(3):431–5.
43. Tchanturia K, Davies H, Roberts M, Harrison A, Nakazato M, Schmidt U, et al. Poor cognitive flexibility in eating disorders: examining the evidence using the Wisconsin Card Sorting Task. PLoS One. 2012;7(1):e28331.
44. Holliday J, Tchanturia K, Landau S, Collier D, Treasure J. Is impaired set-shifting an endophenotype of anorexia nervosa? Am J Psychiatry. 2005;162(12):2269–75.
45. Lang K, Stahl D, Espie J, Treasure J, Tchanturia K. Set shifting in children and adolescents with anorexia nervosa: an exploratory systematic review and meta-analysis. Int J Eat Disord. 2014;47(4):394–9.
46. Shott ME, Filoteo JV, Jappe LM, Pryor T, Maddox WT, Rollin MD, et al. Altered implicit category learning in anorexia nervosa. Neuropsychology. 2012;26(2):191–201.
47. Oberndorfer TA, Frank GK, Simmons AN, Wagner A, McCurdy D, Fudge JL, et al. Altered insula response to sweet taste processing after recovery from anorexia and bulimia nervosa. Am J Psychiatry. 2013;170(10):1143–51.
48. Titova OE, Hjorth OC, Schioth HB, Brooks SJ. Anorexia nervosa is linked to reduced brain structure in reward and somatosensory regions: a meta-analysis of VBM studies. BMC Psychiatry. 2013;13:110.
49. Frank GK, Shott ME, Hagman JO, Mittal VA. Alterations in Brain Structures Related to Taste Reward Circuitry in Ill and Recovered Anorexia Nervosa and in Bulimia Nervosa. Am J Psychiatry. 2013; 170(10):1152–60.
50. Wagner A, Aizenstein H, Venkatraman VK, Fudge J, May JC, Mazurkewicz L, et al. Altered reward processing in women recovered from anorexia nervosa. Am J Psychiatry. 2007;164(12):1842–9.
51. Decker JH, Figner B, Steinglass JE. On Weight and Waiting: Delay Discounting in Anorexia Nervosa Pretreatment and Posttreatment. Biol Psychiatry. 2015;78(9):606–14.
52. Frank GK, Reynolds JR, Shott ME, Jappe L, Yang TT, Tregellas JR, et al. Anorexia nervosa and obesity are associated with opposite brain reward response. Neuropsychopharmacology. 2012;37(9):2031–46.
53. Cowdrey FA, Park RJ, Harmer CJ, McCabe C. Increased neural processing of rewarding and aversive food stimuli in recovered anorexia nervosa. Biol Psychiatry. 2011;70(8):736–43.
54. Fladung AK, Gron G, Grammer K, Herrnberger B, Schilly E, Grasteit S, et al. A neural signature of anorexia nervosa in the ventral striatal reward system. Am J Psychiatry. 2010;167(2):206–12.
55. Frank GK, Bailer UF, Henry SE, Drevets W, Meltzer CC, Price JC, et al. Increased dopamine D2/D3 receptor binding after recovery from anorexia nervosa measured by positron emission tomography and [< sup > 11</sup > C] raclopride. Biol Psychiatry. 2005;58(11):908–12.
56. Broft A, Slifstein M, Osborne J, Kothari P, Morim S, Shingleton R, et al. Striatal dopamine type 2 receptor availability in anorexia nervosa. Psychiatry Res. 2015;233(3):380–7.
57. Cha J, Ide JS, Siciliano F, Biezonski D, Bowman D, Simpson HB et al. Hyperconnectivity of reward circuitry in Anorexia Nervosa: A longitudinal, multimodal MRI study. Human brain mapping. revise and resubmit.
58. Carroll ME, France CP, Meisch RA. Intravenous self-administration of etonitazene, cocaine and phencyclidine in rats during food deprivation and satiation. J Pharmacol Exp Ther. 1981;217(2):241–7.
59. Cadoni C, Solinas M, Valentini V, Di Chiara G. Selective psychostimulant sensitization by food restriction: differential changes in accumbens shell and core dopamine. Eur J Neurosci. 2003;18(8):2326–34.
60. Carroll ME, Meisch RA. Oral phencyclidine (PCP) self-administration in rhesus monkeys: effects of feeding conditions. J Pharmacol Exp Ther. 1980;214(2):339–46.
61. Galvan A, Hare TA, Parra CE, Penn J, Voss H, Glover G, et al. Earlier development of the accumbens relative to orbitofrontal cortex might underlie risk-taking behavior in adolescents. J Neurosci. 2006;26(25):6885–92.
62. Somerville LH, Hare T, Casey BJ. Frontostriatal maturation predicts cognitive control failure to appetitive cues in adolescents. J Cogn Neurosci. 2011;23(9):2123–34.
63. Kaye WH, Fudge JL, Paulus M. New insights into symptoms and neurocircuit function of anorexia nervosa. Nat Rev Neurosci. 2009;10(8):573–84.
64. Keating C, Tilbrook AJ, Rossell SL, Enticott PG, Fitzgerald PB. Reward processing in anorexia nervosa. Neuropsychologia. 2012;50(5):567–75.
65. O'Hara CB, Campbell IC, Schmidt U. A reward-centred model of anorexia nervosa: A focussed narrative review of the neurological and psychophysiological literature. Neurosci Biobehav Rev. 2015;52:131–52.
66. Park RJ, Godier LR, Cowdrey FA. Hungry for reward: How can neuroscience inform the development of treatment for Anorexia Nervosa? Behav Res Ther. 2014;62:47–59.
67. Fladung AK, Schulze UM, Scholl F, Bauer K, Gron G. Role of the ventral striatum in developing anorexia nervosa. Transl Psychiatry. 2013;3:e315.
68. Graybiel AM. Habits, rituals, and the evaluative brain. Annu Rev Neurosci. 2008;31:359–87.
69. Balleine BW, O'Doherty JP. Human and rodent homologies in action control: corticostriatal determinants of goal-directed and habitual action. Neuropsychopharmacology. 2010;35(1):48–69.
70. O'Doherty J, Dayan P, Schultz J, Deichmann R, Friston K, Dolan RJ. Dissociable roles of ventral and dorsal striatum in instrumental conditioning. Science. 2004;304(5669):452–4.
71. Daw ND, Shohamy D. The cognitive neuroscience of motivation and learning. Soc Cogn. 2008;26(5):593–620.
72. Robbins TW, Gillan CM, Smith DG, de Wit S, Ersche KD. Neurocognitive endophenotypes of impulsivity and compulsivity: towards dimensional psychiatry. Trends Cogn Sci. 2012;16(1):81–91.
73. Herholz K, Kreig JC, Emrich HM, Pawlik G, Beil C, Pirke KM, et al. Regional cerebral glucose metabolism in anorexia nervosa measured by positron emission tomography. Biol Psychiatry. 1987;22:43–51.
74. Delvenne V, Goldman S, De Maertelaer V, Simon Y, Luxen A, Lotstra F. Brain hypometabolism of glucose in anorexia nervosa: normalization after weight gain. Biol Psychiatry. 1996;40:761–8.
75. Delvenne V, Goldman S, De Maertelaer V, Lotstra F. Brain glucose metabolism in eating disorders assessed by positron emission tomography. Int J Eat Disord. 1999;25(1):29–37.
76. Krieg JC, Holthoff V, Schreiber W, Pirke KM, Herholz K. Glucose metabolism in the caudate nuclei of patients with eating disorders, measured by PET. Eur Arch Psychiatry Clin Neurosci. 1991;240(6):331–3.
77. Sanders N, Smeets PA, van Elburg AA, Danner UN, van Meer F, Hoek HW, et al. Altered food-cue processing in chronically ill and recovered women with anorexia nervosa. Front Behav Neurosci. 2015;9:46.
78. Walsh BT. The enigmatic persistence of anorexia nervosa. Am J Psychiatry. 2013;170(5):477–84.
79. Steinglass J, Walsh BT. Habit learning and anorexia nervosa: a cognitive neuroscience hypothesis. Int J Eat Disord. 2006;39(4):267–75.
80. Hatch A, Madden S, Kohn M, Clarke S, Touyz S, Williams LM. Anorexia nervosa: towards an integrative neuroscience model. Eur Eat Disord Rev. 2010;18(3):165–79.

81. Godier LR, Park RJ. Compulsivity in anorexia nervosa: a transdiagnostic concept. Front Psychol. 2014;5:778.
82. Marsh R, Maia TV, Peterson BS. Functional disturbances within frontostriatal circuits across multiple childhood psychopathologies. Am J Psychiatry. 2009;166(6):664–74.
83. Foerde K, Steinglass JE, Shohamy D, Walsh BT. Neural mechanisms supporting maladaptive food choices in anorexia nervosa. Nat Neurosci. 2015;18(11):1571–3.
84. Steinglass J, Foerde K, Kostro K, Shohamy D, Walsh BT. Restrictive food intake as a choice-A paradigm for study. Int J Eat Disord. 2015;48(1):59–66.
85. Hare TA, Camerer CF, Rangel A. Self-control in decision-making involves modulation of the vmPFC valuation system. Science. 2009;324(5927):646–8.

Improving the post-meal experience of hospitalised patients with eating disorders using visuospatial, verbal and somatic activities

Emily Griffiths[1], Nicholas Hawkes[2], Sam Gilbert[3] and Lucy Serpell[1,4*]

Abstract

Background: This study compares the effects of different cognitive tasks on post-meal negative affect, positive affect, intrusive thoughts and intrusive images of hospitalised patients with eating disorders.

Methods: Twenty-five participants were recruited from an eating disorder service. Using a within-subjects design, participants performed one of the following tasks for 15 min: the game 'Tetris' (visuospatial), a general knowledge 'Quiz' (verbal), 'Braille' translation (somatic) and 'Sitting Quietly' (control). In total, participants completed each task on three occasions.

Results: The visuospatial, verbal and somatic tasks had beneficial effects on all positive and negative indicators, when compared with 'Sitting Quietly'. Visuospatial and somatic tasks were more effective at reducing intrusive imagery than the verbal task.

Conclusions: The results suggest that certain engaging activities can help hospitalised patients with eating disorders manage the difficult post-meal period.

Keywords: Eating disorders, Affect, Post-meal tasks, Distraction

Background

Mealtimes can be extremely distressing for individuals with eating disorders, resulting in symptoms of anxiety and depression [1–4]. This is likely to be heightened in eating disorder inpatients, who are frequently supervised and restricted in their activities following meals [5]. This study investigates whether visuospatial, verbal, and somatic activities performed in a hospital setting can reduce post-meal distress.

Inpatient eating disorder services vary widely in how they implement mealtimes [6], mostly relying on clinical judgement [7]. Although almost half of services assessed in the UK reported offering a post-meal activity [8] there is limited evidence to support the provision of specific activities during this time (though see [9–11]).

The underlying processes that underpin post-meal distress in people with eating disorders are not fully understood. People with eating disorders report feeling fat [12], which has been associated with distress, negative bodily images/sensations, and negative self-beliefs [13, 14]. One theory suggests that feeling fat results from a misinterpretation of particular emotions of depression, anxiety or guilt and bodily sensations of feeling full, bloated and sweaty [12, 15]. Considering this theory, it is possible that distress after mealtimes is a result of misinterpreting bodily sensations, such as the stomach stretching, which leads to a variety of images such as an overly expanded stomach. This is then viewed as evidence for the feared catastrophe: rapid weight gain. Therefore, one possible way to reduce distress during the post-meal period may involve interrupting the processing of feeling fat either through interrupting

* Correspondence: lucy@serpell.com
[1]University College London, Clinical, Educational & Health Psychology, 1-19 Torrington Place, London WC1E 7HB, UK
[4]Eating Disorders Service, North East London NHS Foundation Trust, London, UK
Full list of author information is available at the end of the article

intrusive imagery, intrusive thoughts or somatic experiences. Studies within the Post-Traumatic Stress Disorder (PTSD) literature have considered a similar approach of interrupting intrusive imagery to reduce later traumatic flashbacks [16, 17].

The aim of this study is therefore to investigate the effects of post-meal visuospatial, verbal and somatic tasks on self-reported positive and negative affect and intrusive thoughts and intrusive imagery, in comparison with a control condition of sitting quietly. This may help to shed light on suitable activities to improve the difficult post-meal experience.

Methods

Participants

Participants were recruited from three hospital units within the same eating disorders service: an inpatient ward, a residential rehabilitation unit and a day hospital. Participants were required to be between 18-65 years old and were excluded if they were unable to speak English fluently, had a moderate to severe learning disability, were on bed-rest or were imminently being discharged.

Procedure

This study used a within-subjects design. Immediately following their meals (breakfast, lunch or dinner) whilst on the unit, participants accessed an online web-based programme using a laptop. This programme administered various questionnaires (see below), and one of four tasks, which lasted for 15 min.

Participants on the ward or rehabilitation unit repeated this procedure following any 12 meals (breakfast, lunch or dinner) of their choice, which they completed within a two week (inpatients) or one month (day patients) period. Each of the four tasks was assigned to three of the sessions in a Latin Square design so that participants could not predict in advance which task they would perform, and each task was equally likely to occur at each of the 12 time points.

Tasks

1. Visuospatial (Tetris). A computerised game requiring participants to use cursor keys to rotate falling geometric blocks (see "http://www.ucl.ac.uk/sam-gilbert/tetris.php").
2. Verbal (Quiz). A computerised general knowledge quiz requiring participants to select answers from four possible choices (see "http://www.ucl.ac.uk/sam-gilbert/quiz.php").
3. Somatic (Braille). A novel task requiring participants to use their fingertips to translate a random list of Braille letters into letters of the English alphabet.
4. Control (Sitting Quietly). Participants were required to sit quietly.

Measures

The Positive and Negative Affect Scale (PANAS; [18]) consists of 10 items of positive affect and 10 items of negative affect, each of which is rated on a scale from 1 (very slightly/ not at all) to 5 (extremely). The measure has been validated among adult samples, with alpha coefficients ranging from 0.84-0.90 [18]. This scale was administered at the beginning of each session (before the participant knew which task they would perform) and again immediately following the task. Any short-term effect of the task during the post-meal period was measured by the change score, where a positive change score on the PANAS negative affect subscale would represent an increase in negative affect over time and a positive change score on the PANAS positive affect subscale would represent an increase in positive affect over time.

Participants were also asked the following two questions after the task had been administered; 'To what extent did you experience intrusive body and fatness related thoughts during the activity?' and 'To what extent did you experience intrusive body and fatness related images during the activity?' These questions were rated from 1 (very slightly/not at all) to 5 (extremely).

Ethical approval

Ethical approval was granted from the local NHS Research Ethics Committee. Informed consent to participate was obtained from all participants.

Results

Of those suitable, 36 (69 %) agreed to take part in the study. Subsequently 11 participants dropped out, defined as completing fewer than 75 % of trials, versus 25 'completers', who were included in subsequent analyses. Participants who dropped out of the study were twice as likely to be White British as completers. No other significant difference was observed between these two groups (see Table 1 for full clinical and demographic data). Outcome measures are shown in Fig. 1.

PANAS

PANAS negative baseline scores did not differ significantly between tasks (Tetris: 23.6; Quiz: 23.9; Braille: 23.5; Sitting Quietly: 24.6; $p = .53$) but there was a significant effect of task on change scores ($p = .002$). PANAS negative was reduced from pre- to post-task in the Tetris, Quiz, and Braille conditions ($p < .03$), but not in the Sitting Quietly condition ($p = .90$). Pairwise comparisons revealed a significant difference between Sitting Quietly and: Quiz ($p = .001$) and Braille ($p = .011$), and a

Table 1 Demographic and clinical data

Demographic	Completers (*n* = 25)	Drop Outs (*n* = 11)	*p* value
Unit (%)			
Inpatient	52.0	90.9	
Rehabilitation	32.0	0	.06[a]
Day Hospital	16.0	9.1	
Age, years: mean (S.D.)	27.4 (9.8)	36.7 (15.0)	.12[b]
Gender: % F	96.0	100	.50 [a]
Ethnicity (% WB)	36.0	72.7	.04 [a]
Employment status (%)			
Unemployed	16.0	63.6	
Student	44.0	27.3	
Non-professional/voluntary	16.0	9.1	.06 [a]
Professional	20.0	0	
Retired	4.0	0	
Diagnosis (%)			
AN-R	64.0	72.7	
AN-BP	24.0	18.2	.88[a]
EDNOS	12.0	9.1	
BMI on admission: mean (S.D.)	15.4 (2.4)	13.9 (1.3)	.08[c]
Duration of illness, years: mean (S.D.)	9.9 (10.4)	20.3 (14.6)	.06[b]
Length of current stay in hospital[d], days: mean (S.D.)	32.2 (49.3)	79.0 (140.9)	.22 [b]
PHQ[e]: mean (S.D.)	17.0 (8.0)	17.1 (7.5)	.97[c]
GAD[f]: mean (S.D.)	13.2 (5.0)	13.8 (5.0)	.74 [c]
EDE-Q[g]: mean (S.D.)			
Restraint	3.7 (2.0)	2.8 (2.6)	.32 [c]
Eating Concern	3.6 (1.6)	3.0 (1.7)	.39 [c]
Shape Concern	4.4 (1.5)	3.8 (0.9)	.30 [c]
Weight Concern	3.9 (1.6)	3.5 (1.3)	.43 [c]
Global	3.8 (1.5)	3.3 (1.3)	.31[c]

Note. *F* female, *WB* White British, *AN-R* Anorexia Nervosa, Restrictive subtype, *AN-BP* Anorexia Nervosa, Binge Purge subtype, *EDNOS* Eating Disorders Not Otherwise Specified, *BMI* Body Mass Index
[a] Categorical data was compared using Chi-squared statistical test. [b] Data not meeting the assumptions for parametric tests was compared using Mann-Whitney U test. [c] Data meeting the assumptions for parametric tests was compared using independent samples *t*-test. [d] Length of current stay calculated from admission into hospital until commencing the study. [e] Patient Health Questionnaire [19]. [f] General Anxiety Disorder assessment [20]. [g] Eating Disorders Examination Questionnaire [21]

trend difference for Tetris ($p = .087$). There was also a difference between Tetris and Quiz ($p = .023$), with the Quiz leading to greater reduction in negative affect. No other significant differences were observed.

PANAS positive baseline scores also did not differ significantly between tasks (Tetris: 16.3; Quiz: 16.7; Braille: 16.2; Sitting Quietly: 16.2; $p = .73$) but again there was a significant effect of task on change scores ($p = .005$). PANAS positive was increased from pre- to post-task in the Tetris and Braille conditions ($p < .01$), did not change significantly in the Quiz condition ($p = .67$), and decreased in the Sitting Quietly condition ($p = .04$). Pairwise comparisons revealed a significant difference between Sitting Quietly and: Tetris ($p = .001$) and Braille ($p = .006$). There was also a difference between Quiz and Tetris ($p = .014$). No other significant differences were observed.

Intrusive thoughts and images

There was a significant effect of task on ratings of both intrusive thoughts and images ($p < .001$). For both ratings, pairwise comparisons between Sitting Quietly and each of the three other tasks were significant ($p < .002$). Compared with Quiz, there was a significant reduction in intrusive images for Braille ($p = .033$) and a trend for Tetris ($p = .08$). Ratings of intrusive thoughts did not differ significantly between the three active tasks.

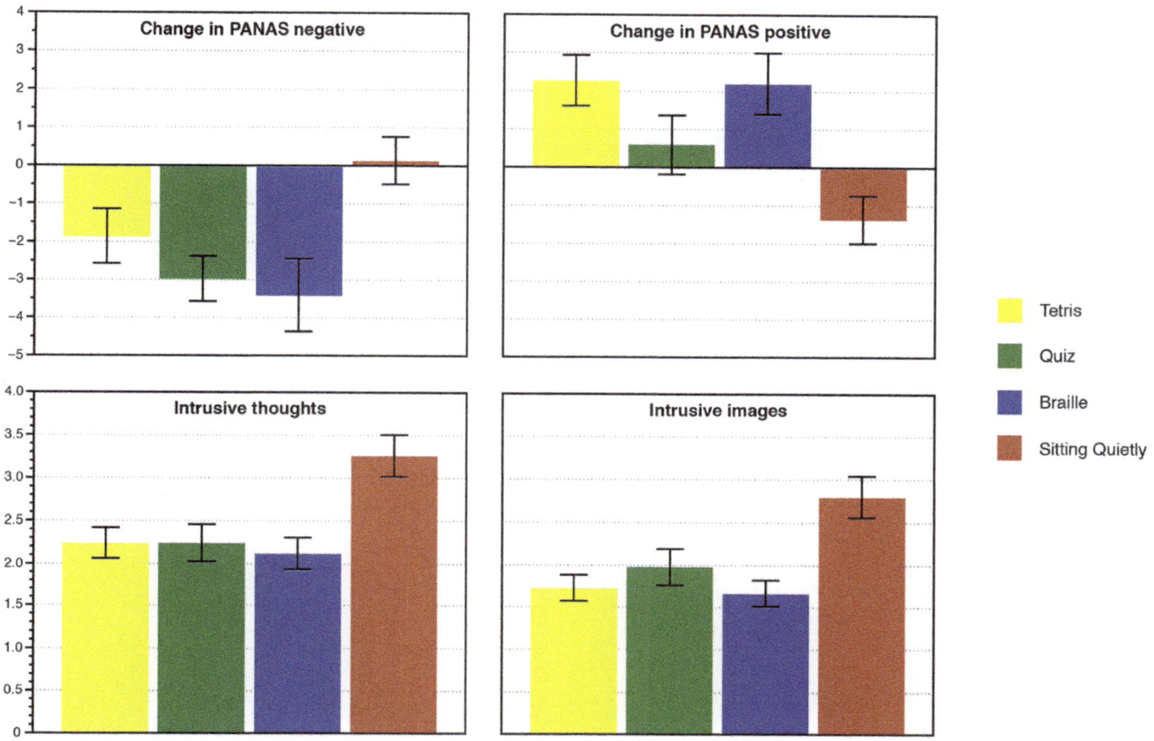

Fig. 1 Changes in PANAS scores, intrusive thoughts and intrusive images following post-meal activities

Discussion

The findings of this study show that engaging in an activity after meals helps to improve the post-meal experience for hospitalised patients with eating disorders. Compared with sitting quietly, all three tasks increased positive affect, decreased negative affect, and decreased intrusive thoughts and images. There was also evidence for nonequivalence between tasks: compared with the Quiz task, Braille was significantly more effective at reducing intrusive imagery and Tetris led to significantly more favourable PANAS positive. However, Quiz was significantly more effective than Tetris for reducing PANAS negative. Thus there is preliminary evidence that post-meal distress may be multidimensional and might be addressed by specific mechanisms beyond general distraction.

The main limitation of this study was that there were key differences between the three units used to obtain participants. They differed in terms of participant illness severity, how much participants were supervised following meals, levels of distraction and whether they could be on their own or not to complete the study. Completers and drop-outs differed significantly in ethnicity and there were marginally significant differences in other measures. In addition, the sample size was relatively small and participants varied in demographic factors and clinical indicators, creating a rather heterogeneous subject group. However, this heterogeneity might suggest that the highly significant effects observed are unlikely to depend critically on small procedural details or highly restricted participant demographics. Studies with more homogenous samples may help detect mediating factors for different cognitive tasks. A further question for future research is to investigate the maintenance over time of the effects reported in this article. It is acknowledged that the high drop-out rate from the study may represent a challenge in using this as an intervention in treatment settings.

Conclusions

These findings add to the scarce literature providing evidence of the benefit of post-meal activities for eating disorders, and are of practical use to patients and supporting services that incorporate mealtimes, in particular hospitals. Improving patients' ability to manage this time has the potential of improving their engagement with hospital treatment and improving clinical outcomes.

Competing interests

The authors declare that they have no competing interests.

Authors' contributions

EG, NH, SG and LS contributed to the conception and design of the study. SG developed the online platform for task administration and data collection with assistance of EG. EG recruited participants and collected the data. EG analysed the results with support from NH, SG and LS. EG drafted the manuscript whilst NH, SG and LS reviewed it critically for accuracy and theoretical integrity. All authors read and approved the final manuscript.

Author details

[1]University College London, Clinical, Educational & Health Psychology, 1-19 Torrington Place, London WC1E 7HB, UK. [2]St Ann's Eating Disorders Service, Barnet, Enfield and Haringey Mental Health NHS Trust, London, UK. [3]University College London, Institute of Cognitive Neuroscience, 17 Queen Square, London WC1N 3AR, UK. [4]Eating Disorders Service, North East London NHS Foundation Trust, London, UK.

References

1. Lawson EA, Holsen LM, Santin M, DeSanti R, Meenaghan E, Eddy ET, et al. Postprandial oxytocin secretion is associated with severity of anxiety and depressive symptoms in anorexia nervosa. J Clin Psychiatry. 2013;74(5):e451–7.
2. Rawal A, Williams JMG, Park RJ. Effects of analytical and experiential self-focus on stress-induced cognitive reactivity in eating disorder psychopathology. Behav Res Ther. 2011;49(10):635–45.
3. Shafran R, Robinson P. Thought-shape fusion in eating disorders. Br J Clin Psychol. 2004;43(4):399–408.
4. Shafran R, Teachman BA, Kerry S, Rachman S. A cognitive distortion associated with eating disorders: thought-shape fusion. Br J Clin Psychol. 1999;38(2):167–79.
5. Geller J, Williams KD, Srikameswaran S. Clinician stance in the treatment of chronic eating disorders. Eur Eat Disord Rev. 2001;9(6):365–73.
6. National Institute for Health and Clinical Excellence. Eating Disorders: Core interventions in the treatment and management of Anorexia Nervosa, Bulimia Nervosa and related eating disorders. Gaskell: The British Psychological Society and The Royal College of Psychiatrists; 2004.
7. Gowers SG, Edwards VJ, Fleminger S, Massoubre C, Wallin U, Canalda G, et al. Treatment aims and philosophy in the treatment of adolescent anorexia nervosa in Europe. Eur Eat Disord Rev. 2002;10(4):271–80.
8. Long S, Wallis DJ, Leung N, Arcelus J, Meyer C. Mealtimes on eating disorder wards: a two-study investigation. Int J Eat Disord. 2012;45(2):241–6.
9. Breiner S. An evidence-based eating disorder program. J Pediatr Nurs. 2003;18(1):75–80.
10. Leichner M, Standish K, Leichner P. Strategies for supporting youths with eating disorders when intensive treatment is needed. B C Med J. 2005;47(1): 49–55.
11. Shapiro JR, Pisetsky EM, Crenshaw W, Spainhour S, Hamer RM, Dymek-Valentine M, et al. Exploratory study to decrease postprandial anxiety: Just relax! Int J Eat Disord. 2008;41(8):728–33.
12. Fairburn CG. Cognitive Behavior Therapy and Eating Disorders. New York, NY: The Guildford Press; 2008.
13. Cooper MJ, Deepak K, Grocutt E, Bailey E. The experience of "Feeling Fat" in women with anorexia nervosa, dieting and non-dieting women : an exploratory study. Eur Eat Disord Rev. 2007a;15(5):366-72.
14. Cooper MJ, Todd G, Turner H. The effects of using imagery to modify core emotional beliefs in bulimia nervosa: an experimental pilot study. J Cogn Psychother. 2007b;21(2):117–122.
15. Murphy R, Straebler S, Cooper Z, Fairburn CG. Cognitive behavioral therapy for eating disorders. Psychiatr Clin North Am. 2010;33(3):611–27.
16. Holmes EA, James EL, Coode-Bate T, Deeprose C. Can playing the computer game "Tetris" reduce the build-up of flashbacks for trauma? A proposal from cognitive science. PLoS One. 2009;4(1):e4153.
17. Holmes EA, James EL, Kilford EJ, Deeprose C. Key steps in developing a cognitive vaccine against traumatic flashbacks: visuospatial Tetris versus verbal Pub Quiz. PLoS One. 2010;5(11):e13706.
18. Watson D, Clark LA, Tellegen A. Development and validation of brief measures of positive and negative affect: the PANAS scales. J Pers Soc Psychol. 1988;54(6):1063–70.
19. Kroenke K, Spitzer RL, Williams JB. The PHQ-9: Validity of a brief depression severity measure. J Gen Intern Med. 2001;16(9):606–13.
20. Kroenke K, Spitzer RL, Williams JB, Monahan PP, Löwe B. Anxiety Disorders In Primary Care: Prevalence, Impairment, Comorbidity, and Detection. Ann Intern Med. 2007;146(5):317–25.
21. Fairburn CG, Beglin SJ. Assessment of eating disorder psychopathology: interview or self-report questionnaire? Int J Eat Disord. 1994;16:363–70.

SCOFF in a general swedish adolescent population

Erika Hansson[1,2], Daiva Daukantaitė[2] and Per Johnsson[2*]

Abstract

Background: Although Disordered Eating Behaviors (DEB) is an ill-defined concept, multiple studies have examined prevalence of DEB and its relations to other variables in various populations. DEB have been shown to predict more serious eating disorders which in turn can lead to death. Mostly girls seem to suffer from DEB, but the question has been raised whether this, at least, partially is due to the methods used for screening. The SCOFF-questionnaire has been suggested as a quick and easily administered tool to assess DEB. However, the psychometric results regarding SCOFF suggest some inconsistencies, and more research is needed in various countries and age samples.

Method: To validate SCOFF, a total of 1265 Swedish adolescents (51.6 % girls) completed self-report questionnaires using the Eating Disorder Examination Questionnaire (EDE-Q) as a reference standard.

Results: The factor analyses show inconclusive results as to whether SCOFF should be regarded as a comprehensive scale; furthermore, the results indicate a correlation between SCOFF and the EDE-Q in both girl and boy samples. Girls scored significantly higher on SCOFF and also had a higher total score, indicating more severe problems than boys.

Conclusions: The results raised questions as to whether the SCOFF might be interpreted and responded to in different ways by girls and boys, risking overlooking boys' DEB and also whether one "yes" answer, instead of the stipulated two, could be sufficient when using SCOFF for screening purposes. In sum, the results challenge the use of SCOFF in a general adolescent population.

Keywords: Subclinical, Disordered eating behaviors, SCOFF

Background

Disordered Eating Behaviors (DEB) is not a unified concept and therefore difficult to study. DEB is used to describe various behaviors or symptoms that can "take many forms" ([3], p. 41). Fasting, the use of diet pills, purging (by vomiting or the use of laxatives), and smoking for weight control are all examples of DEB [16]. DEB is furthermore suggested to have a distinct core psychopathology, with the same mechanisms in men and women, and having to do with an over evaluation of one's own shape and weight [5].

The prevalence of DEB, despite its imprecise definition, has been calculated with frequencies varying from 15 % in boys and 33 % in girls in a study of 1895 11–17 year-old adolescents in a German sample [11] to 30 % in Israeli girls with a mean age of 14.7 years [13] to 17 % in boys and 52 % in girls with a mean age of 14.9 years in a Finnish sample [9]. The results indicate that DEB is a prevalent health problem in both girls and boys. Adolescents with DEB run a high risk of developing a clinical eating disorder [25] which renders high morbidity [12, 27] and therefore, it is of great importance to detect DEB as early as possible, providing appropriate help for adolescents at risk. For early identification of DEB, reliable and valid instruments are needed. The SCOFF-questionnaire [23] which we aim to validate in a Swedish adolescent sample in the present study, addresses core features of both anorexia nervosa and bulimia nervosa and has been used as a screening tool to enable the detection of individuals possibly at risk for an eating disorder [2, 12, 26]. During its development, great effort was made to make the SCOFF brief since it was meant to be used as part of primary care screening, often in addition to other cumbersome measures [12]. By deciding the cut-off to be the answer "yes" to two out of five questions, the researchers maximized the sensitivity of the test, which was considered a priority [12]. In the initial

* Correspondence: per.johnsson@psy.lu.se
[2]Lund University, Lund, Sweden
Full list of author information is available at the end of the article

study by Morgan et al. [23], the test's sensitivity in the sample of adult females already diagnosed with anorexia nervosa or bulimia nervosa was 100 %, whereas in a study by Pannocchia et al. [26], the sensitivity was 97 %. The false positive rates of 12.5 % and 12.7 %, respectively, were claimed to be an acceptable trade-off for the high sensitivity.

A validation of the SCOFF in a non-clinical adolescent sample in Finland demonstrated that 81 % of the students whose eating disorder symptoms were detected by the SCOFF-questionnaire (i.e., answered "yes" to two of five questions) had undetected DEB in a health examination performed by a nurse [10]. Furthermore, the questionnaire has been found to be accurate and reliable with a reported sensitivity of 94.6 % in a sample of students administered the SCOFF and judged to be at high or low risk of an eating disorder by a health professional [8]. Other studies are more moderate in their assessment and consider the SCOFF to have acceptable psychometric properties [15] or to be restricted but feasibly useful for ruling out the presence of eating disorders, according to a study by Lähteenmäki et al. [18] in which none of the participants with current eating disorders scored zero points on the SCOFF-questionnaire.

Thus, although multiple studies have examined the SCOFF, the results suggests some inconsistencies and more research in various samples is needed.

In addition to the SCOFF, the Eating Disorder Examination Questionnaire (EDE-Q) is a widely used instrument to examine DEB. The EDE-Q is a self-reported instrument derived from the Eating Disorder Examination interview [6] and contains questions about shape, weight and eating concerns as well as the practice of food restraint. Although the EDE-Q is a highly reliable and valid instrument in screening for DEB [20, 21], it has lately been criticized for not adequately assessing eating, weight and shape control behaviors in adolescent boys [19]. Furthermore, because of the EDE-Q's length with thirty-six items to be answered both by multiple choice as well as with answers concerning frequencies, shorter and easier administered instruments, such as the SCOFF, which only have five items, have been requested from primary care personnel. Because the EDE-Q assesses a broad range of the specific psychopathologies of DEB, the instrument has been used as a reference in studies examining the validity of the SCOFF. It is expected that those with higher scores on the EDE-Q, indicating DEB, would also answer "yes" to two or more questions of the SCOFF.

In sum, although many of the aforementioned studies advocate the SCOFF as a useful screening tool, the results and conclusions of these studies differ. This contrast could be due to cultural influence, sample age [22], different forms of recruitment [24], or gender diversity. Because earlier adolescent validation studies have been conducted in Finland, Spain and Hong Kong, a validation study in a non-clinical, gender diversified Swedish adolescent setting would add valuable information to research regarding the validity of the SCOFF. Thus, in this study, we aim to examine the validity of the SCOFF by screening for DEB in a Swedish sample using the EDE-Q as a "reference standard". We expect that individuals with high scores on the EDE-Q, which indicates more DEB, will also score higher on the SCOFF. Furthermore, because most validation studies contain few males and mostly adult samples, the present study will focus on adolescent boys and girls since gender differences regarding the SCOFF and its relationships to the EDE-Q also seems to be of great importance. Finally, the limit of two "yes" answers on the SCOFF is questioned, focusing on whether only one "yes" answer could be sufficient for the individual to obtain further examination to rule out DEB.

Method

Measures

Demographic variables

The demographic variables reported by the adolescents included age, gender, country of birth, country of parents' birth, and family composition (e.g., two-parent or single-parent home).

Disordered eating behaviors

SCOFF. The SCOFF questionnaire [23] contains five questions concerning eating habits and attitudes toward weight and body shape: "Do you make yourself sick (vomit) because you feel uncomfortably full?"; "Do you worry that you have lost control over how much you eat?"; "Have you recently lost more than one stone (15 pounds) (ca 6.8 kg) in a 3 month period?"; "Do you believe yourself to be fat when others say you are thin?"; and "Would you say that food dominates your life?". A threshold of two positive answers has been proposed to raise a suspicion of an existing eating disorder [17, 23].

The SCOFF was translated into Swedish by one of the authors by using back translation with help from another Swede competent in English.

EDE-Q. Twenty-two Likert-scale questions of the original 36-item version of the EDE-Q [4] were used in the present study. The questions included in the study are from the following subscales: restraint (e.g., " How many of the past 14 days have you been deliberately trying to limit the amount of food you eat to influence your shape or weight (whether you have succeeded)"); shape concerns (e.g., "How many of the past 14 days have you had a definite desire to have a totally flat stomach"); weight concerns (e.g., "How many of the past 14 days have you had a strong desire to lose weight") and eating concerns (e.g., "How many of the past 14 days have you had a definite fear of losing control over eating"). The questions are answered on a 7-point Likert scale ranging from 0 = "not one day" to 6 = "every day". The questions in each subscale provide subscale scores and a global score can be calculated by summing and averaging the subscale scores. Higher scores are indicative of higher eating disorder psychopathology. In the current study, Cronbach's alpha was .95 for the total scale, .77 for eating concern, .93 for shape concern, .85 for weight concern and .90 for restraint.

Procedure

Both the legal guardians of students below age 15 and the students themselves, irrespective of age, received written information about the study aims, procedures and the possibility to decline participation. The students were further informed on the day of data collection and assured confidentiality. Parents provided passive consent which required them to sign and return a form if they refused to allow their child to participate in research. Students consented actively by completing the questionnaire, which took approximately 1 h. The study was approved by the Regional Ethics Committee in Lund, Sweden.

Statistical analysis

The data for girls and boys were divided into two parts. In one of the parts, an exploratory factor analysis using principal component analysis in SPSS was conducted, and in the other part, a confirmatory factor analysis using program R was conducted to evaluate the structure of the SCOFF. The reliability of the scale was assessed with Kuder and Richardson's formula 20 (KR20). To compare the total SCOFF-score between girls and boys, a Mann–Whitney U test was conducted, and to calculate the correlations between the SCOFF and the EDE-Q and its subscales, point biserial correlations were used. To compare the zero "yes" group of SCOFF to the one and two or more "yes" group, the non-parametric Kruskal-Wallis H test was used due to differences of variances in the groups and non-normal distribution of the scores. The pairwise comparisons were conducted by Mann–Whitney tests, and effect sizes were calculated as suggested by Field [7].

Participants

The manuscript is based on the second wave of data collection in an ongoing longitudinal study in a municipality in southern Sweden and was conducted from January to March in 2014. The sample consisted of 1265 students (M_{age} = 16.19, *SD* = 1.21; 54.5 % female) who were approximately 78 % of the population of 1621 students attending the schools participating in the study. Of the 356 students who did not participate, 62 chose to refrain from participation either on their own or their parents' initiative. The remaining 294 students were absent from school on the day of data collection for unclear reasons.

In total, 83.1 % of the adolescents were born in Sweden or another Scandinavian country, whereas the others were born in another European country (4.7 %), the Middle East (7.9 %), or other parts of the world (4.3 %). The number of foreign-born parents was somewhat higher; specifically, approximately two-thirds of the parents were born in Sweden or another Scandinavian country (mothers: 67.0 %, fathers: 67.7 %), another European country (mothers: 12.9 %, fathers: 12.4 %), the Middle East (mothers: 11.7 %, fathers: 12.0 %), or other parts of the world (mothers: 8.4 %, fathers: 8.0 %).

Approximately three-quarters of the adolescents (74.8 %) lived in two-parent households with both their biological parents, 10.3 % of the children lived in a single-parent household (8.2 % with mother), and 3.7 % lived with a parent and a step-parent (3.1 % with biological mother). One in ten adolescents (9.9 %) lived alternatingly with mother and father, 0.9 % lived with adults other than their parents, and 0.5 % lived alone.

Results

Exploratory factor analysis

To explore the structure of the SCOFF in the Swedish adolescent sample, a principal components factor analysis with direct oblimin rotation was conducted for half of the total sample of girls and boys separately. The Kaiser-Meyer-Olkin measure verified the sampling adequacy for the analysis of the total sample (KMO = .65) as well as for girls only (KMO = .61) and for boys only (KMO = .68). In all samples, the tests showed two factors with eigenvalues over Kaiser's criterion of 1 explaining 56.37 % (girls: 54.61 %, boys: 60.83 %) of the variance. Table 1 shows the factor loadings after rotation for the girl and boy samples. The items that load on the same factor for the girl sample suggest that factor 1 represents thoughts about food and eating, whereas factor 2 represents actions regarding food and eating. In the boy sample, four of the items loaded on one factor and only one item; fast weight reduction, added to a second factor.

Confirmatory factor analysis (CFA)

Based on the EFA results and to further examine the structure of the SCOFF, confirmatory factor analyses were performed to test one-factor (i.e., all SCOFF items comprise one factor) vs. two-factor models (Model 1: items 1 and 3; Model 2: items 2, 4 and 5). The results of the CFA for the second part of the participants are presented in Table 2. For girls, goodness-of-fit statistics indicated good fit for both 1-factor and 2-factor models, whereas for boys, a 1-factor model showed excellent fit with non-significant chi-square, zero value of RMSEA and high values for CFI and TLI.

Table 1 Factor Loadings for Exploratory Factor Analysis with Direct Oblimin Rotation of Items of the SCOFF-scale

	Rotated factor loadings			
	Girls (n = 329)		Boys (n = 258)	
	Factor 1 Thoughts about food	Factor 2 Acts in regard to food	Factor 1	Factor 2
Do you make yourself sick (vomit) because you feel uncomfortably full?	. 23	.65	.62	.05
Do you worry that you have lost control over how much you eat?	.79	−.01	.83	−.10
Have you recently lost more than one stone (15 pounds) (ca 6.8 kg) in a 3 month period?	−.18	.84	−.01	.98
Do you believe yourself to be fat when others say you are thin?	.68	.12	.82	−.14
Would you say that food dominates your life?	.64	−.08	.53	.19

Based on the CFA results, the SCOFF was used as a 1-factor scale in further analyses in the present article. The reliability of the SCOFF-scale, assessed with Kuder and Richardson's formula 20 (KR20), was .48 in the current study and considered acceptable for screening tests [28].

Gender differences of the SCOFF

To compare the total SCOFF-score between girls and boys, a Mann–Whitney U test was conducted. The girls (*Md* = *.000, n* = *684*) revealed higher scores, indicating higher DEB than in the boys (*Md* = *.000, n* = *559*), $U = 146907.5$, $z = -8.54$, $p = <.001$, $r = .24$.

Table 3 shows the number and percentages of girls and boys answering "yes" and "no" to the single SCOFF-items. Large and significant gender differences indicating more "yes" answers by girls were found for all items except item 3, regarding weight loss.

Relationships between SCOFF and EDE-Q

Table 4 shows the point biserial correlations between the SCOFF and EDE-Q subscales. The results indicate strong relationships between the SCOFF and all EDE-Q subscales, with the highest relationship being eating concern for girls, $r = .63$, $p = < .001$, and weight concern for boys, $r = .58$, $p = < .001$. Although the results show significantly stronger relationships between the SCOFF and eating restraint and eating concern for girls than for boys, the differences are not large.

Table 2 Summary of Confirmatory Factor Analyses for Two SCOFF Models for Girls and Boys Separately

	Girls		Boys
Goodness-of-fit statistics	1-factor model	2- factor model	1-factor model
χ^2	8.13	4.41	4.44
df	5	4	5
p	.15	.35	.49
RMSEA	.028	.018	.00
CFI	.98	.99	1.00
TLI	.97	.98	1.02
r		.61	

Gender differences in frequency of one "yes" answer to the SCOFF

The threshold of two "yes" answers to the SCOFF was established for further investigation of eating disorders [23]. However, one "yes", especially on particular items (e.g., vomiting or losing a substantial amount of weight during a short period of time), may be a significant indicator of DEB risk. In the present sample, 168 of 689 girls and 85 of 575 boys answered "yes" to the SCOFF once. As Table 5 shows, one "yes" answer was rarely found on the first item regarding vomiting, indicating a non-healthy eating behavior. No significant gender differences were found on this item. More boys than girls answered "yes" on items regarding eating behavior (i.e., items three and five), whereas more girls than boys answered "yes" on items regarding losing weight and appearance.

To further investigate differences among those with different numbers of "yes" answers to the SCOFF, girls and boys were divided into three SCOFF groups representing a group with no "yes" answers (Group 0), a group with one "yes" answer (Group 1) and a group with two or more "yes" answers (Group 2). Group differences were examined on the total EDE-Q scale and subscales, and Kruskal-Wallis' tests were conducted to examine group differences. Pairwise comparisons were made with the Mann–Whitney test. The results are presented in Tables 6 and 7 for girls and boys, respectively. In girls, significant differences were found between all groups on all studied variables, and the effect-sizes were large when comparing group 0 to group 2. When comparing group 0 to group 1 and group 1 to group 2, the effect-sizes for the girls were in the medium range, indicating a moderate difference between the groups. The girls with one "yes" answer differed from the girls with zero "yes" answers, with effect sizes ranging from .22 for restraint to .30 for eating and weight concern. In boys, smaller effect sizes were found. However, group 1 differed significantly from both group 0 and group 2 on all EDE-Q subscales.

Table 3 The number (in parenthesis) and percentages of girls and boys answering "yes" and "no" to the SCOFF items, respectively

	Total		Girls		Boys		
	"Yes"	"No"	"Yes"	"No"	"Yes"	"No"	Z
Do you make yourself sick (vomit) because you feel uncomfortably full?	(41)	(1238)	(33)	(645)	(8)	(545)	3.33**
	3.3 %	96.7 %	4.9 %	95.1 %	1.4 %	98.6 %	
Do you worry that you have lost control over how much you eat?	(152)	(1090)	(126)	(552)	(25)	(532)	7.52***
	12.2 %	87.8 %	18.6 %	81.4 %	4.5 %	95.5 %	
Have you recently lost more than one stone (15 pounds) (ca 6.8 kg) in a 3 month period?	(75)	(1158)	(41)	(633)	(34)	(518)	−.055
	6.1 %	93.9 %	6.1 %	93.9 %	6.2 %	93.8 %	
Do you believe yourself to be fat when others say you are thin?	(154)	(1078)	(126)	(544)	(27)	(528)	7.35 ***
	12.5 %	87.5 %	18.8 %	81.2 %	4.9 %	95.1 %	
Would you say that food dominates your life?	(180)	(1045)	(120)	(547)	(58)	(493)	3.67 ***
	14.7 %	85.3 %	18.0 %	82.0 %	10.5 %	89.5 %	

** $p = < .001$, ***$p = < .0001$

Discussion

The aim of this study was to explore the validity of the SCOFF questionnaire [23] in a Swedish community sample of adolescents of both genders. The confirmatory factor analysis showed good fit concerning a one-factor model for girls, replicating results by Pannocchia et al. [26] and excellent fit regarding a one-factor model for boys, who were not included in the Pannocchia et al. [26] study. However, the exploratory factor analysis was not as permissive, and the results indicated that the SCOFF scale should be interpreted with some caution. Notably, the result of the exploratory factor analysis in which the scale for girls was divided into two factors ("thoughts about food" and "acts in regard to food") resembled the two-factor model suggested by Muro-Sans et al. [24] in which the girl sample (11–17 years) loaded on the same two factors as the girl sample of the present study. Another two-factor model including girls as well as older adolescents of both genders showed a slightly better fit than a uni-factorial model [10]. The results combined indicate that although the confirmatory analysis showed good as well as excellent fit, there might be pitfalls if treating the SCOFF questionnaire as uni-factorial.

Table 4 Point biserial correlations divided between genders in regard to the SCOFF Total and EDE-Q scales

	SCOFF TOTAL		z
	Girls	Boys	
EDE-Q Total	.66 ($n = 559$)	.60 ($n = 476$)	1.61 ns
EDE-Q Restraint	.55 ($n = 619$)	.39 ($n = 521$)	3.37**
EDE-Q Eating Concern	.63 ($n = 617$)	.52 ($n = 520$)	2.86*
EDE-Q Weight concern	.58 ($n = 607$)	.58 ($n = 518$)	0.00 ns
EDE-Q Shape concern	.59 ($n = 595$)	.55 ($n = 509$)	1.05 ns

Note. All reported correlations are significant at the $p = .001$ level (two tailed)
*$p = < .01$ ** $p = < .001$

The results of the present study also showed that, consistent with earlier studies [9, 11], girls scored significantly higher on the total SCOFF and that they were over-represented in frequency in the group with 2 or more "yes" answers to the SCOFF, indicating more severe DEB. Furthermore, more girls than boys answered "yes" to the SCOFF questions concerning "lost control" and "feelings of being fat", which implies that these questions are either indicators of more pronounced problems in girls or that the questions are interpreted differently by girls and boys. More boys than girls answered "yes" to the question whether food "dominates your life", which may also be a question of interpretation as in either "eating all the time", like many healthy growing adolescent boys experience that they are doing, or as constantly thinking about food and planning each calorie-intake.

Because DEB are most common among girls and the SCOFF primarily has been validated in female samples, it is possible that boys do not sufficiently adhere to the items the scale uses and that screening questionnaires in general may be missing pertinent questions for boys who might express specific "male risk behaviors" ([29] p. 448). Mond et al. [19] suggested that boys (and girls) might perform excessive exercise to lose weight. This factor could be one example of a question missing in the SCOFF. However, the question about losing a substantial amount of weight during a 3 month period might be related to this behavior. This item was also one of the questions in which girls and boys did not differ in their answers, posing the idea that this item is fairly "gender neutral". Although hard to administer in a screening milieu, the SCOFF might benefit from a girl and boy version like the works of Kopp and Gillberg [14], investigating autism spectrum disorders in gender specific ways.

When comparing SCOFF to the EDE-Q scale, the SCOFF and the global EDE-Q were found to correlate

Table 5 Table showing the answers posed by those answering" yes" to only one of the SCOFF questions

	Total sample		Girls		Boys		z
	"Yes"	"No"	"Yes"	"No"	"Yes"	"No"	
Do you make yourself sick (vomit) because you feel uncomfortably full?	(10)	(244)	(8)	(160)	(2)	(83)	.93
	3.9 %	96.1 %	4.8 %	95.2 %	2.4 %	97.6 %	
Do you worry that you have lost control over how much you eat?	(47)	(206)	(19)	(149)	(24)	(61)	−3.39**
	18.7 %	81.4 %	11.3 %	88.7 %	28.2 %	71.8 %	
Have you recently lost more than one stone (15 pounds) (ca 6.8 kg) in a 3 month period?	(43)	(211)	(39)	(128)	(8)	(77)	2.67*
	16.9 %	83.1 %	23.4 %	76.6 %	9.4 %	90.6 %	
Do you believe yourself to be fat when others say you are thin?	(55)	(196)	(45)	(121)	(10)	(74)	2.74*
	21.9 %	78.1 %	27.1 %	72.9 %	11.9 %	88.1 %	
Would you say that food dominates your life?	(102)	(149)	(39)	(107)	(42)	(42)	−4.22*
	40.6 %	59.4 %	35.5 %	64.5 %	50 %	50 %	

*$p = < .01$ ** $p = < .001$*** $p = < .0001$

strongly in both girls and boys. This evidence is consistent with the results reported by Leung et al. [15] using a sample of Hong Kong high school students. In evaluating the subscales of the EDE-Q, girls showed higher correlations between the SCOFF and the EDE-Q subscale restraint, which taps items concerning areas as making oneself sick. Girls also showed higher correlations than boys in regard to eating concern, which detects issues of losing control over eating and of preoccupation with food, eating and calories. Leung et al. [15] used only the global EDE-Q and therefore no further comparisons can be made; however, the results revealed in this study by the use of the EDE-Q subscales imply that when using the EDE-Q as a

Table 6 Kruskal-Wallis Test with pairwise comparisons for the girl sample divided into three groups (Group 0 = 0 "yes"-answers to the SCOFF scale, Group 1 = 1 "yes" answer to the SCOFF-scale and Group 2 = 2 or more "yes" answers to the SCOFF scale)

Girl Sample	Kruskal –Wallis Test	N	Mdn	M(SD)	Pairwise comparisons	z***	ES
EDE-Q Total	H(2) = 174.74 ***	0 = 330	.41	.65(.68)	0–1	−6.15	.28
		1 = 137	1.09	1.32(1.10)	0–2+	−12.88	.63
		2 = 92	2.89	2.78(1.28)	1–2 +	−6.63	.44
		559					
EDE-Q Restraint	H(2) = 130.19***	0 = 361	.20	.48(.74)	0–1	−4.94	.22
		1 = 155	.40	.96(1.20)	0–2+	−11.21	.52
		2 + = 103	1.90	2.25(1.68)	1–2 +	−6.12	.38
		619					
EDE-Q Eating concern	H(2) = 188.72***	0 = 364	.00	.25(.49)	0–1	−6.73	.30
		1 = 154	.40	.76(.91)	0–2+	−13.29	.62
		2 + = 99	2.0	1.96(1.39)	1–2 +	−6.67	.42
		617					
EDE-Q Weight concern	H(2) = 170.85***	0 = 355	.40	.81(.96)	0–1	−6.66	.30
		1 = 154	1.40	1.72(1.44)	0–2+	−12.58	.59
		2 + = 98	3.20	3.11(1.45)	1–2 +	−6.14	.39
		607					
EDE-Q Shape concern	H(2) = 167.74***	0 = 352	.75	1.09(1.05)	0–1	−6.06	.27
		1 = 145	1.63	2.03(1.55)	0–2+	−12.61	.59
		2 + = 98	4.13	3.72(1.54)	1–2 +	−6.44	.41
		595					

*** $p = < .0001$

Table 7 Kruskal-Wallis Test with pairwise comparisons for the boy sample divided into three groups (Group 0 = 0 "yes"-answers to the SCOFF scale, Group 1 = 1 "yes" answer to the SCOFF scale and Group 2 = 2 or more "yes" answers to the SCOFF scale)

Boy Sample							
	Kruskal –Wallis Test	N	Mdn	M (SD)	Pairwise comparisons	z	ES
EDE-Q Total	H(2) = 71.87***	0 = 383	.13	.28(.44)	0–1	−5.03***	.24
		1 = 70	.45	.72(.79)	0–2+	−7.26***	.36
		2 + = 23	1.71	2.06(1.35)	1–2+	−3.77***	.39
		476					
EDE-Q Restraint	H(2) = 65.99***	0 = 419	.00	.27(.70)	0–1	−4.83***	.22
		1 = 76	.20	.76(1.25)	0–2+	−6.96***	.33
		2 + = 26	1.4	1.76(1.60)	1–2 +	−3.55**	.35
		521					
EDE-Q Eating concern	H(2) = 84.01***	0 = 420	.00	.11(.35)	0–1	−6.18***	.28
		1 = 77	.20	.37(.53)	0–2+	−7.30***	.35
		2 + = 23	1.2	1.31(1.23)	1–2 +	−3.35*	.34
		520					
EDE-Q Weight concern	H(2) = 68.03***	0 = 415	.20	.39(.65)	0–1	−3.88***	.18
		1 = 77	.60	.84(.97)	0–2+	−7.61***	.36
		2 + = 26	2.8	2.75(1.65)	1–2 +	−4.67***	.46
		518					
EDE-Q Shape concern	H(2) = 62.51***	0 = 408	.13	.43(.70)	0–1	−4.29***	.20
		1 = 74	.5	.92(.98)	0–2+	−7.03***	.34
		2 + = 27	2.25	2.59(1.85)	1–2 +	−3.80***	.38
		509					

*p = < .01 ** p = < .001*** p = < .0001

validation instrument, the use of the subscales would be recommended.

Although the "cut-off" for the SCOFF in an attempt to maximize both sensitivity and specificity [23] has been set at two "yes" answers, the question of whether only one "yes" might indicate DEB and warrant further investigation was assessed. As results of the present study showed, eight girls and two boys answered "yes" to the question about whether they had made themselves sick after eating too much. Although the number of adolescents who replied "yes" to the question was low, a healthy eating behavior does not involve any vomiting. Furthermore, thirty-nine girls and eight boys answered "yes" to the SCOFF question about losing 6.8 kg during a 3 month period. The answers of these two questions could be due to measuring errors but still ought to be highlighted due to the severity of the behaviors and their proximity to the DSM-V criteria of anorexia nervosa and bulimia nervosa [1], as opposed to the maybe less severe "thoughts" about food measured by the other questions. The sensitivity is undoubtedly heightened by using only one "yes" answer as cut off [8, 18, 24] but naturally, it lowers specificity. The question is whether the cost of lowered specificity is acceptable in the matter of adolescent screening.

In dividing the adolescents into three groups (zero, one and two or more "yes" answers to the SCOFF), all groups differed from each other concerning all subscales of the EDE-Q. Notably, the individuals who reported one "yes"-answer differed significantly from those reporting zero and two "yes"-answers, again indicating the importance of monitoring the "one yes" group for DEB. If the one "yes"-answer group would be investigated further this would certainly heighten the rate of false positives and perhaps lead to an attenuated questionnaire. On the other hand, since the point of SCOFF is to raise the suspicion of DEB, to hopefully get ahold of adolescent boys and girls before they develop full-blown eating disorders, this goal stands a greater chance of being fulfilled if adolescents are identified and questioned as early as possible.

Strengths and limitations

The strengths of the present study are the large sample size and the gender diversity which provide valuable information on boys' adherence to the SCOFF and risk of DEB as well as the differences between girls and boys in this specific area.

A limitation is that the cross-sectional design of the study only shows the scores of the SCOFF during one point in time. However, a longitudinal study using the SCOFF scale as a screening instrument might not be optimal considering the possible fluctuation of these behaviors during adolescence [10]. Still, the individuals with zero "yes" answers and those with one "yes" answer could change into two "yes" answer individuals with more severe DEB [25].

Additional limitations are the self-report format and the back translation, which was not reviewed by the original authors for face validity.

Conclusions

Despite the above mentioned limitations, the results of the present study, in which SCOFF was highly correlated to the EDE-Q, indicate that the SCOFF is a fairly good measure of DEB. However, the exploratory and confirmatory factor analyses differed in regard to factors to be extracted and also showed different response-patterns for boys and girls.

Girls scored significantly higher on the SCOFF and also had a higher total score, indicating more severe problems than those of boys, which is consistent with the findings of earlier research. Furthermore the results raised the questions whether the SCOFF items might be interpreted differently by girls and boys and whether one "yes"-answer might be "enough" when using the SCOFF for screening purposes. Future studies should consider whether a one "yes" answer should lead to follow up questions for a more thorough screening.

Although several researchers [2, 8, 12, 26] have noted the benefits of this "simple" five-item screening-questionnaire, our results suggest that the SCOFF needs further evaluation and probably requires revision to be valid screening instrument, especially among boys. Significant gender differences on item level further indicate that more profound research is needed to reveal whether any of the questions are too blunt, vague or difficult to relate to and in which way the questions could either be reworded to fit a more gender-diversified group or entirely exchanged to fit a group of adolescent boys [19]. This information should be of interest to obtain a broader view of boys' DEB, which might be less common but also might be undetected. Further studies are also needed to investigate whether some of the SCOFF items are critical, in which even one "yes" on the item might signal DEB risk.

Competing interests

The authors declare that they have no competing interests.

Authors' contributions

EH designed the study, carried out the data collection, performed the statistical analysis and wrote the paper. DD designed the study and performed the statistical analysis. PJ designed the study and gave conceptual advice. All authors discussed the results and implications and DD and PJ commented on the manuscript at all stages. All authors read and approved the final manuscript.

Author details

[1]Kristianstad University, Kristianstad, Sweden. [2]Lund University, Lund, Sweden.

References

1. American Psychiatric Association. Diagnostic and statistical manual of mental disorders. 5th ed. DC: Washington; 2013.
2. Botella J, Sepulveda AR, Huang H, Gambara H. A meta-analysis of the diagnostic accuracy of the SCOFF. Span J Psychol. 2013;16:E92. doi:10.1017/sjp.2013.92.
3. Combs JL, Pearson CM, Zapolski TC, Smith GT. Preadolescent disordered eating predicts subsequent eating dysfunction. J Pediatr Psychol. 2013;38(1): 41–9. doi:10.1093/jpepsy/jss094.
4. Fairburn CG, Beglin SJ. Assessment of eating disorders: interview or self-report questionnaire? Int J Eat Disord. 1994;16(4):363–70.
5. Fairburn CG, Harrison PJ. Eating disorders. Lancet. 2003;361(9355):407–16.
6. Fairburn CG, Wilson GT, Schleimer K. Binge eating: Nature, assessment, and treatment. New York: Guilford Press; 1993.
7. Field A. Discovering statistics using IBM SPSS statistics: Sage. 2013.
8. Garcia FD, Grigioni S, Chelali S, Meyrignac G, Thibaut F, Dechelotte P. Validation of the French version of SCOFF questionnaire for screening of eating disorders among adults. World J Biol Psychiatry. 2010;11(7):888–93. doi:10.3109/15622975.2010.483251.
9. Hautala L, Helenius H, Karukivi M, Maunula AM, Nieminen J, Aromaa M, et al. The role of gender, affectivity and parenting in the course of disordered eating: a 4-year prospective case-control study among adolescents. Int J Nurs Stud. 2011;48(8):959–72. doi:10.1016/j.ijnurstu.2011.01.014.
10. Hautala L, Junnila J, Alin J, Gronroos M, Maunula AM, Karukivi M, et al. Uncovering hidden eating disorders using the SCOFF questionnaire: cross-sectional survey of adolescents and comparison with nurse assessments. Int J Nurs Stud. 2009;46(11):1439–47. doi:10.1016/j.ijnurstu.2009.04.007.
11. group, B. S, Herpertz-Dahlmann B, Wille N, Holling H, Vloet TD, Ravens-Sieberer U. Disordered eating behaviour and attitudes, associated psychopathology and health-related quality of life: results of the BELLA study. Eur Child Adolesc Psychiatry. 2008;17(Suppl 1(S1)):82–91. doi:10.1007/s00787-008-1009-9.
12. Hill LS, Reid F, Morgan JF, Lacey JH. SCOFF, the development of an eating disorder screening questionnaire. Int J Eat Disord. 2010;43(4):344–51. doi:10.1002/eat.20679.
13. Kaluski DN, Natamba BK, Goldsmith R, Shimony T, Berry EM. Determinants of disordered eating behaviors among Israeli adolescent girls. Eat Disord. 2008; 16(2):146–59. doi:10.1080/10640260801887303.
14. Kopp S, Gillberg C. The autism spectrum screening questionnaire (ASSQ)-revised extended version (ASSQ-REV): an instrument for better capturing the autism phenotype in girls? a preliminary study involving 191 clinical cases and community controls. Res Dev Disabil. 2011;32(6):2875–88.
15. Leung SF, Lee KL, Lee SM, Leung SC, Hung WS, Lee WL, et al. Psychometric properties of the SCOFF questionnaire (Chinese version) for screening eating disorders in Hong Kong secondary school students: a cross-sectional study. Int J Nurs Stud. 2009;46(2):239–47. doi:10.1016/j.ijnurstu.2008.09.004.
16. Loth KA, MacLehose R, Bucchianeri M, Crow S, Neumark-Sztainer D. Predictors of dieting and disordered eating behaviors from adolescence to young adulthood. J Adolesc Health. 2014;55(5):705–12. doi:10.1016/j.jadohealth.2014.04.016.
17. Luck AJ, Morgan JF, Reid F, O'Brien A, Brunton J, Price C, et al. The SCOFF questionnaire and clinical interview for eating disorders in general practice: comparative study. BMJ. 2002;325(7367):755–6.
18. Lähteenmäki S, Aalto-Setälä T, Suokas JT, Saarni SE, Perälä J, Saarni SI, et al. Validation of the finnish version of the SCOFF questionnaire among young adults aged 20 to 35 years. BMC psychiatry. 2009;9(1):5.
19. Mond J, Hall A, Bentley C, Harrison C, Gratwick-Sarll K, Lewis V. Eating-disordered behavior in adolescent boys: eating disorder examination questionnaire norms. Int J Eat Disord. 2014;47(4):335–41. doi:10.1002/eat.22237.
20. Mond JM, Hay PJ, Rodgers B, Owen C, Beumont PJ. Temporal stability of the eating disorder examination questionnaire. Int J Eat Disord. 2004;36(2):195–203. doi:10.1002/eat.20017.
21. Mond JM, Hay PJ, Rodgers B, Owen C, Beumont PJ. Validity of the eating disorder examination questionnaire (EDE-Q) in screening for eating

disorders in community samples. Behav Res Ther. 2004;42(5):551–67. doi:10.1016/S0005-7967(03)00161-X.
22. Mond JM, Myers TC, Crosby RD, Hay PJ, Rodgers B, Morgan JF, et al. Screening for eating disorders in primary care: EDE-Q versus SCOFF. Behav Res Ther. 2008;46(5):612–22. doi:10.1016/j.brat.2008.02.003.
23. Morgan JF, Reid F, Lacey JH. The SCOFF questionnaire: assessment of a new screening tool for eating disorders. BMJ. 1999;319(7223):1467–8.
24. Muro-Sans P, Amador-Campos JA, Morgan JF. The SCOFF-c: psychometric properties of the catalan version in a spanish adolescent sample. J Psychosom Res. 2008;64(1):81–6. doi:10.1016/j.jpsychores.2007.06.011.
25. Neumark-Sztainer D, Wall M, Guo J, Story M, Haines J, Eisenberg M. Obesity, disordered eating, and eating disorders in a longitudinal study of adolescents: how do dieters fare 5 years later? J Am Diet Assoc. 2006;106(4):559–68. doi:10.1016/j.jada.2006.01.003.
26. Pannocchia L, Fiorino M, Giannini M, Vanderlinden J. A psychometric exploration of an Italian translation of the SCOFF questionnaire. Eur Eat Disord Rev. 2011;19(4):371–3. doi:10.1002/erv.1105.
27. Smink FR, van Hoeken D, Hoek HW. Epidemiology of eating disorders: incidence, prevalence and mortality rates. Curr Psychiatry Rep. 2012;14(4):406–14. doi:10.1007/s11920-012-0282-y.
28. Streiner DL. Starting at the beginning: an introduction to coefficient alpha and internal consistency. J Pers Assess. 2003;80(1):99–103. doi:10.1207/S15327752jpa8001_18.
29. Waaddegaard M, Davidsen M, Kjoller M. Obesity and prevalence of risk behaviour for eating disorders among young Danish women. Scand J Public Health. 2009;37(7):736–43. doi:10.1177/1403494809105794.

Permissions

All chapters in this book were first published in JED, by BioMed Central; hereby published with permission under the Creative Commons Attribution License or equivalent. Every chapter published in this book has been scrutinized by our experts. Their significance has been extensively debated. The topics covered herein carry significant findings which will fuel the growth of the discipline. They may even be implemented as practical applications or may be referred to as a beginning point for another development.

The contributors of this book come from diverse backgrounds, making this book a truly international effort. This book will bring forth new frontiers with its revolutionizing research information and detailed analysis of the nascent developments around the world.

We would like to thank all the contributing authors for lending their expertise to make the book truly unique. They have played a crucial role in the development of this book. Without their invaluable contributions this book wouldn't have been possible. They have made vital efforts to compile up to date information on the varied aspects of this subject to make this book a valuable addition to the collection of many professionals and students.

This book was conceptualized with the vision of imparting up-to-date information and advanced data in this field. To ensure the same, a matchless editorial board was set up. Every individual on the board went through rigorous rounds of assessment to prove their worth. After which they invested a large part of their time researching and compiling the most relevant data for our readers.

The editorial board has been involved in producing this book since its inception. They have spent rigorous hours researching and exploring the diverse topics which have resulted in the successful publishing of this book. They have passed on their knowledge of decades through this book. To expedite this challenging task, the publisher supported the team at every step. A small team of assistant editors was also appointed to further simplify the editing procedure and attain best results for the readers.

Apart from the editorial board, the designing team has also invested a significant amount of their time in understanding the subject and creating the most relevant covers. They scrutinized every image to scout for the most suitable representation of the subject and create an appropriate cover for the book.

The publishing team has been an ardent support to the editorial, designing and production team. Their endless efforts to recruit the best for this project, has resulted in the accomplishment of this book. They are a veteran in the field of academics and their pool of knowledge is as vast as their experience in printing. Their expertise and guidance has proved useful at every step. Their uncompromising quality standards have made this book an exceptional effort. Their encouragement from time to time has been an inspiration for everyone.

The publisher and the editorial board hope that this book will prove to be a valuable piece of knowledge for researchers, students, practitioners and scholars across the globe.

List of Contributors

Carolyn Black Becker and Chelsey Werchan
Department of Psychology, One Trinity Place, Trinity University, San Antonio, TX 78212, USA

Phillippa C Diedrichs and Glen Jankowski
Center for Appearance Research, University of the West of England, Coldharbour Lane, Bristol BS16 1QY, UK

Matthew Fuller-Tyszkiewicz, Ben Richardson, Helen Skouteris, David Austin, Millicent Holmes and Jaclyn Broadbent
School of Psychology, Deakin University, 221 Burwood Highway, Burwood, VIC 3125, Australia

David Castle
Psychiatry Department, University of Melbourne, Melbourne, VIC, Australia
St Vincent's Hospital, Melbourne, VIC, Australia

Lucy Busija
Faculty of Health, Deakin University, Burwood, Australia

Britt Klein
DVC-Research & Innovation Portfolio; the School of Health Sciences; and the Collaborative Research Network, Federation University, Ballarat, Australia
National Institute for Mental Health Research, The Australian National University, Canberra, Australia

Terri A Nicely
Penn State College of Medicine, 500 University Drive, 17033 Hershey, PA, USA

Susan Lane-Loney, Emily Masciulli and Rollyn M Ornstein
Division of Adolescent Medicine and Eating Disorders, Penn State Hershey Children's Hospital, 905 West Governor Road, Suite 250, 17033 Hershey, PA, USA

Christopher S Hollenbeak
Departments of Surgery and Public Health Sciences, Penn State College of Medicine, 500 University Drive, 17033 Hershey, PA, USA

Suzana Drobnjak, Semra Atsiz and Ulrike Ehlert
Department of Psychology, Division of Clinical Psychology & Psychotherapy, University of Zurich, Binzmuehlestrasse 14/26, Zurich 8050, Switzerland

Beate Ditzen
Department of Psychology, Division of Clinical Psychology & Psychotherapy, University of Zurich, Binzmuehlestrasse 14/26, Zurich 8050, Switzerland
Institute of Medical Psychology in the Center for Psychosocial Medicine, University Hospital Heidelberg, Bergheimer Str. 20, Heidelberg 69115, Germany

Brunna Tuschen-Caffier
Department of Psychology, Division of Clinical Psychology & Psychotherapy, Albert-Ludwigs University, Engelbergerstrasse 41, Freiburg 79106, Germany

Anne Werner, Katrin E Giel and Stephan Zipfel
Department of Psychosomatic Medicine and Psychotherapy, University Hospital Tübingen, Osianderstr, 5, 72076, Tübingen, Germany

Ansgar Thiel and Jochen Mayer
Institute of Sports Science, Tübingen University, Tübingen, Germany

Sven Schneider
Mannheim Institute of Public Health, Social and Preventive Medicine, Medical Faculty Mannheim, Heidelberg University, Mannheim, Germany

Charles F Saladino
Department of Chemistry and Biochemistry, Misericordia University, Dallas, PA 18612, USA

Kate Churruca, Janette Perz and Jane M Ussher
Centre for Health Research, University of Western Sydney, Locked Bag 1797, Penrith South 2751, Australia

Elin Monell
Department of Clinical Neuroscience, Karolinska Institute, Norra Stationsgatan 69 7th floor, 113 64 Stockholm, Sweden
Centre for Research & Development, Uppsala University/Region Gävleborg, Uppsala, Sweden

Louise Högdahl, Emma Forsén Mantilla and Andreas Birgegård
Department of Clinical Neuroscience, Karolinska Institute, Norra Stationsgatan 69 7th floor, 113 64 Stockholm, Sweden

Helene Sauer, Anna Krumm, Katja Weimer, Björn Horing, Nazar Mazurak, Stephan Zipfel, Paul Enck and Aydin Demircioglu
Department of Psychosomatic Medicine and Psychotherapy, University Medical Hospital, Tübingen, Germany

Marco D Gulewitsch
Department of Psychology, Clinical Psychology and Psychotherapy, University of Tübingen, Tübingen, Germany

Frank Hellmond, Dirk Dammann, Walter Binder and Peter Linse
Fachkliniken Wangen i.A., Children Rehabilitation Hospital for Respiratory Diseases, Allergies and Psychosomatics, Wangen i.A., Germany

Stefan Ehehalt
Public Health Department of Stuttgart, Department of Pediatrics, Dental Health Care, Health Promotion and Social Services, Stuttgart, Germany

Gerhard Binder
Department of Pediatric Endocrinology and Diabetology, University Children's Hospital, Tübingen, Germany

Eric R Muth
Department of Psychology, Clemson University, Clemson, South Carolina, USA

Isabelle Mack
Department of Psychosomatic Medicine and Psychotherapy, University Medical Hospital, Tübingen, Germany
Department of Psychosomatic Medicine and Psychotherapy, University of Tübingen, Medical Hospital, Frondsbergstrasse 23, 72070 Tübingen, Germany

Carolyn Black Becker and Kaitlin Hill
Department of Psychology, Trinity University, One Trinity Place, San Antonio, TX 78212-7200, USA

Rebecca Greif
Rutgers University, GSAPP, New Brunswick, NJ, USA

Hongmei Han and Tiffany Stewart
Pennington Biomedical Research Center, Baton Rouge, LA, USA

Kerstin Ekeroth, David Clinton and Andreas Birgegård
Resource Center for Eating Disorders/ Center for Psychiatry Research Stockholm, Department of Clinical Neuroscience, Karolinska Institutet, Stockholm, Sweden
Stockholm Centre for Eating Disorders, Stockholm County Council, Stockholm, Sweden

Claes Norring
Resource Center for Eating Disorders/ Center for Psychiatry Research Stockholm, Department of Clinical Neuroscience, Karolinska Institutet, Stockholm, Sweden
Stockholm Centre for Eating Disorders, Stockholm County Council, Stockholm, Sweden

Eric M Stephen, Jennifer S Rose, Lindsay Kenney and Ruth Striegel Weissman
Department of Psychology, Wesleyan University, 207 High Street, Middletown, CT 06459, USA

Francine Rosselli-Navarra
Department of Psychology, Manchester Community College, Great Path MS#4, PO Box 1046, Manchester, CT 06040, USA

Jasmijn de Vos, Georgia Katsaragaki, Elske van de Berg and Jack Dekker
Arkin Mental Health Institute, Klaprozenweg 111, PO Box 75848, 1070, AV, Amsterdam, the Netherlands
De Viersprong Mental Health Institute, Bergen op Zoom, the Netherlands

Laura Houtzager
Arkin Mental Health Institute, Klaprozenweg 111, PO Box 75848, 1070, AV, Amsterdam, the Netherlands
De Viersprong Mental Health Institute, Bergen op Zoom, the Netherlands

Pim Cuijpers
Vrije Universiteit, Amsterdam, the Netherlands

Jonathan M Mond
Research School of Psychology, Australian National University, Canberra ACT 0200, Australia

Marit Danielsen and Sigrid Bjørnelv
Department of Neuroscience, Faculty of Medicine, Norwegian University of Science and Technology, 7491 Trondheim, Norway
Eating Disorder Unit, Department of Psychiatry, Levanger Hospital, Hospital Trust Nord-Trøndelag, NO-7600 Levanger, Norway

Øyvind Rø
Regional Department for Eating Disorders, Division of Mental Health and Addiction, Oslo University Hospital, Oslo, Norway
Division of Mental Health and Addiction, Institute of Clinical Medicine, University of Oslo, Levanger, Norway

Ulla Romild
Department of Research and Development, Levanger Hospital, Hospital Trust Nord-Trøndelag, NO-7600 Levanger, Norway

Marsha Rowsell and Jacqueline C. Carter
Department of Psychology, Memorial University of Newfoundland, St. John's, NL A1B 3X9, Canada

Danielle E. MacDonald
Department of Psychology, Ryerson University, Toronto, Ontario M5G 2C4, Canada
Department of Psychiatry, University Health Network, Toronto, Ontario M5G 2C4, Canada

Colleen Stiles-Shields
Department of Preventive Medicine, Northwestern University Feinberg School of Medicine, Chicago, IL, USA

Bryony H. Bamford
The London Centre for Eating Disorders and Body Image, London, UK

Stephen Touyz
University of Sydney, School of Psychology, Sydney, Australia

Daniel Le Grange
Department of Psychiatry, University of California, San Francisco, San Francisco, CA, USA
Department of Pediatrics, University of California, San Francisco, San Francisco, CA, USA

Phillipa Hay
Centre for Health Research, School of Medicine, Western Sydney University, Sydney, Australia

Hubert Lacey
St. George's, University of London, Eating Disorders Research Group, London, UK

Sarah Greer
Richmond Hospital, 7000 Westminster Hwy, Richmond, BC V6X 1A2, Canada

Myra Cooper
Isis Education Centre, University of Oxford, Warneford Hospital, Oxford OX3 7JX, UK

Joanna E. Steinglass and B. Timothy Walsh
1051 Riverside Drive, Unit 98, New York, NY 10032, USA

Emily Griffiths
University College London, Clinical, Educational & Health Psychology, 1-19 Torrington Place, London WC1E 7HB, UK

Nicholas Hawkes
St Ann's Eating Disorders Service, Barnet, Enfield and Haringey Mental Health NHS Trust, London, UK

Sam Gilbert
University College London, Institute of Cognitive Neuroscience, 17 Queen Square, London WC1N 3AR, UK

Lucy Serpell
University College London, Clinical, Educational & Health Psychology, 1-19 Torrington Place, London WC1E 7HB, UK
Eating Disorders Service, North East London NHS Foundation Trust, London, UK

Erika Hansson
Kristianstad University, Kristianstad, Sweden
Lund University, Lund, Sweden

Daiva Daukantaitė and Per Johnsson
Lund University, Lund, Sweden

Index